SOUTH ONTARIO BRANCH LIBRARY

W9-DEW-803

The
Eye Book

A Johns Hopkins Press Health Book

ONTARIO CITY LIBRARY

DEC - - 1998

ONTARIO, CA 91764

THE
EYE
BOOK

A Complete Guide to Eye Disorders and Health

GARY H. CASSEL, M.D.
MICHAEL D. BILLIG, O.D.
HARRY G. RANDALL, M.D.

THE JOHNS HOPKINS UNIVERSITY PRESS
Baltimore & London

Note to the Reader: This book is not meant to substitute for professional eye care, and decisions about treatment should not be based solely on its contents. Instead, treatment must be developed in a dialogue between the individual and his or her eye care professional. Our book has been written to help with that dialogue.

© 1998 The Johns Hopkins University Press
All rights reserved. Published 1998
Printed in the United States of America on acid-free paper
9 8 7 6 5 4 3 2

The Johns Hopkins University Press
2715 North Charles Street
Baltimore, Maryland 21218-4363

A catalog record for this book is available from the British Library.

Library of Congress Cataloging-in-Publication Data

Cassel, Gary H., 1953–
  The eye book : a complete guide to eye disorders and health / Gary H. Cassel, Michael D. Billig, Harry G. Randall.
      p.   cm. — (A Johns Hopkins Press health book)
  Includes bibliographical references and index.
  ISBN 0-8018-5835-6 (alk. paper). — ISBN 0-8018-5847-X (pbk. : alk. paper)
  1. Eye—Diseases—Popular works. 2. Eye—Popular works. I. Billig, Michael D., 1956–   . II. Randall, Harry G., 1934–   . III. Title. IV. Series.
RE51.C34 1998
617.7—dc21   97-35348
                                                                               CIP

Illustrations by Jacqueline Schaffer

A webpage for this book and an e-mail link to the authors are located within the Johns Hopkins University Press website at www. press.jhu.edu.

This book is dedicated to all our patients, who over the years have helped us realize that caring is one of the most important aspects of eye care.

Contents

Figures

Foreword

As the consumerism movement has flourished in the United States, so too has the need increased for more personal participation in health care decisions. Individual responsibility for understanding one's own health is an obvious component of this process. Numerous self-help periodicals and books have appeared to meet the growing demands of the public for health information of all kinds.

Drs. Cassel and Randall, experienced community ophthalmologists and part-time faculty members of the Wilmer Eye Institute at Johns Hopkins, along with their respected colleague, Dr. Billig, now publish *The Eye Book: A Complete Guide to Eye Disorders and Health* within this educational framework. It is an exceptionally useful book for the public because it dispels myths and offers practical guidelines in a very readable style. It covers the routine (for example, eyeglasses) and the serious (for example, macular degeneration). The authors are appropriately cautious about recommending new, but unproven, treatments.

We are entering a golden age of knowledge about heretofore perplexing and sometimes blinding diseases, and futuristic techniques, ranging from optoelectronics to genetic engineering, promise bright prospects for our aging population. Medical and scientific institutions such as the Wilmer Institute at Johns Hopkins are actively continuing the search for better treatment techniques; simultaneously, they continue their dedication to the clinical care of routine and complex eye disease as well as to the education of doctors and researchers—and the general public. For the good health of your own eyes and vision, I encourage you to read and consult this helpful book for information, and to seek the assistance of highly experienced eye care specialists for diagnosis and treatment.

Morton F. Goldberg, M.D., F.A.C.S.
Director, Wilmer Eye Institute
The Johns Hopkins Medical Institutions
Baltimore, Maryland

Preface

The eye, responsible for one of our most vital senses, is one of the most important organs in the body. When all is well, most of us take our eyes for granted. But as you no doubt know from experience, when your vision is blurred, or your eyes are itchy and watery, or it feels like there's something "sticking" in there, it's hard to concentrate on anything *but* your eyes. When something's not right with your eyes, then nothing's right with the world. As eye care specialists, we devote our working hours to helping people with eye problems of all kinds. And we have written this book to help the many people who have such problems, or who are worried about their eyes or the eyes of someone they care about.

It's remarkable and humbling to consider how far the field of ophthalmology—the medical specialty covering the anatomy, functions, pathology, and treatment of the eye—has progressed over the last three decades, a period when we have seen our patients helped by innovations in every aspect of eye care that were unheard of only a short time ago. New antibiotics and medications, safer cataract surgery with shorter recovery time, better glaucoma treatments, refined surgical techniques for mending retinal detachments and clearing vitreous hemorrhages, and retinovitreous treatments—not to mention a revolution in lens-making materials and technology—have helped thousands of people to see better longer.

In this book we describe all of these recent innovations and offer information and advice about what you and your eye doctor can do together to safeguard your vision, and your general health. We describe the eye's anatomy and what changes occur naturally over time, as well as what changes are not natural and may be dangerous—and tell you what to do about them. We demystify the eye examination, describe how eyeglasses and contact lenses work (and how to tell what will work best for you), and take up the controversial vision-corrective surgery called refractive surgery.

Cataracts, glaucoma, and age-related macular degeneration are the three major diseases of the eye that rob older people of good vision. Knowing the signs and symptoms of these diseases and how to get proper checkups and screening are crucial first steps; once the diagnosis is made, treatment options must be weighed and decisions made. The three chapters in the second part of the book discuss each of these problems in detail.

In part 4 of the book we continue the discussion of eye problems, beginning from the front of the eye, at the lids and lashes, and ending up at the back, with the optic nerve. Explanations of problems ranging from the annoying ("floaters and flashes," for example, or a twitching eyelid) to the more serious (uveitis, or arthritis of the eye) may be found here.

In the final section of the book we have collected chapters on topics that are important for anyone wishing to have a better understanding of what happens to our eyes as we age. Eye trauma and emergencies are discussed so that readers will be able to take better care of their eyes and know how to recognize an eye emergency and what to do. A thorough explanation of how such diseases as diabetes, high blood pressure, and migraine headaches affect the eyes should be helpful to anyone coping with these problems. A chapter on low vision describes helpful devices and services and offers useful tips for people with declining visual acuity. Our final chapter looks at how common medications like antibiotics and blood pressure medications can affect the eyes, while in an appendix we describe the side effects of specific eye medications.

This book is designed to offer reliable and current information. We hope that it will help you understand your own eyes, your vision, and any problems you may be having. If you are facing a decision about eye treatment, you may want to take this book with you to your doctor's office, to discuss information that you find useful. As helpful as we hope this book will be, however, we know that only you and your doctor can make decisions about your treatment, based on your specific situation.

Finally, as in other aspects of life, many myths have sprung up around the area of vision, and they have been passed on from generation to generation, causing confusion and sometimes fear. Before turning to part 1, let's explore some of these bits of accepted wisdom as good examples of the bad information we hope to replace with this book.

VISION MYTHS

Reading in dim light can hurt your eyes.

Picture Anne Sullivan, the dedicated, selfless teacher of Helen Keller, night after endless night, reading in half-light, straining her own eyes to the breaking point. Makes you wish for indoor flood lamps, doesn't it? And yet, although inadequate light *can* cause temporary eye fatigue, it can't permanently damage your eyes. If it could, Abe Lincoln, who studied by candlelight—as did every scholar in the centuries before Edison—would have had poor vision. But why do it? Everyone ought to use good lighting—especially as we get older, when cataracts and other problems can dim our vision. Also, good lighting always makes it easier for your eyes to focus on what you are reading and helps to lessen fatigue.

Eye exercises can improve vision.

Sadly, for almost all of us, this one isn't true either. There are muscles in the eye, but they don't "shape up" like a flabby belly on a regimen of sit-ups. Only a small percentage of eye problems respond to eye exercises. Also, eye exercises can't prevent you from ever needing eyeglasses. *Note:* If an eye doctor recommends a course of eye exercises for you, please seek a second opinion; these ocular workouts are useful in some circumstances, but they have their limitations.

Wearing the right sunglasses can prevent cataracts.

Many products—natural foods, herbal medicines, expensive lens coatings, special eye drops, high-tech sunglasses—have been marketed as means of preventing cataracts, and there's some science to back this up: ultraviolet toxicity can harm the eyes, but not nearly as commonly or easily as sunlight damages the skin and causes skin cancer. But we also have to note that most people have some cataract development as they get older. In some people, cataracts develop quickly and need treatment; in others, they don't. Thus—because the sheer numbers are so great—statistically, any product that claims to prevent, or at least slow, cataract development will appear to work fairly often. Do they really? Probably not.

It's entirely reasonable to ask what practical steps can be taken to prevent your vision from deteriorating, but the bottom line is that many eye problems are simply the luck of the genetic draw. For example, myopia, like heart disease, has a major genetic component. If your family reunion looks like a LensCrafters commercial, then you probably ought to resign yourself to the fact that myopia runs in your family. But there are some things you can do: Try to avoid injuries. Take care of your general health—especially if you have diabetes or high blood pressure. And get regular eye exams throughout your life. Many eye problems are highly treatable, but only if they are caught in time.

Eating carrots helps you see better (so rabbits must see great).

Carrots are rich in vitamin A, which is indeed important for eyesight. But carrots haven't cornered the market on vitamin A; many other foods—green vegetables and yellow squash, for instance—are also rich in it. And we don't need that much Vitamin A, anyway; a well-balanced diet, with or without carrots, provides all the nutrients we need for good vision.

However, severe *lack* of vitamins A, C, and E—a problem often found in people living in underdeveloped countries—can lead to serious eye disease. And one recent study has also suggested that macular degeneration, a common cause of visual difficulty in many older people, may be due to another dietary deficiency: a lack of trace metals (such as zinc). The message here: Take your vitamins in reasonable doses (not megadoses). Take one multivitamin daily. And eat your vegetables.

Sitting in front of a computer screen for hours on end can damage your eyes.

Well, it sure doesn't do them any good, but fortunately the eyestrain and fatigue caused by overuse of computers and video display terminals (VDTs) is only temporary. Eyestrain and fatigue can be unwelcome by-products of *any* close-up task that requires prolonged use of the eye muscles. What can you do to relieve the strain? Take frequent breaks. Rest your eye muscles by periodically looking up or across the room. Keep the monitor twenty-four inches away. You may find it helpful to use a pair of "computer glasses," so that your eyes don't have to work so hard. (See your eye doctor.)

If you look cross-eyed long enough, your eyes will stay that way.

They won't.

PART I

Introduction

1

A Guide to the Adult Eye

No matter how hard we fight it, certain unavoidable things happen to the body over time. Our skin starts to sag, for example; our bones begin to thin; so does our hair.

And inevitably, just like the rest of the body, our eyes age, too. But because these changes are often much more subtle and incremental—in other words, because the eyes staring back at us in the mirror still *look* about the same as always—it's difficult for most people to detect them immediately.

This chapter is designed to help acquaint you with the parts of the eyes and how they work together so that we can see. In the next chapter we'll take a look at what's been happening to your eyes over the years, and later in the book we'll cover specific problems—and what you can do about them—in much more detail. Now, let's begin with a quick review of the eye's basic anatomy and the changes that most of us can expect to encounter as time goes by.

THE ORBIT

First, imagine a ping-pong ball. That's about how big your eye is. But unlike a simple ping-pong ball, your eye is wonderfully complex and intricately layered. Now, think of your eyelids as movable curtains on a stage. What we see of the eye is just the front surface that's visible between the opened lids; backstage in the eye is just as important and interesting. As you read the following description of the anatomy of the eye, you may find it helpful to refer to figure 1.1, panels A, B, and C.

A.

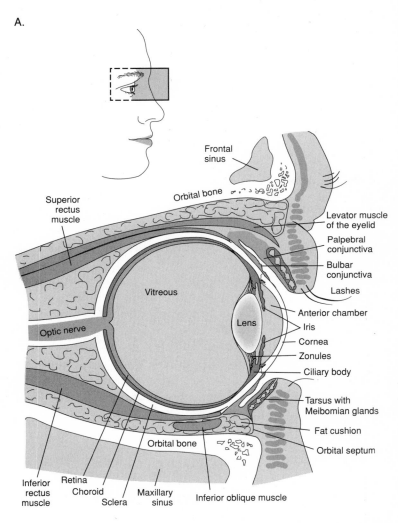

Fig. 1.1. Anatomy of the eye: (A) side view; (B) top view; (C) front view

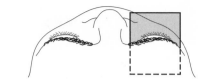

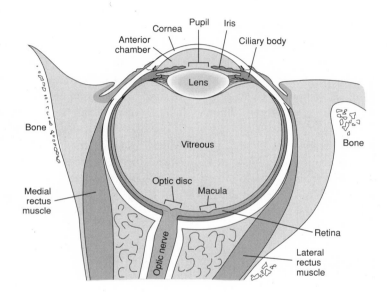

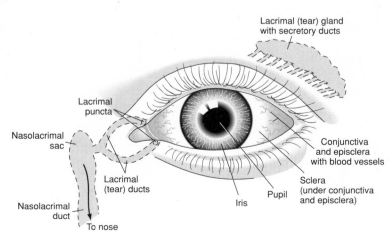

Nature provided the soft, vulnerable eye with excellent protection—a layered cradle, or socket, of bone called the *orbit*. The orbit has heavy bone on its outer edges, thinner bone on the inner (nasal) surfaces, and also a pillow of fat, which cushions the eye. This cavity also contains the muscles and nerves that allow your eyes and eyelids to move; blood vessels, which nourish and sustain eye tissue; and the *lacrimal gland*, which produces the tears that lubricate the eye. (Imagine how difficult and painful it would be to move your eyes back and forth, or open and close your eyelids, without this moisture!) The lacrimal gland is also part of the eye's defense system: in response to the sting of chemicals or onions, or to such irritants as dust or pollen, it turns on the faucet to dilute and wash away anything that might harm the eye. (For other reasons not entirely understood, this tear gland also responds to grief, great joy, and other strong emotions.)

Fortunately, unlike other bones, orbital bone—which is comparably thin to begin with—is not susceptible to osteoporosis: it does not thin or weaken significantly with aging. In very elderly persons, the cushion of orbital fat sometimes atrophies, or shrinks, causing the eyes to sink noticeably back into the skull—which may pose an aesthetic problem, but not a functional one. In other people the orbital fat may herniate forward into the eyelids, causing abnormal puffiness or even "bags" under the eyes (see chapter 10).

THE EYELIDS

The *eyelids* are covered on their inner aspect with a sheet of thin, slippery membrane called *conjunctiva*, which folds back and connects to the front surface of the eye. Over this lining, and giving the eyelid some rigid support structure and strength—like a tab insert in a collared shirt—is a tough, fibrous plate of connective tissue called the *tarsus;* then come layers of muscle and skin. A thinner layer of fibrous tissue, called the *orbital septum*, connects the tarsus to the *periosteum*, the outermost layer of bone covering the orbit. The orbital septum is a thin fence that keeps the previously mentioned layer of orbital fat confined inside the bony orbit. As the orbital septum weakens over time, a few chunks of orbital fat can poke through this fence, making unsightly lumps in the skin under the eyes. (*Note:* Such lumps are "bad" only in that they're not terribly attractive. For many people these lumps present only a temporary problem, because they can be, and often are, removed surgically.)

As the skin of the eyelids ages—just like the skin on the face or arms—it tends to lose its suppleness and begins to droop. Sometimes the skin of the upper lid can sag enough to interfere with vision. (In the lower lid, this drooping skin—"bags under the eyes"—does not interfere with seeing, although again, some people consider it a cosmetic problem.) Sagging, excess skin on either or both eyelids can be taken care of with minor surgery, a procedure called *blepharoplasty* (see chapter 10).

At the edges of the eyelids are ducts for glands that secrete an oily substance, which helps keep tears from oozing out of the eyes and onto the skin. Here also are the bases of the eyelashes: delicate, efficient filters that protect our eyes from dust and myriad other foreign objects. Our eyelashes tend to become more sparse as we get older. Interestingly, they become lighter, but rarely do they turn white with age.

THE SCLERA AND CORNEA

The "white" of the eye visible between the lids is the front portion of the *sclera*, a thick, protective sheath that encircles the eye, with a porthole at its very front. At this porthole, sitting like a watch glass on its casing, is the cornea. The *cornea* is normally transparent, like a camera lens; through it you can see the iris and pupil. The cornea has no blood vessels, while the conjunctiva and episclera (two tissue layers that cover the sclera) do—a major difference and important for understanding the discussion of corneal neovascularization later in this book (see chapter 5).

The back surface of the sclera is connected to the tough outer covering of the optic nerve, the cable that links the eye with the brain. (If you think of the eye as a kind of TV camera, the brain is where the electrical signals are sorted out and transformed into an image that makes sense.) Sometimes the white sclera of the eye develops dark areas (a condition called *focal senile translucency* of the sclera). Don't worry—these dark areas are of no significance. They're caused by calcium deposits, which cause the sclera to lose its normal white color, allowing the dark pigment inside the eye to show through. (Oddly, calcium in the cornea causes the same problem in reverse: the cornea loses its transparency and turns white.)

The domed cornea is like a cake with five layers: the epithelial, or outer-lining, cells (the icing, if you will, on this cake); Bowman's layer; the tough but transparent stroma, the bulk of the cornea (the cake itself); Descemet's membrane; and a single layer of endothelial, or inner-lining, cells.

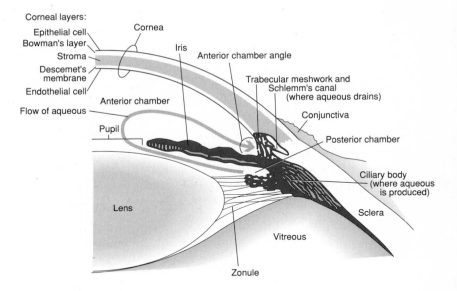

Fig. 1.2. The cornea, iris, pupil, and lens

The inner endothelial cells tend to decrease in numbers and become thin with age. If too many endothelial cells are lost, through old age or injury, the cornea becomes cloudy, but fortunately the endothelial cells usually last a lifetime. As people get older, the outer cornea tends to develop a white ring called *arcus senilis*. This corneal ring is composed of cholesterol and its derivatives, but it is not usually related to an older person's blood cholesterol level. In some people the ring is very obvious, but the condition is so common as to be virtually normal, and it is of no significance.

The cornea is more than a window; it is a converging lens. As in a camera, it takes light rays and bends and focuses them to the back of the inside of the eye, the *retina*. The power of the cornea changes during growth but stays relatively constant in adults, with minor fluctuations in curvature causing slight shifts in our eyeglass prescription.

THE IRIS AND PUPIL

The *iris*, visible through the cornea, is composed of connective tissue and muscle with a hole in the middle. The color of the iris is actually due to the amount of pigment in the iris connective tissue layer. Brown eyes have a lot of pigment, blue eyes very little. (In the colloquial sense, if you have brown eyes, your iris is brown, and so on. No one knows why irises come in such a fascinating variety of colors and patterns.) The *pupil* is the hole in the iris, which allows light to reach the retina. The iris uses one muscle to constrict the pupil and another to actively dilate, or enlarge, it. Like an f-stop on a camera, the pupil is wider in a darkened room and narrower in full sunshine. The iris characteristically loses pigment and thins with aging, resulting in the surprisingly bright "China blue" color of the eyes of some older people. The pupil tends to become smaller with age.

Around the iris, hidden by the sclera, is the *ciliary body*, the ring or tether that holds the lens in place, connected in back with the *choroid*, a bolstering, nourishing layer of blood vessels between the sclera and the retina. Normal aging changes the choroid, but usually not in any remarkable way. The ciliary body produces the *aqueous*, a watery solution that bathes the lens; manufactured behind the iris, it travels through the posterior chamber and the pupil and leaves the eye through a drain in the *anterior chamber angle*, where the iris meets the cornea. (This fluid must get out of the eye, and trouble can arise when its exit is blocked. An important job of the eye's plumbing is to keep the pressure in the eye from becoming too high.) The aqueous is secreted by one group of cells and eventually leaves the eye through a drain or meshwork created by other cells. This balance maintains what's called the *intraocular pressure*—and this, like the pressure in a balloon, is essential for maintaining the shape of the eye (and particularly for preserving the curvature of the cornea). (See chapter 8, on glaucoma, which is a problem that develops when eye pressure isn't normal.)

THE LENS

Behind the iris is the *lens*—about the size and shape of an M&M candy—fastened to the ciliary body by thin fibers called *zonules*. The lens is elastic: to focus, it stretches and snaps back into place. In the job of focusing light on the retina, the cornea does about three-quarters of the work and the lens about one-quarter; but the cornea has *fixed* focus power and the lens *variable* focus power—at least for a while. This brings us to a universally recognized signpost of aging, which arises when our eyes develop trouble mastering a task called *accommodation*. Accommodation takes place when a muscle in the ciliary body contracts, relaxing the tension on the

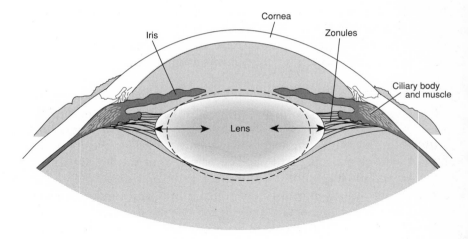

Fig. 1.3. The lens, showing accommodation for fine-tuning focus

zonules, thus allowing the lens to become less flattened and more spherical. Accommodation begins to diminish at about age ten, but the change is usually not noticeable until about age forty, when reading the small type in the phone book suddenly isn't as easy as it used to be. What happens? The muscle of the ciliary body continues to work as well as ever, but the lens grows harder and less elastic; it no longer changes shape when the tension is relaxed. The result? The dawn of a sobering new phase in adulthood: dependence on reading glasses.

THE RETINA

Inside the sclera is the vascular choroid; inside the choroid is the *retina*, the reason for being of everything else in the eye. The exquisitely complicated retina does far more than merely register an image like a bit of photographic film. Indeed, cells in the retina break down an image into countless elements—brightness, position, color, movement—then encode all these elements as electrical signals and transmit them to the brain. Remarkably, all of this is done not only faster—literally—than the blink of an eye, but faster than we can even comprehend without the help of highly specialized scientific instruments.

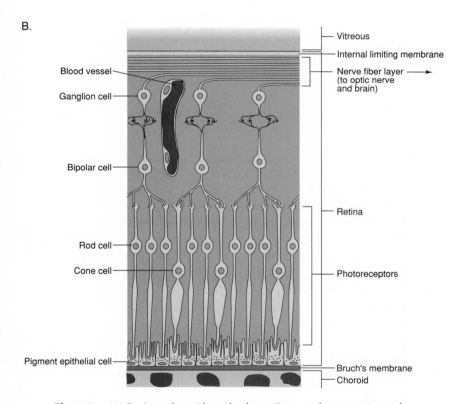

Fig. 1.4. (A) Retina, choroid, and sclera; (B) neural connections of
the cells in the retina

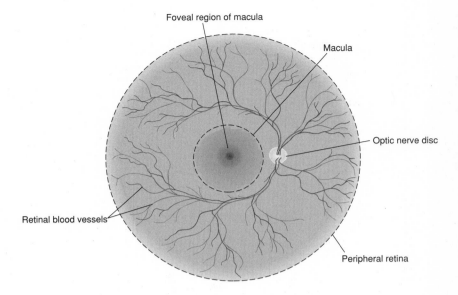

Foveal region of macula

Macula

Optic nerve disc

Retinal blood vessels

Peripheral retina

Fig. 1.5.   A view of the retina inside the eye

The intricate structure and function of the retina could be the subject of an entire book in themselves, but briefly: First, layers of *rods* and *cones* receive the basic units of light, triggering a photochemical reaction in these cells. Then *bipolar cells* apparently receive, organize, and transmit this information to *ganglion cells*, which send these signals to the brain through a collection of nerve fibers called the *optic nerve*. Though many diseases affect the retina, normal aging does not affect the retina in a predictable manner. This is especially true in the *macula*, the area of the retina responsible for central vision, which is needed for such functions as reading and fine visual acuity. The macula, the most significant part of the retina, is located next to the optic nerve and is responsible for our *central vision* (as opposed to our *peripheral vision*). The macula is composed mostly of cones and is also an important part of color vision.

Most of the interior of the eye is filled with *vitreous*, a nearly transparent substance that resembles Jell-O in texture. Vitreous is supported by scaffolding, a meshwork of collagen fibers, and a gel of hyaluronic acid. In normal aging, this gel slowly liquefies, allowing the meshwork to collapse and clump. The meshwork is thicker against the retina, at a site called the *posterior vitreous membrane*, attached at the optic nerve, the ciliary body, and

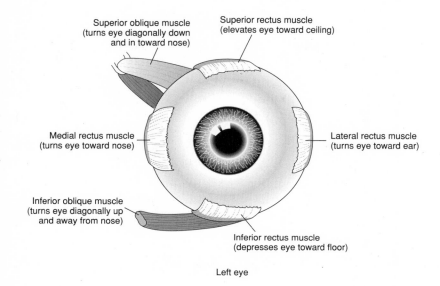

Fig. 1.6. The muscles of the eye

various other places in the retina. Sometimes, as the gel liquefies and the meshwork collapses, the posterior vitreous membrane can slide or suddenly pull off from its attachment with the retina or optic nerve, resulting in visual floaters or flashes—a condition known as a *posterior vitreous detachment* (see chapter 15).

The Muscles

Part of the process of aiming the eyes to see an object is turning the body and moving the head. But the eyes can also move independently; in other words, you can move your eyes without turning your head. To keep the eyes correctly focused on a moving object, like a baseball, while the body is running and turning, is truly an impressive bit of engineering. There are six *extraocular muscles* fastened to the eye (in addition to muscles such as the ciliary muscles, which are inside the eye). The extraocular muscles are a *medial* and *lateral rectus*, mostly for horizontal movement, and *superior* and *inferior rectus* and *oblique* muscles, for vertical and torsional (twisting) movements. Understanding the actions of individual muscles in different eye positions gets complicated; there is a sophisticated feedback

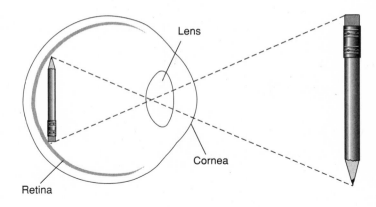

Fig. 1.7.   How we see an object

What Happens When We See

Figure 1.7 illustrates what happens when we see something. Light, bounced off an object, reaches the eye and is refracted by the cornea and lens and focused into an image on the retina. But the eye's workings are like a camera's, which means that the image made on the retina is upside down and reversed. It's up to the brain to make sense out of it.

You may be aware that the left side of the brain controls the right hand and vice versa. Well, many functions of vision operate under this same confusing crossover system. With your eyes, in other words, the *right* half of the visual field in each eye goes to the *left* half of the brain. As figure 1.8 indicates, the right half of the visual field corresponds to the left half of each retina. The fibers from the left retina of the left eye go to the left half of the brain. The fibers from the left retina of the right eye cross over to the left brain via the optic chiasm (from chi, the Greek letter *X*).

system in the brain to keep the eyes focused together, to maintain binocular vision (that is, two eyes working together), and avoid double vision (diplopia). Unless you have a specific muscle disease or some damage to the brain areas that control eye movements, the coordinated movement of your eyes shouldn't be affected by aging (see chapter 2).

AS THIS BRIEF OVERVIEW INDICATES, the eye is one of the most complicated structures in the body, and its function—vision—is one of the most impor-

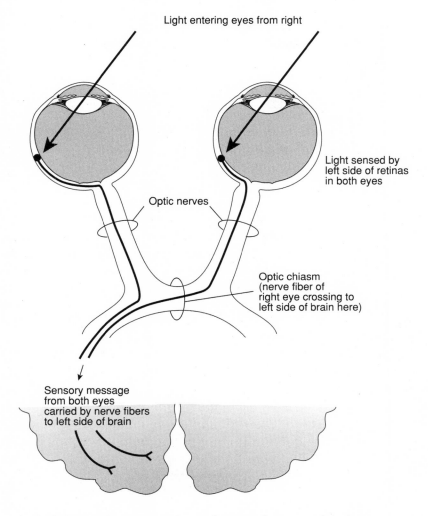

Fig. 1.8.   The crossover system between the eyes and the brain

tant. What goes on with the eyes when we age can affect our vision just a little bit, or more seriously. Any disease, injury, or infection in the eyes, of course, can cause even more problems, affecting vision and also causing discomfort or pain. We'll get to these specific problems later in the book. For now, let's turn in the next chapter to a discussion of how *everyone's* vision changes over time, and how these changes matter.

2

How Our Vision
Changes over Time

When we're children, most of us see well enough on our own without needing glasses. But by the time we reach our forties, that's no longer the case; many of us need *something*—glasses or contact lenses—to help us see better. Even then, it can be frustrating. Every few years our prescriptions change; we all wonder when our eyes will finally settle down. Well, guess what? They never do! From a vision standpoint, our eyes are in a constant state of flux our entire lives. Even after we're fully grown, our eyes keep right on changing. Some of these fluctuations cause a shift in our prescriptions. Some of them cause a change in our vision, due to age-related eye disease.

CHANGES THAT AFFECT OUR PRESCRIPTIONS

What changes our prescriptions? To answer this question, let's take a minute to review how we actually see. (You may want to refer back to figure 1.1A.) It may help to picture the eye as a camera. The *cornea*, the front surface of the eye, acts as a converging lens: it takes rays of light and bends and focuses them. Next, the light is focused more finely still by the *lens*, which sits just behind the *iris* (the colored part of the eye).

In a perfect eye, all of this focused light is then beamed back to the *retina*—what you might call the eye's "film." The elegant, complicated retina processes all the information it receives, breaking it down into countless elements, and then transmitting these elements in the form of electrical signals to the brain.

But as we get older, our eyes become less than perfect. Both the cornea and the lens change shape over time. Accordingly—inevitably—our prescription changes, too.

Changes in the cornea: When we're born, our upper eyelids are nice and tight and tend to press on our corneas. It has been suggested that this snug fit eases over time, and as it does, the cornea starts to reshape itself. What results is a mini-domino effect. The loosening of the eyelids causes the corneas to alter their contour, changing the way our eyes focus light—and, consequently, changing the prescription we need to correct this focus. Often this also causes us to have an increase in astigmatism (a focusing problem; see below) as we reach our forties and fifties.

Changes in the lens: Another issue is that the lens within the eye also changes throughout our lives, starting even before we're born. As it grows, layer after layer of cells—like the rings of a tree or the skins of an onion—add themselves to the front surface of the lens. This growth pattern too has an impact on our prescription. Older layers of cells within the center of the lens become more compacted, making the lens nucleus more dense and the lens in general less flexible. Eventually these changes affect our ability to focus on near objects. (An increase in lens density is also the most common cause of cataracts. For more on this, see chapter 7.)

REFRACTIVE ERRORS

When you need to wear corrective lenses in order to achieve clear vision, you have what's called a *refractive error*. *Refraction* is a physics term that refers to how light is bent as it passes through a lens. When your eye doesn't do a good job of bending and focusing light onto your retina—and thus allowing you to see—then there's an error in the eye's "refraction ability." (*Refraction* also describes the technique doctors use to determine what your glasses prescription should be.) Refractive errors for the eye are myopia, hyperopia, astigmatism, and presbyopia.

Myopia

Myopia means "nearsightedness." A nearsighted eye can focus better on close objects than on distant objects. But this is a relative term, meaning that the degrees of nearsightedness vary considerably. Without corrective lenses, someone who is extremely nearsighted really only sees clearly at too close a distance to be functional, while people who are only mildly near-

A.

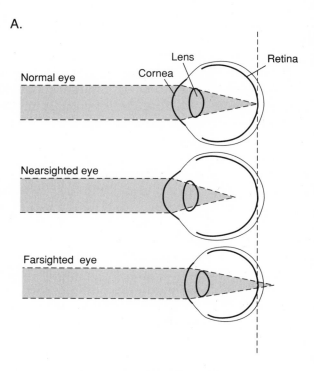

Fig. 2.1. (A) Normal eye, nearsighted eye, and farsighted eye;
(B) nearsighted eye with and without corrective lens;
(C) farsighted eye with and without corrective lens

sighted can generally see well enough to perform most of their daily tasks.

The myopic eye is actually an eye that has *too much* focusing power. There are three possible reasons for this excess power: either the cornea has too much curvature, or the eye is too long from front to back, or the lens within the eye is focusing excessively. In all of these instances, light is focused *in front* of the retina (in other words, it undershoots its mark). Your prescription is designed to have the opposite effect, so that your corrective lens offsets the eye's high power and allows the light to focus directly on the retina. Eyeglass prescriptions written for someone who's nearsighted have a minus sign in front of the lens power. This indicates that the lens of the eyeglasses is effectively *taking away* the excess power of the eye. A nearsighted eye is not weak; instead, it's too strong.

B.

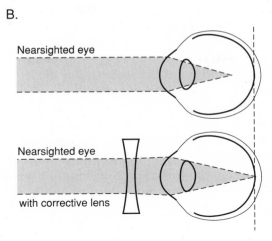

Nearsighted eye

Nearsighted eye

with corrective lens

C.

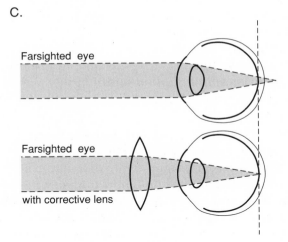

Farsighted eye

Farsighted eye

with corrective lens

Hyperopia

Hyperopia is the technical term for farsightedness. As you might expect, a hyperopic eye is the opposite of a myopic eye in that it doesn't have *enough* power to focus light precisely on the retina. Either the cornea or the lens doesn't have enough curvature, or the eye is too short for light to be focused appropriately. The term *accommodation* refers to the way the eye muscle and lens work together to focus on something nearby—a book, for example, or a makeup mirror. Farsighted people use this same accommodative system to compensate for their lack of focusing power, in order to see at a distance. When farsighted people try to read, however, they must focus for their hyperopia as well as for the reading distance—an effort that requires significantly more eye muscle power. For farsighted people, then, vision is relatively clearer at a long distance than up close, because it takes less muscular effort. For someone who is extremely farsighted, the world really is blurry at all distances. The hyperopic prescription is the opposite of the myopic prescription: there's a plus sign before the lens power, indicating that the eyeglass or contact lens is adding more power to the eye.

Astigmatism

Astigmatism may be one of the most misunderstood and misused terms in our field; we've heard patients use it to describe everything from lid twitches to floaters. Actually, astigmatism is a refractive problem in which an eye doesn't focus light evenly.

A short lesson in physics may help illustrate this. Imagine that you have a tiny light bulb, the size of a pinpoint. This light sends rays out equally in all directions, forming a sphere of light. If this light is focused through a lens that is also spherical—in other words, if it's curved equally in all directions like a basketball—then this light, when focused onto a flat surface such as a wall, forms a circle, just like the round spot of light you create when you shine a flashlight at a wall.

A lens that has astigmatism isn't curved evenly in all directions. Instead of a basketball, it's like a football. In an eye that has astigmatism, usually the corneal curvature is greatest in one direction and least in the opposite direction. A football has less curvature across the ball than around it. Both directions—across the ball and around the ball—have some curvature, but it's not evenly distributed, as it is on the basketball.

If you focus a pinpoint of light through a football-shaped lens, the light gets focused more around the lens than across the lens, and it exits as a stretched-out circle or oval. Because the eye's variations in curvature are much more delicate, you really can't see this football shape. But this subtle difference in curvature tends to blur images that we see, so that the world looks stretched out, just like that contorted circle of light.

If you have astigmatism, a good way to demonstrate this distortion is for you to look at the taillights on a car in front of you at night without your

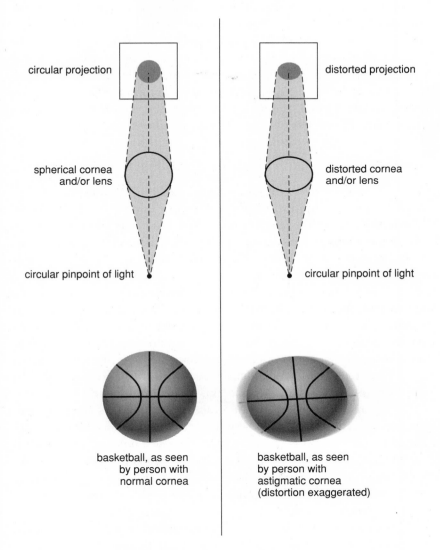

Fig. 2.2.   How astigmatism distorts vision

glasses (while someone else is driving, of course!). The red taillights will send off streamers in the same direction as your astigmatism. These streamers will diminish when you put your glasses back on, but they won't fully go away, because of some scattering of the light at the edges of your glasses.

In eyeglasses, an astigmatic prescription is designed to create the opposite of the eye's curvature, so that light is focused evenly onto the retina. In an astigmatic prescription, the power is referred to as *cylinder power*. The *axis* is specified to tell the optician at what angle to direct the cylinder power (either horizontally, vertically, or somewhere in between).

Presbyopia

The word *presbyopia* is derived from Latin and translates literally— though rather unflatteringly to those of us who develop it—as "old eyes." The term describes the phenomenon that eventually befalls everyone: the loss of our ability to focus up close. Presbyopia generally starts anywhere from age thirty-five to fifty. You may first notice it when you're trying to read the label on a bottle of aspirin or the fine print of a magazine ad.

This is what happens: Remember the accommodative system, the muscle and lens system within the eye that enables us to focus on near objects? The ciliary muscles, part of this system, sit just behind the iris. When these muscles contract, they cause the lens to bulge forward and change the focus of the eye, so that we can see something up close (see figure 1.3).

Now, remember how the lens in our eye is always growing? Well, by the time we reach our mid-thirties, this constant thickening has taken its toll; the lens has lost the flexibility needed to adjust its shape. Consequently, we can't accommodate—in other words, we can't see close up— nearly as well as we used to. Over time, the *closest* point at which the eye can focus moves farther and farther away—which is why one day we start holding the newspaper at arm's length to read it. But our arms are only so long, and eventually they're just not long enough to let us read without the help of corrective lenses.

Because presbyopia is part of the normal growth and development process of the lens, it isn't really what we think of as an "age-related degenerative change" to our body. That is, the ciliary muscles aren't weakening, and no tissue is breaking down. This ongoing evolution of the lens is simply an inevitable part of aging, something we can't change or control. There are no exercises or treatments that can stave off presbyopia, or even slow it down.

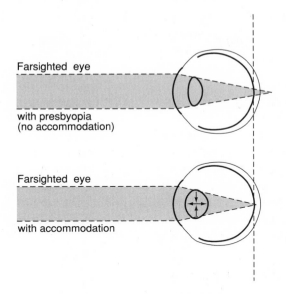

Fig. 2.3.   Farsighted eye with presbyopia, with and without accommodation

How will presbyopia affect you? It depends. If you're mildly to moderately nearsighted, presbyopia means you can read comfortably without your glasses, because your myopia does the job of focusing for a near object in place of your ciliary muscle and lens system. Because you can read more easily without glasses, presbyopia might not even trouble you until your late forties or early fifties. If you're farsighted, problems with presbyopia will likely occur much sooner; your ciliary muscles already have extra work just compensating for the hyperopia as well as focusing on objects up close. People with astigmatism often compensate by bringing reading material closer, which makes it relatively larger and easier to see. When presbyopia begins, you probably won't be able to compensate as well for your astigmatism, and you might need a presbyopic prescription sooner.

The presbyopic prescription is described as the *lens addition* or the *add*, and it's usually the same in both eyes. That is, your distance prescription (if you need one) balances out your vision, so that you see as well as you can with either eye by itself and with both eyes together. Because both eyes receive the same message from the brain to accommodate for up-close viewing, once your distance vision is balanced, you'll probably need an even amount of lens power added to both eyes to help you see to read. You can think of the distance prescription as the basic foundation for an eyeglass correction. The reading prescription is added on to this to give the eyes the extra power they need to see up close.

REFRACTIVE CHANGES THAT OCCUR WITH AGE

With each of the refractive errors discussed above, the changes in eyeglass prescriptions that occur throughout our lives tend to follow certain basic patterns. However, no two people are exactly alike; in fact, no two eyes are exactly alike! That's why, even though both eyes follow the same general trends as we get older, it's not unusual for one eye to change at a different pace than the other. But here are some changes you can expect, depending on your particular eyesight.

Aging and Nearsightedness

Here is the typical lifetime course of myopia: As our eyes grow, over the first twenty-five years or so, nearsighted people tend to become more nearsighted. Also, because so much of these early years is spent in school, the many hours a day spent reading and focusing up close probably add to the problem. All of the accommodation (discussed above) necessary for this focusing creates a situation in which the ciliary muscles are constantly contracted and the lens is constantly focused at near; eventually the eye can adapt to that contracted state—in other words, by getting used to focusing mostly at a reading distance—and become still more myopic.

Between ages twenty-five and thirty-five, the nearsighted prescription usually doesn't change much. However, as you might expect, those of us whose work involves extensive reading, writing, or other up-close focusing may still need increasingly stronger prescriptions during this time.

After about age thirty-five, the eye changes that cause accommodation problems begin to affect our degree of nearsightedness as well. As the up-close focusing system starts to fail, myopia that was brought on by excessive accommodation actually starts to get better; often this trend continues into our late fifties and early sixties. However, because this decrease in nearsightedness is a sign of diminishing accommodation, this seemingly happy turn of events may simply turn out to be the first step on the road to needing bifocals. Thus, for many people in their sixties there comes, after years of enjoying milder prescriptions, a reality check of sorts: becoming more nearsighted again. The most common type of cataract, nuclear sclerosis, is a consequence of years of growth and subsequent hardening of the lens. (For more on cataracts, see chapter 7.) In people with myopia this hardening of the lens at first may tend to *increase* its focusing power, and once again we start getting more nearsighted.

Aging and Farsightedness

With hyperopia, again, there's a typical lifetime cycle of progression. Up to about age twenty-five, farsightedness sometimes gets better on its own, as our eyes grow and develop. (If, for instance, the problem is that the eye is too short for light to be focused appropriately, this might resolve itself when the eye simply gets *bigger*.) Often there's no need to correct this problem in someone younger than twenty-five, because the accommodative system has a tremendous ability to compensate for this kind of anatomical shortcoming.

But the eye changes that cause us to need bifocals can manifest themselves much earlier in someone who's farsighted, and they can begin to affect our ability to read and focus up close as early as our twenties. As we get into our late thirties and early forties, when we begin holding the newspaper at arm's length, we also begin to lose the ability to accommodate for our hyperopia. We begin having trouble with our distance vision and may require corrective lenses to help us to see better. Glasses prescriptions for distance vision often get stronger in our late fifties and early sixties.

For farsighted people the dawn of cataract formation may cause the opposite effect of the change that occurs with nearsighted people: a shift in the power of the lens within the eye causes an *increase* in the eye's focusing power, which results in a *decrease* in hyperopia. That is, in a farsighted person, distance vision without eyeglasses can actually improve with early cataracts. This is known as *second sight* (see below and chapter 7).

Aging and Astigmatism

Astigmatism doesn't change as much with age as myopia or hyperopia do. After the eye stops growing, astigmatism levels off; decades may go by before you need a new prescription. Then along comes presbyopia—

and this plus changes in lid tension across the cornea can cause changes in astigmatism that may be for better or worse, depending on your particular case. Early cataract formation can also cause changes, as the cataract subtly changes the shape of the lens within the eye.

Aging and Presbyopia

After its onset, presbyopia produces a classic pattern of change over the next fifteen to twenty years. Initially your glasses prescription is doing part of the focusing for you. As your accommodative system changes, the glasses prescription increases, until eventually the prescription does *all* of the focusing for you.

Usually the first symptom of presbyopia is that we can't seem to bring an object as close to our eyes, *and keep it in focus*, as we used to. Also, it takes longer to bring a near object into focus and then to shift our focus to look at something across the street or even across the room. (The cause of this delay is the ever-thickening, increasingly less flexible lens, which doesn't do its job as fluidly and effortlessly as it once did.)

As presbyopia progresses, the point at which we can focus moves farther and farther away, until eventually anything inside of twenty feet looks blurry. While your presbyopia progresses to the point where your reading addition to your distance prescription does 100 percent of the focusing for you, your near range of focus tends to diminish until your vision is really only clear from about twelve to twenty inches.

What's happening is that as you need more lens power in your glasses to compensate for your presbyopia, your ciliary muscles and lens are less flexible for range of vision, and your near working distance keeps inching closer, to where the spectacle lens focuses.

Those of us who spend a lot of time viewing objects at intermediate distances of twenty to forty inches—the computer monitor, for example— often need additional lens prescriptions. For many people the best solution is either a progressive addition, "no-line" bifocal that allows for multiple working distances, or a trifocal that adds another lens to your spectacles, designed particularly for intermediate-distance viewing.

Early cataract formation, or nuclear sclerosis, also affects presbyopia. Because this causes a shift in vision that can make people either more nearsighted or less farsighted, some of us suddenly find ourselves able to read without our bifocals (a delightful phenomenon often referred to as *second sight*). Unfortunately, this is a short-term improvement; as the cataract progresses, vision at all levels tends to get worse.

BINOCULAR FUSION

Besides refractive errors, the eye is also subject to other changes that affect our vision. Remember, we don't see with our eyes alone but with our eyes *and brain* (see chapter 1). Everything we see—image information beamed into each eye—is transmitted to the brain. In turn, the analyzed information from *both* eyes is then processed by the brain to allow us to view the world, as eye doctors put it, "binocularly." The term *binocular vision* refers to our ability to use both eyes together to provide an enhanced, in-depth view of the world. (Most of us see better with both eyes together than with either eye alone.)

This ability for our eyes to work together is harder than it sounds, and it requires extensive coordination. Messages from the brain enable both eyes to move together when viewing and tracking the movement of any object. When our eyes work together in this manner, it's called *binocular fusion*. Binocularity is a combination of *motor* and *sensory* fusion. Motor fusion is the mechanical ability of the eye muscles to work together; sensory fusion is how well the brain can turn these visual messages from both eyes into one coherent image.

Because the eye muscles from both eyes are rarely perfectly coordinated, it's the sensory fusion that helps fine-tune any slight mechanical misalignment. As we age, our ability to maintain good motor fusion, or mechanical alignment, tends to weaken; the muscles start to weaken in the eyes, just as they do elsewhere in the body. If your eyes tend to cross, for example, this tendency can increase as you get older and the sensory fusion system starts to labor harder than usual to help keep your eyes working together. When this happens, unfortunately, people are all too aware of it. Headaches located in or around the eyes can become common; so can symptoms of the eyes "pulling" together, plus overall fatigue and eyestrain with any big visual chore such as a long time spent behind the wheel of a car or in front of a book. Finally, if the sensory fusion system becomes too overburdened—if it can no longer compensate for misaligned eye muscles by keeping the images fused—the result is double vision.

The most common fusion problem with age is also a consequence of

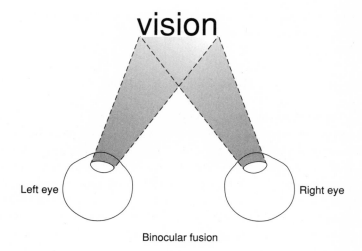

Binocular fusion

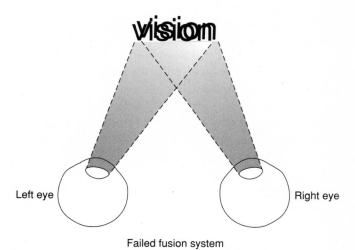

Failed fusion system

Fig. 2.4.   Binocular fusion system

presbyopia. When you read, both eyes have to turn in slightly, in order for them to focus together on the page. This process is called *convergence*. The simple act of looking at something up close, like a book, sets off a series of actions in the brain and eyes just so that you can focus the lens within your eye, to make the book appear clear, and to converge your eyes, so that the words appear single.

Remember the accommodation process that enables our eyes to change shape so that we can see up close? Each amount of accommodation is matched by the same amount of convergence to maintain clear and single vision. In other words, it's not enough just to focus on something up close; the eyes must also be *coordinated* enough that we see a single, understandable image. With presbyopia, as we discussed above, this ability to accommodate diminishes. Also, the signal the brain sends—to tell the muscles to converge what we see into a single image—gets weaker over time. The sensory fusion system tries to overcome this problem and keep our eyes working together.

By the time our presbyopia reaches the point where our reading prescription does 100 percent of our focusing, the motor convergence system is basically kaput; for some people who had an underlying convergence problem before they developed presbyopia, the sensory fusion system isn't up to the task of maintaining single vision at near viewing distances. The result? Reading becomes an arduous grind. The print swims, runs together, and doubles.

But there is hope. Fusion problems can be treated with eyeglasses, eye exercises, eye muscle surgery, or a combination of any of these. Eye exercises have proven helpful in increasing sensory fusion in some people, but often the sensory system can't be built up enough to overcome the increasing weakness of the eye muscles. Eye muscle surgery is often a last resort, when all other attempts have failed to restore binocularity. Often the best solution is to incorporate into the glasses prescription a lens correction called *prism*. This isn't the prism you might have played with as a child—the long, triangle-shaped glass that spun rainbows when light shone through it. In spectacle lenses, prism is used to bend and redirect the light coming through the lenses without changing the lenses' ability to refract the light. That is, the prism doesn't change the power of the prescription; it just helps compensate for the misalignment of the eye muscles. Prism can be ground into an eyeglass prescription so that it can't be seen in the lens, and your view of the world with either eye by itself doesn't change. But with it, your view of the world with both eyes together is much more comfortable and clear; the prism boosts the motor fusion system, so that your eye muscles don't need to work as hard. At the same time, the prism eases the sensory fusion system, so that the images of both your eyes come together more completely for clear single vision.

Some Questions You May Have about Changes in Your Vision

It seems like my eyes keep getting worse. Will I just keep getting more nearsighted until I'm blind?

Relax. Most of the increases in nearsighted prescriptions occur during the growth and development phase of life. Then the changes slow down. It might seem that every time you go to the eye doctor you need something stronger, but that trend usually reverses itself between the ages of thirty-five and sixty. Myopia typically stops progressing and actually starts to *reverse* with the onset of presbyopia. However, early cataract formation (also called *nuclear sclerosis*, discussed above) sometimes causes a shift in the prescription, which can make your myopia worse.

You may have heard about a rare condition called *pathological myopia*, in which a nearsighted eye can progress to the point of blindness. The blindness occurs because the eye becomes so large and the retina becomes so stretched and distorted that it may eventually degenerate. The people most likely to develop pathological myopia are those who were very myopic as young children. But again, this is a *very rare* condition and is far from the normal course of the aging eye.

I never used to wear glasses when I was younger. What's wrong with me now? Why do I keep needing stronger glasses every time I come in, and why can't I see as well without my glasses?

This question is usually asked by someone who is hyperopic, or farsighted. (For a discussion of farsightedness, see above.) As your focusing system, which involves your ciliary muscles, begins to lose its ability to "accommodate" for reading, it also becomes less able to compensate for your hyperopia. If you're farsighted, you've probably been using these ciliary muscles all your life to compensate for this relative eye weakness. Because of this, when you're younger the ciliary muscles tend to stay somewhat contracted; as a result, any early eyeglass prescriptions you may have are weaker than you might need if these muscles were fully relaxed.

As you get older and—like everyone else—develop presbyopia, the muscle tone in these ciliary muscles starts to decrease. (Basically, these muscles get out of shape because they don't have much luck trying to push an aging, inflexible lens to focus.) As this muscle tone becomes more lax, the prescription for distance vision increases as the latent hyperopia—which was there all along, but masked by the efforts of the ciliary muscles—begins to express itself.

Even if you don't progress beyond a certain distance prescription for hyperopia, you may still notice a deterioration of your vision at a distance without your glasses. As the accommodation system (for a discussion, see above) fails and your vision without glasses is not compensated for by the ciliary muscles and lens system, you'll probably find yourself relying on your glasses more and more to see at a distance. You might not need stronger glasses over time, but you just won't see as well without them.

This is great! I used to need my glasses for reading, but now I don't. Did my eyes get better?

Well, the best answer may be, Enjoy it while it lasts! The earliest onset of age-related cataracts, or nuclear sclerosis (discussed above), causes a shift in the focusing ability of the eyes. This shift tends to make nearsightedness worse and farsightedness better for a time.

But sadly, as noted above, this "second sight" is a relatively fleeting phenomenon. Eventually the cataract takes its toll on our vision; we notice that, with or without our glasses, we don't see as well as we used to, and once again we need a new prescription or perhaps cataract surgery (see chapter 7).

It's official: I'm a senior citizen. Should I worry about my ability to drive?

Yes. For many of us, however much we hate to admit it, getting older means we don't see as well to drive as we used to.

Relax—we're not suggesting that you turn in your driver's license the first time you have trouble seeing a traffic light or road sign. But your ability to drive is something you'll need to consider, with unflinching honesty, from now on. Next to the notorious sixteen- to twenty-four-year-old age group, drivers older than sixty-five are second in the number of auto accidents per vehicle-mile traveled. Nobody knows exactly how many of these accidents are due to poor vision, but it has to be a factor.

Currently, more than thirteen million American drivers are age seventy or older—and this is just a drop in the bucket compared with what's going to happen over the next two decades, as more baby boomers hit the bifocal and cataract years. By the year 2020 an estimated thirty million drivers will be over age seventy.

Most states (forty-two so far) require vision testing for a driver's license renewal; most likely, all states will adopt such policies soon. A recent study showed that between 1985 and 1989, states that *did not* require vision testing for driver's license renewal had significantly more fatalities each year among older drivers than states with mandatory vision screening.

What does this mean to you? Mainly, just be careful and use your common sense. If you have any trouble seeing at night, limit your driving to daytime. If your peripheral vision is not great—from glaucoma or diabetic retinopathy, for example—do your best to avoid busy intersections, where side vision can be particularly important. If glare is a problem, consider purchasing glasses with special antireflective coatings (see chapter 4).

Why do I see double, and is there any help for me?

Double vision is often a result of the weakening of the extraocular eye muscles, the muscles that move the eyes. These muscles can lose their ability to keep the eyes working together as they should. When this happens, your right and left eyes aren't working well together; each eye sees a slightly different image. The brain can't put these two images together, and you see double. *Close one eye;* if you can lose one of the images by closing either eye, then your double vision is caused by this kind of muscle imbalance.

In rare circumstances certain diseases can affect the positioning of the eyes. An overactive thyroid gland, for example, can cause the eyes to shift within their sockets, resulting in a misalignment of the eye muscles. Certain tumors can affect the nerves in the brain that control eye muscle movements, and this may also lead to double vision.

If you still see double after closing one eye, then your double vision is caused by one of three other factors besides the relatively common muscle imbalance and the rare diseases that affect vision.

First, your double vision might be caused by cataracts, which occasionally develop at an inconvenient spot within the lens of the eye so that light that enters the lens is scattered by the cataract and splits into two images (see chapter 7).

The second possible reason is a sudden increase in astigmatism, which can also happen with the development of a cataract. Uncorrected astigmatism distorts an image so that it's stretched in one direction. Occasionally this will appear as a clear image with a second "ghost image" next to it—kind of like what you see when you have bad TV reception.

The third reason can be the most serious of the three: age-related changes within the macula, the center of the retina that provides our best vision, can also cause a splitting of the image.

If you have double vision—even if it goes away for a time—*seek immediate attention!* Usually the problem is indeed related to the eyes; however, it's also extremely important to rule out any other problems that may be jeopardizing your general health.

What does 20/20 vision mean?

The top number 20 refers to the testing distance of the eye chart. *Optical infinity* is a term that describes the minimum distance that an object needs to be from your eye so that it can be seen without any accommodation effort, or focusing of your eye muscles. Twenty feet is the minimum distance between an object and the eye to be effectively at optical infinity; that's why this has become a standard testing distance for eye charts. The bottom number represents the size of the letter or target that you view. Years of research have yielded an average-size letter that you should be able to see at a given testing distance if your eyes have normal vision. (Technically, a 20/20 letter subtends 5 minutes of arc at 20 feet.) This letter size was given the designation 20. When you mathematically divide 20 (the size of the letter) by 20 (feet) you get a result of 1, so that 20/20 vision becomes an index of normalcy. If, for example, you have 20/40 vision, then 20 divided by 40 equals ½, and it could be said that your vision is *half as good* as it should be. Another way to interpret 20/40 vision is to say that you need to double the size of a 20/20 letter, or double the visual angle that a 20/20 letter makes, in order for you to be able to read that letter at twenty feet. Very simply, a person with 20/40 vision can see an object clearly from twenty feet that a person with "normal" eyes can see clearly all the way from forty feet.

Eye charts were designed by analyzing all of the letters in the alphabet and categorizing each letter according to how difficult it is to read at the testing distance. The letter *L*, for example, is not confused with many other letters and is therefore easy to spot at a distance. The letter *E*, however, can look like a *B, F, P, R, S,* or *Z* at a distance, and it's usually the first letter that is missed on a line. Each line on an eye chart contains letters from easy and hard categories, so that if you misread a letter on a line, the specialist performing the test can determine the significance of your error. Missing a hard letter like E is not as significant as missing an easy letter.

PART II

Getting to 20/20

3

The Eye Exam

Getting your glasses and your eyes checked can be a fairly simple prospect or a very complicated one, depending on the problem—and, of course, on who's doing the checking (in other words, on how in-depth an exam you receive). Routine eye examinations can be performed by ophthalmologists and by optometrists, and parts of routine eye exams can be done by technicians who may or may not have a specific degree or certification. Before we cover the specifics of eye examinations, though, let's take a moment to discuss the professionals who perform them.

EYE CARE PROFESSIONALS

Ophthalmologists

An ophthalmologist is a medical doctor, a graduate of an accredited medical school with an M.D. degree—which means that you can expect him or her to have a pretty good understanding of the illnesses that can befall the *rest* of your body, and the ramifications of such ailments (diabetes, for instance) for your eyesight. Ophthalmologists can also be doctors of osteopathic medicine (D.O.). In addition, a board-certified ophthalmologist must have completed at least three years of residency training beyond the M.D. degree and passed extensive written and oral examinations in diseases and surgery of the eye.

Many ophthalmologists provide total eye care, beginning with the comprehensive medical eye examination: they prescribe glasses and contact lenses, diagnose eye diseases and disorders, and perform the appropriate medical, surgical, and laser procedures necessary to treat them. Other ophthalmologists perform eye exams and diagnose and treat diseases of the eye but limit themselves to a fairly narrow range of surgical procedures, refer-ring patients needing different procedures to other ophthalmic subspecial-ists. And some subspecialists—doctors who concentrate on treating specific diseases and performing certain procedures (literally, they're specialists *within* a specialty)—don't perform routine eye exams at all.

Like many other branches of medicine, ophthalmology has become increasingly subspecialized over the last twenty years. Although some pol-icymakers are fond of making the blanket statement that "there are just too many specialists," the undisputed fact is that *anyone* (even, one suspects, those policymakers) who needs a surgical procedure wants the operation to be done by a surgeon who has performed *that very same procedure* many times—someone who does it every day, or at least several times a week, someone who is deeply familiar with every detail of the operation, and with every nook and cranny of that particular body part—rather than by a gen-eralist whose job is to know a little bit about everything, who might have done that procedure only a few times before. (Which means, and we'll make this point again in later chapters, that if and when you need a surgi-cal procedure, consider *getting a second opinion*, and find the best, most ex-perienced physician you can to perform it. Think about it: it's your pre-cious vision at stake here, and your one chance to get the job done right.) It's also true that most surgeons want to do only the operations that they do really well. The situation is complicated, and it keeps changing.

Optometrists

An optometrist is someone who has earned a doctor of optometry (O.D.) degree after completing four years of post-graduate-level optome-try school, following a four-year undergraduate college degree. Optometry school covers the structure and function of the eye, mechanisms of vision and optics, and the diagnosis and treatment of eye disease. Some optome-try schools have even developed collaborative arrangements with medical schools to give optometry students the opportunity to develop a better understanding of how the eye relates to the human body and its overall condition.

Optometrists traditionally limited their scope of practice to nonmed-ical treatment of eye problems. This included prescribing glasses and con-tact lenses to improve the quality of vision and the use of vision therapy to improve the overall functioning of the visual system. Optometrists were taught how to diagnose eye diseases and look for signs of associated systemic ("whole body") diseases so that the patient could be referred to the appropriate physician. Currently, however, many optometrists are learning how and being licensed to treat noncomplicated eye disease and how to manage surgery patients along with ophthalmologists.

Opticians

An optician is an eye care professional licensed to fit, adjust, and dispense eyeglasses and other optical devices following the written prescription of an ophthalmologist or optometrist. In some states opticians can also fit and dispense contact lenses.

RECENTLY, CONTROVERSIAL LEGISLATION in many states concerning the use of diagnostic and therapeutic eye drops and procedures by optometrists has heightened the public's awareness of the differences in training among ophthalmologists, optometrists, and opticians. Most eye care professionals, however, agree that each of these specialists has a separate yet complementary role in eye care—and in the future, you're likely to see these three groups settling their differences and working more closely together. This will allow for a more comprehensive approach to eye care, one that can also be cost-efficient for patients and their insurance companies, as well as for eye care providers.

HOW OFTEN SHOULD YOU GET YOUR EYES CHECKED?

This is what the American Academy of Ophthalmology recommends.

If you're between ages forty and sixty-five: If everything's fine—if you have no symptoms and are at low risk for eye disease—you should get a comprehensive baseline medical eye examination, to establish a point of reference for future checkups, and then go back for follow-up checkups every two to four years.

If you're over sixty-five: Again, if everything's fine—if you have no symptoms and are at low risk for eye disease—you should have a comprehensive eye exam every one to two years. Why the need for more frequent checkups as you get older? Because, as with other ailments, your risk of developing certain eye problems such as cataracts, glaucoma, and macular degeneration goes up slightly with each passing year, and your best odds of maintaining good vision lie in catching any problems early, at the first signs of trouble.

If you have any symptoms of eye trouble: Even if you've just had your regular eye examination, it's very important to get any new symptoms checked out right away. Symptoms of blurred vision, for example, can mean much more than that you just need to change your eyeglass prescription. Therefore, waiting for the next routine examination—especially if it's two years away—is not a great idea. By then you might have some permanent vision damage from a problem that could have been much less serious if caught in time.

If you have other health problems or a family history of eye disease: In this case you'll probably need more frequent eye exams. Remember, the eye isn't immune from the repercussions of systemic medical conditions (hypertension and diabetes, for instance, can be particularly hard on the eyes). Also, if you have a family history of eye disease—glaucoma, cataracts at an early age, retinal detachment, or macular degeneration, for example—then your own risk of developing these is higher, and your doctor will want to be on the lookout for early signs or symptoms as you get older.

What You Can Expect at a Routine Eye Examination

To begin the exam, the doctor or a member of the staff will take your medical history, asking a series of basic questions, beginning with your age (see box).

Visual Acuity Tests

After taking your medical history, the doctor will usually test your *distance visual acuity* and *near visual acuity*—how well you're able to read letters correctly across the room, and how well you read them up close. (In years past, the distance test was always done at a length of twenty feet, but today the test chart distance is generally downsized with mirrors, and visual acuity can be measured at a distance of sixteen or even fourteen feet, so don't worry if the examining room seems small!) The classic "20/20" visual score measure means that at twenty feet, *with or without corrective lenses,* you can read the same letters that a person lucky enough to have perfect vision

Your Medical History: Ten Important Questions about Your Health

Your eye examination will begin with your ocular history, followed by a few basic, important questions about your general health, beginning with your age. Although the questions may vary, you can probably expect to answer at least the following:

- What eye problems are you having now?
- What eye problems have you had in the past?
- How is your vision?
- Do you wear glasses? If so, do they work?
- Have you ever had eye surgery?
- How old are you, and how is your general health?
- What medical problems do you have?
- Do you take any medicines?
- Do you have allergies?
- Has anyone in your family had eye trouble or eye disease such as glaucoma?
- Has anyone in your family had diabetes, hypertension, heart disease, or thyroid disease?

can read at twenty feet (see chapter 2). So a score of 20/40 on this test means that you see *less well* than normal (you must stand at twenty feet to read the same letters a person with perfect vision can read from forty feet), whereas 20/15 means your vision is *better* than normal (you can read from twenty feet away the same letters a person with perfect vision can only read at fifteen feet).

Usually, visual acuity, both distance and near—near acuity is measured at the usual reading distance of fourteen to sixteen inches—is recorded for each eye separately and for both eyes together. Some of these measurements may be skipped, depending on how much the doctor already knows about you. For example, in someone young enough to have normal accommodation, or focusing power, who has no trouble reading, recording near acuity may not really be useful.

Refraction

Refraction is the process by which the doctor determines the lens combination that helps you to see the best. Refraction can be done in several ways. One is for the doctor to hold up lenses and ask you questions (this is called *subjective refraction* or *manifest refraction*). Another is to shine a light into your eye and neutralize the movement of the light with lenses (a process called *retinoscopy*). Or your doctor may prefer to use one of several types of automatic refractors—computerized machines that estimate the lens combination that's best for you. Subjective refraction is then often used to fine-tune your prescription, using your response to questions. After all, you are the best judge of how you really see.

All of these methods of refraction are useful under certain conditions, but none of them can be counted on in every circumstance or for every patient, which means that your doctor will need to determine which one is most accurate for you. For example, retinoscopy is invaluable for determining proper corrective lens strength for children or adults who cannot cooperate in subjective refraction. While most twelve-year-old children can participate in subjective refraction, only some ten-year-olds, and fewer still eight-year-olds, can do so. Automatic refractors are wonderful time-savers and do almost as good a job as subjective refraction. However, most of us who use the subjective refraction process are sure we do at least a little better than the machines. (And most of us are more interesting to talk to!)

Note: Just because the eye doctor can find a lens combination that provides the best possible visual acuity for you does not automatically mean that you must wear those lenses—or any lenses. Other than children with lazy-eye problems, no one has to wear glasses just because the doctor says so. People need to wear glasses only in order to correct *the problems that bother them.* Eye doctors are often surprised by the vision problems that people will tolerate in order to avoid wearing glasses. Going without glasses may seem silly to some people, but after all, they're *your* eyes; even though you may squint a lot or not see as well as you could, it doesn't hurt your eyes *not* to wear glasses, and it is ultimately your decision.

External Examination

After vision and refraction comes the external examination—what your doctor can learn simply by looking at your eyes without any specialized instruments. We may not write all of the observations down, or may do so very briskly, but we do pay attention to the following:

- The appearance and symmetry of the face
- The skin of the eyelids

- The edges of the lids and the lashes
- The position of the lids, and how well they open and close
- The clarity and shininess of the cornea, the irises, and the pupils, and their reaction to light
- The color, texture, and moisture of the conjunctiva (the slippery membrane on the front surface of the eye)
- The position, movements, and coordination of the eyes

This external exam can be done quickly. If there's anything abnormal-looking or anything that needs to be looked at more carefully and in more detail, we generally notice it during the exam, even if we don't always comment on it. If you think that your doctor missed something, or if you have a particular concern, by all means, ask! If, for example, you say, "What did you think of the black spot on my right eye?" your doctor may need to take another look—but more likely he or she has already formed an opinion about it.

Pupillary Testing

The pupil is the black area of the eye, the part that is surrounded by color (the iris). All images must pass through the pupil before they are processed by the retina and perceived by the brain. The pupil, just like the aperture of a camera, opens and closes in response to light. In bright light the pupil gets small. In dim light it opens wide to allow more light to the back of the eye, to enhance the visual image. The shape and symmetry (or asymmetry) of your pupils and the way they react to light can give your doctor a lot of information about how you are seeing. Since the nerves that control pupil function have a relatively long course, including a circuitous route through the neck, abnormal pupil function can also provide clues about disease and other problems taking place elsewhere in your body, such as tumors, aneurysms, and vascular disease.

Examination of Important Structures within the Eye

Next, your doctor will examine your eyes with a *slit lamp*—a microscope with magnification of ten times (10x) to forty times (40x) or even higher. This lamp has a light source that can be used either to provide illumination or to produce a thin, controlled sheet of light. The intense line of light produced by this "slit" can illuminate a thin section of the cornea, the

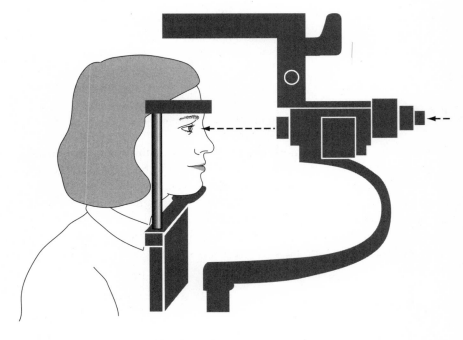

Fig. 3.1. Slit lamp biomicroscope

anterior chamber, or the lens. (For a look at these parts of the eye, see chapter 1.) These important structures of the eye are relatively transparent, so, like someone peering through a windowpane, we can look *through* one of them to focus on another. The slit lamp can also magnify and illuminate the iris, the conjunctiva, and the lids. With special stains and color filters, the slit lamp can reveal abnormalities of the cornea and conjunctiva from injuries or infections, or it can point out a deficiency of lubricating tears. With additional optics the slit lamp can also be used to examine the vitreous and retina.

Measurement of Intraocular Pressure

The measurement of intraocular pressure (pressure within the eye) is a routine part of the exam for adults, and often for younger patients as well. To measure intraocular pressure, the doctor must use a specially calibrated device. Several instruments have been designed for measuring intraocular pressure. Some use weights and look like small food scales, and others

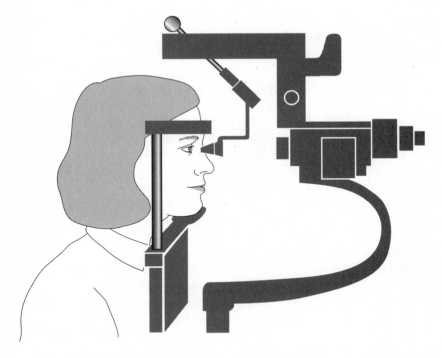

Fig. 3.2.   Slit lamp biomicroscope with applanation tonometer

shoot a puff of air at the eye. The most commonly used instrument, however, is the *applanation tonometer*, which is mounted on the slit lamp. (This tool can swing out of the way when the slit lamp is being used to look at the eye.) Before using the applanation tonometer, the doctor will put a local anesthetic in the eye, as well as a dye called *fluorescein*, either separately or together. (These may sting briefly.)

When a cobalt blue filter is put on the light source, the fluorescein glows (or "fluoresces") a bright, otherworldly green. The doctor or technician looks through the tonometer and turns a dial until the tonometer tip flattens a given amount of corneal surface. The amount of pressure in the eye is calculated using the relationship between (1) the force required to flatten the cornea and (2) the area of cornea flattened. During this process the smooth plastic tonometer actually touches the front of the cornea, but the local anesthetic keeps the patient from feeling any discomfort. Finally, the doctor reads the dial of the applanation tonometer to find out how hard the tonometer had to work to flatten the cornea. This reading, the intraocular pressure, is registered in millimeters of mercury. The tonometer is an extremely useful instrument that makes it easy for ophthalmologists and optometrists to measure pressure within the eye.

Examination of the Retina

The slit lamp can also be used to illuminate the retina, but most doctors prefer an *ophthalmoscope* for this important part of the examination. There are two basic varieties. The *direct ophthalmoscope* is a hand-held instrument; the doctor holds it up to his or her own eye and then shines the light into the patient's eye. The *indirect ophthalmoscope* looks like the classic miner's lamp, with the light fastened to a headband. This light shines through a lens, held by the doctor in front of the patient's eye. The lens focuses the light reflected *back out* of the patient's eye into an optical image. The indirect ophthalmoscope can explore a larger area of retina, allowing the doctor to see farther into the peripheral retina, and in three dimensions. Ophthalmoscopes can reveal most abnormalities of the retina; in addition, they're used to examine the optic nerve, the vitreous, and the blood vessels of the retina. (For a description of these structures, see figure 1.5.)

The retina is best viewed through a dilated pupil. Pupils are dilated by instilling dilating drops (see Appendix) into the patient's eyes and waiting fifteen to thirty minutes for the drops to be fully effective. (In people whose irises are a dark color, this may take longer.) These drops affect each person differently and last longer for some people than for others, depending on the type and strength of the drop or drops used. In general, pupil dilation will also be accompanied by a loss of accommodation, or the ability to see things up close. Most people maintain adequate distance vision, so they can see to drive home; but they will need to wear their distance glasses if they usually do so for driving. Sunglasses may also be necessary, especially on a bright day.

If you are uncertain about how dilating drops will affect you, the safest approach is to bring someone along with you to the eye examination—a designated driver. Usually the effects of the dilating eye drops wear off after a few hours, but in very rare instances these effects can take days to go away. Eye doctors must be very careful when using drops to dilate the pupils, since these drops can bring on acute closed-angle glaucoma in people with a narrow anterior chamber angle (see chapter 8).

ADDITIONAL TESTS YOU MAY NEED

What we've just covered are the basic parts of the standard eye examination: your medical history, the measurement of visual acuity, refraction, the external examination, examination of the internal structures, the measurement of intraocular pressure, and the retinal exam. Remember the beginning of this chapter, where we said that an eye exam could be fairly simple or more involved? Well, of all the many tests that can be done on eyes, some, like these, are done always and are considered routine.

Some additional tests, however, are done often but not always; many others are done only occasionally, unless the doctor has a special interest in, or specializes in diagnosing and treating, a specific type of problem.

This second group of tests—those that are done often but not always—includes measurement of visual fields, gonioscopy, exophthalmometry, and tests of tearing, of eye coordination, and of color vision. Let's go over these.

Measurement of Visual Fields

Your visual field is pretty much what it sounds like: the total area, up, down, and sideways, that you can see with one eye. It is also the drawing or diagram that represents what you can see. A visual field drawing indicates what size or color object you can see, at what distance from straight ahead, diagramed as odd-shaped circles. To get a better idea of how this works, see figure 3.3. People see best straight ahead, with the macula, and then less well the farther the object is from "fixation," or dead center—in other words, at the outer edges of our visual field, or what we can glimpse from "the corner of the eye."

Like nearly everything else in our high-tech world, visual field testing has become much more complicated and expensive over the last decade or so—but also better, in this case with the use of automated, computerized "perimeters," or visual-field-testing machines. These usually measure how high or how bright a light has to be in order for you to see it at a given position. Some of the more elaborate tests, involving hundreds of spots of light, can be tiring, but most are reasonably brief. Your doctor can also measure your visual field by having you observe a light at a certain spot getting brighter, or a light of fixed size moving in from the periphery toward your center of vision.

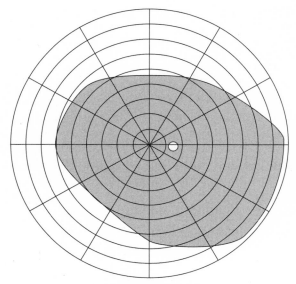

Visual field of right eye

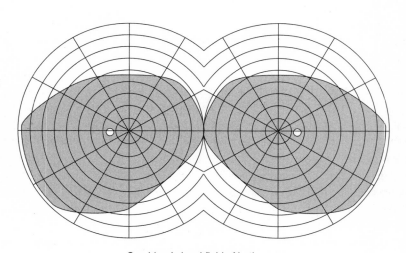

Combined visual field of both eyes

Fig. 3.3.   Visual fields

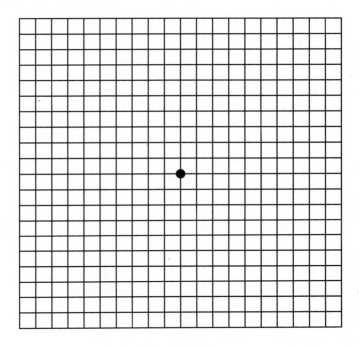

Fig. 3.4. Amsler grid

As a means of quick screening, to see whether someone's visual field warrants further study, a simpler test can be done. In this test your eye doctor might ask you to focus on his or her face and then would note at what point you're able to see a pencil or finger coming into view from below, above, and the sides. This type of "confrontation" field is a good way of determining whether your visual fields are normal or not. However, tests of this type are useless for detecting glaucoma; and because such tests do not accurately diagram any abnormality, they can't tell us anything about whether a specific condition is getting worse.

Another, specialized type of visual field test, called an *Amsler grid*, is a square with a pattern of small squares (like a piece of graph paper) and a dot in the middle (see figure 3.4). It was designed by Professor Marc Amsler as a rapid self-test to detect changes in the central 20 degrees of the visual field. The test is particularly helpful at identifying diseases of the macula and optic nerve that affect vision.

Here's how it works: First, you'll be asked to focus your gaze (using one eye at a time) on the dot in the center of the square. Now, some questions. How does the pattern of small squares look to you? Does any part of it seem to be missing, distorted, blurred, or warped? Which part? Distortion is an important warning sign; in most cases the distortion a patient sees matches a problem in the corresponding area of the retina.

Amsler grids can be administered at home as self-tests by patients who are considered likely to develop retinal problems. (Particularly at risk, for instance, are patients who have already had retinal trouble in one eye. For a more detailed discussion of retinal problems, see chapters 9 and 15.) Here's how to use the grid at home: Post it someplace where you can easily see it every day—some hard-to-miss spot like the refrigerator door or bathroom mirror. It's designed to be looked at, *in modest light*, from a distance of about a foot. If you wear glasses, contacts, or bifocals for reading, use them for this test, too.

It's simple to use. First, cover one eye and study the grid with your other eye. Look *straight ahead at the central dot and nowhere else!*

Now, answer these questions:

- Can you see the dot in the center?
- Can you see all four corners of the grid?
- Are all the small squares the same size?
- Are all of the lines straight, or are some of the lines wavy? Are any parts of the graph missing?
- Is there any movement? Any color aberration?

Now, repeat the test using the other eye. If you notice any changes—distortion, blurring, discoloration, or a complete absence of any part of the grid—contact your eye doctor *immediately* for an examination. If you're at high risk for macular or optic nerve problems—if you have advanced macular degeneration, for example—you should test yourself daily. Other people should consult their eye care specialist for a recommendation about how often they should perform this test.

Gonioscopy

A *gonioscope*, or *gonioprism*, is a device, about the size and shape of a thimble, that fits against the cornea. With the help of an anesthetic eye drop and a gooey drop to keep out air bubbles, the doctor can use this instrument to detect some kinds of glaucoma. An angled mirror inside the gonioscope—similar to the one your dentist uses—allows the slit lamp to focus "around a corner" into the space where the back of the cornea meets the front of the iris. (For more on these parts of the eye, see chapter 1.) This space is called the *angle of the anterior chamber*, and the angle itself is important: a narrow chamber angle may signal glaucoma.

Exophthalmometry

An *exophthalmometer*—one of our real tongue twisters—is a ruler with two arms that rest on the outer rims of the patient's orbits. Its angled mirrors enable the doctor to check, basically, whether the eye sticks out, or projects, farther than it should. The exophthalmometer is used most often to measure the amount of abnormal eye protrusion (also known as *exophthalmos*) associated with thyroid disease, but it is also used to monitor other causes of protrusion of the eyes.

Tests of Tearing

Do you have dry eyes? (The problem of dry eyes is discussed in chapter 13.) Would artificial tears help you? There are several tests available to help us answer these questions. One of these tests for diagnosing "deficiency of lubricating tears"—in other words, dry eyes—involves using paper strips to measure tear production, often along with an anesthetic drop (which helps decrease reflex tear production during the test). This is called the *Schirmer test*. One end of each paper strip is bent to fit inside the lower lid; the rest of the strip hangs down over the cheek. The amount of the strip wetted by tears is measured after two to five minutes. *Note:* There's a surprising amount of disagreement among ophthalmologists about the accuracy and usefulness of the paper strip test.

The *rose bengal dye test* provides another gauge of whether the patient has dry eyes and will find artificial tears useful. In this test a drop of dye is put inside the lower lid. The dye usually stings and is usually applied after application of anesthesia. If someone has a tearing deficiency, the dye leaves tiny pink-stained dots on the cornea and conjunctiva. The dots are visible with the slit lamp and represent areas where the corneal epithelial cells are either devitalized or missing. The doctor can tell by the patterns of dye staining whether there's a problem with dry eyes. (*Note:* While these dots are not permanent, there is in this test a possibility of spilling the dye on clothing, where it probably *is* permanent, so be careful not to rub your eyes immediately after the test, and make sure your doctor carefully rinses this dye from your eyes before sending you home.)

Tests of Eye Coordination

Most people see a little better with *both* eyes than with either eye alone. When this seems not to be the case, the problem usually has to do with the coordination of the two eyes—how well they work together. The brain uses a highly sophisticated feedback system to keep our eyes coordinated and avoid double vision. This system can correct large amounts of horizontal drift, quite small amounts of vertical drift, and almost no amount of rotational drift (see chapters 1 and 2).

As with any complicated system, some problems are more fixable than others. A few examples: If it's an eye muscle problem making someone see objects as level with one eye but tilted with the other eye, about all we can do is patch one eye and hope the other one will get better; or we can perform eye muscle surgery in an attempt to level the tilted eye. Much more common—and much more easily correctable—are small but annoying amounts of horizontal or vertical muscle imbalance. Such muscle imbalances are usually not detectable with an external exam, but we can distinguish them with tests such as the *cover-uncover test*, the *alternate cover test*, and a *red glass test*. Here's how the red glass test works: When you look at a light, your brain knows you're seeing just one light, and it works hard (but not cheerfully) to keep single vision. If, however, you hold a red glass in front of one eye, the brain relaxes its effort, and the white image seen by one eye separates from the red image seen by the other eye. The amount of this separation can be measured by the amount of prism necessary to line the two images up together. A prism lens can bend light in predictable amounts to compensate for eyes that cannot line up visual images by themselves. Putting a portion of the calculated amount of prism into the patient's glasses is often very helpful in solving such problems of muscle imbalance.

Tests of Color Vision

Tests of color vision are mainly used to diagnose inherited genetic defects of color vision. Such testing is rarely done in adults but may be used in diagnosing some optic nerve and retinal problems completely unrelated to inherited color blindness (for example, in checking for possible toxicity—in other words, too much of a drug in the system—from Plaquenil, a drug used to treat rheumatoid arthritis). These tests consist of asking the patient to identify colored numbers lying in a field of another color, or arranging various color samples in a specified order (as at the paint store, when we are trying to find the perfect shade of blue for the living room walls). If someone has trouble distinguishing different colors, the tests will reveal the problem and identify the problem range—red and green, for example—in the color spectrum.

OTHER, LESS COMMON, TESTS

Still other diagnostic tests, used much less commonly, are *retinal photography* and *retinal fluorescein angiography*. As with angiography of the heart, this is a series of pictures of the blood vessels—in this case, those within the retina—taken using a luminous dye. Pictures are taken as this dye, injected into the vein of the arm, moves through the arteries, capillaries, and veins of the eye. These pictures can reveal specific problems inside the eye such as age-related macular degeneration and diabetic retinopathy.

Another test occasionally needed is an *ultrasound examination of the eye*. This painless, noninvasive test—just like the ultrasound imaging commonly used in pregnancy—creates a picture with sound waves. When used in the eye, it can detect abnormalities such as tumors or retinal detachments (when, for example, bleeding in the eye or a dense cataract makes them impossible to detect during an optical examination). Examinations of the eyes by other imaging means, including X-ray, computerized tomography (CT) scans, or magnetic resonance imaging (MRI), can also be helpful in some cases. If one of these tests is necessary, it will usually be performed by a subspecialist, preferably someone recommended by your ophthalmologist or internist.

IN SUMMARY: Most eye exams are quick and simple; a few are long and complicated. Knowing which tests to do under specific circumstances requires the doctor to be well educated and trained, to listen well, and to consider carefully what's best for the patient.

Some Questions You May Have about Eye Exams

I'm getting my eyes dilated today. Will I be able to drive myself home?

Probably. Most people are able to drive after getting their eyes dilated, but everyone reacts differently.

Dilating drops work by enlarging your pupils and relaxing your *accommodation* (see chapter 2). If you're nearsighted, or if you don't normally wear glasses, you may have trouble with bright sunlight and glare, especially if there's snow on the ground. (If you need them, your doctor will probably provide a pair of plastic sunglasses to help cut the glare.) Also, this temporary loss of accommodation usually makes such up-close work as reading a bit more challenging. (If you need to read soon after getting your eyes dilated, it might help to remove your glasses or contacts.) But you probably won't have trouble driving; the eye drops shouldn't hamper your distance vision.

If you're farsighted, however, you may have some trouble temporarily—just for an hour or two, depending on the particular eye drops and their strength. Because the drops affect the eye's ability to accommodate, and your eyes work by using accommodation to see things far away, it's possible that your distance vision could be disrupted for a short while.

If you're concerned about your ability to drive home, discuss this beforehand with your eye doctor. This part of the exam may not be necessary, or you may be able to postpone it to another visit. Or you could bring a "designated driver" to help you get home.

My husband's doctor said that he's legally blind. What does that mean?

Legal blindness is a confusing term. It's not so much a particular diagnosis as a purely legal definition that enables sight-impaired people to qualify for helpful services—many of which are free—including "low-vision" assistance, occupational therapy, and tax benefits.

Every state has its own guidelines for legal blindness. To learn more about these, and to explore the range of services for which you may be eligible, call your state's Department of Social Services.

According to federal guidelines, you're "partially blind" if your vision *in the better eye,* when *best corrected* with glasses or contact lenses, is 20/200 or worse. For example, if you have macular degeneration with a visual acuity of 20/200 in one eye and 20/400 in the other, this would apply to you. (If, however, your vision is terrible in both eyes without glasses *but you see 20/20 with glasses*, then you'd be ineligible.) If your vision is better than 20/200 but your field of vision (see above) is severely limited—as if, with no peripheral vision, you were constantly looking at the world through a tube or tunnel—you may also be considered legally blind.

If your spouse is classified as legally blind, they may be eligible to receive an extra deduction on their federal income taxes. To qualify for a legal-blindness deduction on their federal income taxes, they'll need to attach to their tax return a written statement from their eye doctor, indicating their visual acuity or field of vision. (They should be sure to keep a copy for their own records as well.) If their condition will never improve, they can file an eye doctor's statement to this effect with the Internal Revenue Service. This will be on permanent record for all future tax returns.

Are headaches often due to eye problems?

Not as often as you might think. Headaches (see chapter 18) come in many forms. Some are mild, some severe; some are fleeting, while others linger for days. Some go away with a couple of aspirin; others require much stronger, prescription medication. *But very few of these are actually caused by eye problems.* Discomfort around the eyes can be related to eyestrain and the need for glasses, but this usually results from using your eyes for long periods—especially for close work—and is often relieved by a simple change in activity or by an over-the-counter pain reliever.

Note: If you're having frequent or severe headaches, see your eye doctor and your family physician or internist. They will want to rule out other health problems. Other factors that can cause headaches include tension, allergies, sinusitis, and temporal or giant cell arteritis (see chapters 17 and 18); migraines and other systemic disorders may also need to be considered.

4

All about Eyeglasses

Many of us are all too familiar with the concept of a "vision correction"—usually eyeglasses or contact lenses, but increasingly refractive surgery as well—because we've dealt with less-than-perfect eyesight for years. But there are just as many first-timers out there who are new to all this: adults, often in their forties and fifties, who suddenly find themselves needing extra help to see better. This prospect and all that it might represent, including the inevitability of growing older, can be, at the very least, unsettling.

But take heart. Your timing couldn't be better! Never before has there been such a wide and remarkable range of options, including choices that might have seemed like science fiction even twenty years ago.

Major technological advances in the way eyeglasses and contacts are manufactured now allow us to *see better* with *fewer compromises* to lifestyle and appearance. Today surgery is a possibility for correcting some vision problems that even a few years ago could be compensated for only by those thick, uncomfortable, Coke-bottle lenses.

So, faced with all these choices, what do you do now? If you've never before needed anything to help you to see better, how do you go about deciding what's right for you? What factors are important in making this decision? First you'll need to consider carefully your own needs, your lifestyle, job, and hobbies, and then weigh them against the general health of your eyes and the particular vision correction you require. Also, know that you certainly don't have to decide things all by yourself; that's where this book—and, of course, your own eye doctor and optician—can help. In this chapter we'll discuss all of these options and, we hope, help you narrow down your choices and come to an appropriate decision.

HOW TO FIND WHAT'S BEST FOR YOU: YOUR GUIDE TO LENSES AND FRAMES

Eyeglasses are the most frequently used means of correcting vision. Until about twenty-five years ago they were strictly functional and, as anyone whose face has ever been dwarfed by huge black horn-rims can attest, not much of a fashion statement. Now, with literally thousands of frames and hundreds of lens designs available, the selection can be overwhelming.

What's best for you? The physical attributes of your face may be one limiting factor; obviously, not all frames will look good on everyone. Your prescription may be another; a bifocal prescription or a very strong prescription might not fit well into a certain type of frame. A frame that doesn't fit your face won't do you much good, either; stylish but ill-fitting glasses won't allow the prescription to align properly over your eyes, and as a result your vision won't be clear or comfortable.

Ask for help. Your doctor and optician can guide you to the best selection of frame and lens design. Then, you and they can work together to make a decision. Discuss your concerns with your doctor at the time of your eye examination. Be sure to mention any specific visual needs—if you spend a lot of time reading, for instance, or using a computer—and ask what type of lens design would best suit those needs. Then, consult with your optician. Ask what type of frame is best suited for your face and the prescription. Lenses that provide the same function can be manufactured in numerous ways, some of them better for your needs than others.

First, the Lenses

Configurations

Eyeglasses are made in two basic configurations: *single-vision* and *multifocal.* As the names suggest, single-vision glasses have only one prescription, or lens power, whereas multifocals have more than one power within each lens. Traditionally, single-vision lenses were used by people who didn't need more than one prescription—someone who needed eyeglasses only for driving, perhaps, or just for reading. Or maybe someone needed glasses for both activities but used the same lens power for both. Single-vision eyeglasses sometimes work better for specific activities, such as viewing a computer screen at a fixed distance.

Multifocals may be bifocals, trifocals, or progressive addition lenses. These lenses address more than one need and often allow people to perform various visual tasks wearing the same pair of eyeglasses.

Bifocals have two prescriptions within the same lens, one for distance and one for reading. Bifocals may have a line across the entire width of the lens, with the reading portion on the bottom, or they may contain the reading area within a small part of the lens. Today bifocals can be made without a noticeable line, thanks to a sophisticated polishing technique. These "blended" bifocals—not to be confused with progressive bifocals, discussed later—may look better cosmetically. However, there's a drawback: the seamless line leaves a wide area of distortion where the two lens powers meet, and this shrinks the size of the available reading area. This blend is also noticeable—and, to some people, a nuisance—whenever you shift your gaze from distance viewing to near viewing. That is, although others see no line in your glasses and probably won't realize that you're wearing bifocals, *you* see a line, and it's fairly wide.

Trifocals add a third lens for intermediate vision, for viewing distances of about two to three feet. The intermediate lens has to be positioned just below the pupil, so that the reading portion can still sit high enough in the lens for you to use it comfortably. Because the intermediate lens sits up so high, the line is much more noticeable than with a bifocal, but trust us, you *will* get used to it, and your awareness of the line will diminish greatly as you do.

Progressive addition lenses are seamless multifocals. These lenses are much more functional than the blended bifocals. Their design offers a smooth transition from the distance portion of the lens into the reading portion. With progressive addition lenses you can't see a line from behind the lens. But as your eye moves from the top of the lens through the *intermediate channel* and into the reading area, the power of the lens gradually increases, or *progresses*. With this type of technology there's an appropriate lens power for every viewing distance. Say, for example, you need to view a computer monitor at thirty inches but you're working from a sheaf of papers just sixteen inches away; all you need to do is look *just slightly higher* in the lens to bring the computer monitor into view. Because these lenses include an appropriate part for *all* viewing distances, your vision often seems more natural. For example, say you're using standard bifocals to peruse the contents of a file cabinet drawer. How well can you see what you're doing? The files at the back of the drawer are somewhat in focus through the distance half of your lenses, and you can see the files at the front pretty well, using the near portion of the lens. But what about the files in between? To see them requires that you move your head, either closer to the drawer or farther away from it. Kind of awkward, isn't it? The beauty of the progressive addition lens is that you should be able to see the *entire* drawer, all in focus, all at once.

The drawback to such lenses is that in creating the progressive optics, a small part of the lens becomes unusable and the sides of the lenses become distorted. Still, the technology for crafting these lenses has improved greatly since the late 1970s, when they were first made, and the peripheral distortions are much milder in current lens designs. And, as with other kinds of lenses, you do grow accustomed to the slight inconveniences. At first, when you glance to the side with your progressive addition lenses, your vision will appear wavy, and you'll probably find yourself looking at things with your whole face, pointing your nose toward whatever you're observing. However, after you fully adapt to your new lenses, you'll hardly notice these distorted areas.

Glass or Plastic?

Here's another big decision: selecting the lens material. Sure, lenses are made from either glass or plastic, but that's just the tip of the iceberg. Many more choices lie within these two major categories.

Glass lenses tend to be more scratch-resistant than plastic lenses, but you pay the price: they're also twice as heavy. Plastic lenses are usually the lens of choice because of the weight difference; also, with special coatings, they can become more scratch-resistant. Plastic lenses have other advantages as well. They're more impact-resistant than glass. As a result, they're less likely to shatter or break. And because they're less brittle than glass, plastic lenses are easier to work with, which means that they can be machined to fit into more types of frames than glass lenses.

Also, manufacturers can tint plastic lenses simply by dropping them into a vat of heated dye, where they soak up the tint like a sponge. The amount of tint can be varied by the amount of time the lens is left in the dye. And later, if you decide that your lenses are too dark, the tint can be bleached out. On the other hand, glass lenses that are tinted must usually have a coating applied to the lens surface, like tinted car windows in sunny climates. This coating can scratch off the lens. Until recently, *photochromic* lenses, which get darker when exposed to sunlight, were available only in glass. Although the newer plastic photochromics have improved greatly,

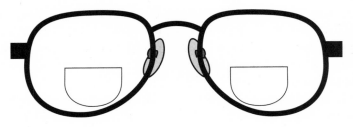

Bifocals for distance and near vision

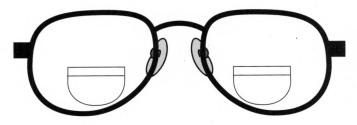

Trifocal lenses for distance, intermediate and near vision

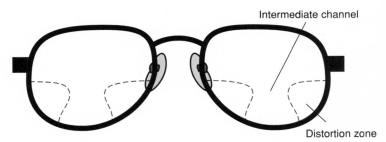

Intermediate channel

Distortion zone

Progressive addition lenses for smooth transition of all visual ranges

Fig. 4.1.   Bifocals, trifocals, and progressive addition lenses

many opticians still feel that the glass ones work better (in terms of how dark the lenses get and how quickly they change).

Other Options

Both glass and plastic lenses can be made in *high index*. Made of denser material, a high-index lens can bend light more powerfully. The result is a thinner—and, to some, a more aesthetically appealing—lens. High-index lenses made of glass tend to be almost as heavy as regular glass lenses. But when they're made of plastic, especially polycarbonate lenses, the lenses are much more lightweight than standard plastic ones.

Other coatings and dyes can be added to lenses to improve both vision and safety. *Antireflective coatings* reduce the amount of light reflected off the front and back surface of the lens as well as light reflected *within* the lens itself. Why is this important? For people with early cataracts, glare can be debilitating and even dangerous. The antireflective coatings can make a tremendous difference in vision, especially for driving at night.

UV protection: Plastic lenses can also be treated with a screening dye to filter out ultraviolet light before it has a chance to enter the eye. Ultraviolet (UV) light, the ultra-short wavelength of light that causes skin damage and sunburn, may also contribute to certain cataracts and retinal problems. *Therefore, UV protection is especially important for sunglasses.* Sunglasses should have 100 percent filtering for UV-A and UV-B light, the two wavelengths of ultraviolet radiation that affect the eyes. If you're buying over-the-counter sunglasses, look for ones with labels that say "100 percent UV-A and UV-B filtering," or "100 percent absorbing below 400 nm" (which means that they filter out all light below the wavelength of 400 nanometers).

Specialty Eyeglasses

If you're shopping for *safety eyeglasses*, look for frames with side shields and for more impact-resistant lens materials such as polycarbonate or glass that is at least one and a half times thicker than standard glass lenses. Polycarbonate lenses are a good choice for people with one eye who wear glasses, since they provide protection for the remaining eye.

Occupational lenses are custom-designed to match specific needs with particular activities. Say you need to look above your head at something close up—as a mechanic does, for instance—and you wear bifocals. The object will be blurry through the distance portion of your lens. An occupational bifocal can be made with a second bifocal segment placed in the *top* of the lens—just like the one at the bottom of the lens—so that you can focus on what you need to see close up. One of the most common uses for occupational eyeglasses is for the computer. With bifocal computer eyeglasses, you can look at your computer screen through an intermediate-vision prescription at the top of the lens and still see your keyboard through a near-vision prescription in the bottom of the lens.

Next, Finding the Perfect Frames

So many decisions already, and we haven't even tackled the issue of frames yet! Again, the range of choices can be overwhelming. It's not unusual for people to spend hours trying on frames, looking in the mirror and soliciting opinions from total strangers. Why is this? Why do we agonize so? One big reason is the long-term commitment involved here. After all, we're not talking about a pair of shoes or a new hat; most of us wear the same pair of eyeglasses all day, every day, for years. Therefore, we find ourselves in the quandary of attempting to find the perfect frames, ones to match our entire wardrobe (or, a tougher assignment, ones to match our every mood).

First of all, relax. You don't have to go through every single pair of frames in the store. The optician can usually help narrow down your choices, and lighten your burden considerably, by guiding you to a selection that will look best with your particular prescription and facial structure. *Note:* Don't let anybody talk you into buying huge frames—that is, unless you want them—simply because "your prescription is so strong." In fact, if you have a very strong prescription you'll probably want to choose a frame as small as possible to help reduce the thickness and weight of your lenses. Other considerations are the shape of your face and nose. If you have a round face, for instance, you probably won't want to choose a perfectly round frame that exaggerates this. If the bridge of your nose is uneven, metal frames may fit better than plastic ones; metal frames typically have nose pads that can be *individually adjusted* for each side of your nose. Lifestyle is an issue as well. For instance, if you perspire a lot, because you exercise strenuously or live in a hot, swampy climate, you may prefer plastic frames; salt, produced by sweat, can be corrosive to metal frames, damaging the frame and causing skin irritation wherever the frame touches the face.

Our advice? Because this is a decision you'll most likely have to live with for some time, take a trusted friend or family member with you. *Note:* Some understanding opticians will allow you to purchase a frame to take home, try on for everyone, and return for credit toward another frame if your family and friends don't like your new look.

Finally, the Right Fit

Thank goodness! You've run the gauntlet of frames and lenses and made your selections. Now it's time for the fitting.

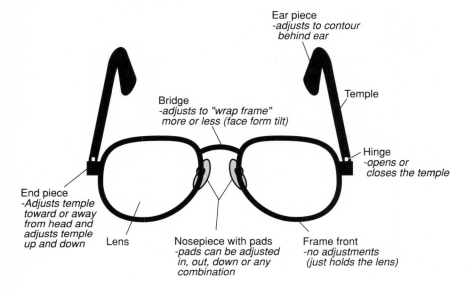

Fig. 4.2.   Eyeglass adjustments: all of these parts of the eyeglasses can be
adjusted to improve comfort and vision

First, the optician needs to measure the physical attributes of your
eyes. This is to make sure that the lenses will be properly centered over
your pupils, and that when the lenses are centered for your eyes, they'll still
fit appropriately in the frame. If you wear a multifocal, the optician needs
to measure where the intermediate and near portions of the lens should be
placed within the frame. Sometimes the optician will examine your old
eyeglasses to see how those measurements compare. Good opticians often
try to match anything that was unusual about your old glasses to make your
transition to the new ones as smooth as possible. The eyeglasses are then
sent to a lab so that the lenses can be ground and set into the frame.

When your new glasses are completed, the optician will shape the
frame to fit the bridge and temples to your face, for optimal comfort and
vision. Keep in mind that there's almost always an adjustment period for
new eyeglasses; this may last from days to weeks. (Most likely, even if your
new eyeglasses aren't a new prescription, you'll still experience a brief period of adaptation just because of the new frame and fit.) It's definitely not
unusual to experience a few aches in your eyes at first. *However, these aches
should not be unbearable, and they should diminish over time.* Often a quick trip

back to the optician to readjust the frame can make all the difference in the world. But if this doesn't help—and if your vision is clear with the new prescription and the comfort level is bearable—try to stick with the frames for two weeks before returning to your doctor to recheck the prescription. Give your eyes time to adjust.

The need to adapt to new eyeglasses is especially demanding, and often annoying, for those who wear multifocals. One of the easiest and most pleasant ways of adjusting, if you're getting used to multifocals for the first time, is simply to curl up with a good book. As you read, occasionally look up across the room. This will help your eyes to learn to move smoothly *through* the lens. Then, once you feel comfortable with reading, give yourself and your eyeglasses new challenges. Take a walk around your home. Because moving around with new bifocals—as you may soon find out—is often easier said than done, practicing in a familiar environment makes the adjustment easier. Finally, know that your predicament is only temporary. You really will get used to your new glasses. After you do, you won't spend your time thinking about "how to use them"; you'll just live your life and do what you need to do, and you'll see better than you did before.

WHEN SOMETHING GOES WRONG

Okay. Having said all that, we also need to address the fact that sometimes in the world of eyeglasses, as in life, there are glitches. So, you've just picked up your new eyeglasses and they're less than great. Something doesn't seem right. You had such high hopes: you thought that you would see better, that the world would look and feel better than it had in a long time. And that's not the case at all. What happened?

The first thing to do is check with your optician and make sure these glasses were made to the doctor's prescription. Frankly, this is almost always a formality; almost invariably the optician will tell you that the lenses are the correct power and that you'll need to return to your doctor to have the prescription rechecked.

However, there's much more to seeing clearly and comfortably than just the power of your new lenses.

When eyeglasses are made for you, the frames and lenses need to be measured and fit to tailor the glasses to your face and eyes. Every lens has an *optical center,* the part of the lens where the prescription is the purest and most precise. *The optical center should be located exactly over your pupil,* and this can happen only if the frame fits properly and the lenses within that frame are perfectly aligned.

When you have a problem with your new glasses that doesn't go away over time and the optician tells you that the eyeglasses are made "to the doctor's prescription," you need to return to your doctor to have both the eyeglasses and your prescription rechecked. You may understand the problem better if you arm yourself with some working knowledge of "optical jargon." To that end, we've included a brief primer to help you translate some key terms often bandied about the optical shop.

An "Optical Jargon" Primer

"PD": PD stands for "pupillary distance," the distance between the centers of your two pupils. This measurement can be taken with a ruler, but it's most accurately calculated with an instrument called a *corneal reflex pupillometer*, or CRP. Using the lights, lenses, and prisms on the CRP, your optician can shine a precise point of light at the center of your pupil. First, the optician will place the CRP over your eyes and ask you to look at a light inside. Then, using that light's reflection off your cornea as a means of alignment, the optician can measure the distance from each eye to the center of the bridge of your nose. Because most people are not perfectly symmetrical, it's not unusual for one eye to be closer to the bridge of the nose than the other. (This becomes important when measuring for progressive addition lenses, where the optical center of each lens must be exactly over each pupil.)

Induced prism: When you look through a lens that is a prism, whatever you see through that lens is displaced. Say, for instance, you're looking at a ball. The ball may appear to be in one place, but it's actually located a few inches or feet over. The ball looks perfectly normal—the size and clarity don't change, in other words—it's just shifted a little. If problems with your eye muscles hinder your eyes from working together precisely, prisms can make a world of difference. They can realign the images each eye sees so that your brain can interpret the world as one image instead of two.

However, sometimes the problem isn't your eyes at all but your glasses. If the optical centers of your glasses aren't properly calibrated over your pupils—when, as opticians say, the PD is not correct—this too can create prism. Oops! When prism isn't intentional—to clear up an eye muscle problem, for instance—your vision can be distorted or doubled. This is called *induced prism.* The farther your pupils are from these optical centers, the greater the "shift"; with stronger prescriptions, the prism problem is even more noticeable. For example, say two people have their new glasses made incorrectly, with the optical centers of their lenses made just 5 millimeters wider than the actual distance between the pupils (5 millimeters may not seem like much, but in this precise science, every millimeter counts). The person with the stronger prescription will have the worse case of prism misalignment. (Prism is discussed in more detail in chapter 2.)

Refraction: This is a physics term describing the way light bends as it passes through a lens. (*Refraction* also describes the procedure your doctor performs when determining your prescription.) When you wear glasses, the lenses bend the light to correct your eyes' refraction problems and refine your ability to focus. (Refraction is discussed in more detail in chapter 2.)

Reflection: This term denotes the bouncing of light off a surface. Light that reflects off your eyeglasses can create glare.

Diffraction: Another physics term, this refers to how light scatters when it meets a surface (think of sunshine on a lake, for instance). On a bright day, light can scatter at the edge of your eyeglass frames and create glare. Cataracts can create the same problem: by diffracting the light that enters your eye, they can cause glare *within the eye* and make your vision seem hazy.

Base curve: Think geometry here. Base curve is the curvature of the front surface of a lens. The total power of a lens equals the sum of the *front surface curvature* and the *back surface curvature* of the lens. You can vary the lens curvatures for a given prescription but keep the power of the lens constant. For any prescription, the lens can be made with many different base curves. (For more on how an incorrect base curve can cause problems, read on.)

Pantoscopic tilt: This term describes how the top of your frame angles away from your face. The frame should be fit with a slight pantoscopic tilt to compensate for a downward posturing of the eyes while reading. Too much pantoscopic tilt, however, will move the optical center farther from the pupil and thereby change your prescription!

Retroscopic tilt: This is the opposite of pantoscopic tilt, when the *bottom* of your frame is angled away from your face, making the top of the frame sit closer than it should. Retroscopic tilt is a bad thing because it distorts vision for both distance and near viewing.

Face form tilt: This term refers to how your frame wraps around your face. Too much face form tilt effectively changes the position of the optical centers of the lenses and results in a distorted view of the world.

Progressive addition lenses: Discussed above, this is the most common type of no-line bifocal, featuring a progressive change in power from the top to the bottom of the lens. The top of the lens, of course, is for your distance vision. The middle of the lens is referred to as the *intermediate channel;* this provides vision at distances of approximately two to six feet. As you gradually look down into the reading portion of your lens, objects that are closer to you come into focus. These lenses do a great job except when you glance to the side, where the world can appear wavy or even tilted. This is entirely normal, the price of the progressive optics, and simply part of the nature of these lenses. *Note:* In recent years major strides have been made in decreasing the size of this distorted area.

Blended bifocals: They're not as common as progressive addition lenses, but blended bifocals are also used to create a no-line bifocal. The concept here is basically that of a lined bifocal, except that the line is smoothed out for cosmetic purposes. Someone looking at your eyeglasses can't see any telltale bifocal line, but you yourself aren't so lucky. You actually see much more of a line than with regular lined bifocals. In smoothing the line, the blending process seems to widen it, leaving a wide area of distortion in the lens.

Seg height: That's "seg" as in "segment." Seg height is where the bifocal segment sits in a lens. For most people who wear lined bifocals, this line of demarcation is at the top margin of the lower eyelid. In progressive addition lenses, the optical center of the distance part of the lens is placed over the pupil, and the amount of seg height is predetermined by the manufacturer of the lens.

Vertex distance: The distance at which your frame holds the lens from the eye is the vertex distance. If you push your eyeglasses in or pull them down on your nose, the prescription will shift away from what it's supposed to be. Your doctor's prescription usually assumes that your frame will sit 7 to 10 millimeters from your eye.

High-index lenses: All lens materials have what's called an *index of refraction:* how much light is bent, or refracted, when it passes through the lens. A high-index lens bends light much more powerfully than a standard lens of the same curvature and thickness—which means that, compared with a standard lens, the high-index lens is thinner (and, to some, more cosmetically appealing).

Polarizing filters: When a light wave bounces off a surface, it becomes polarized: it splits into horizontal and vertical components. The horizontal component of the light wave is what we see as glare. Glasses can be made with a filter that screens out *only* the horizontal light waves to reduce glare.

Such filters are especially helpful for people who spend a lot of time driving or on the water.

Surfacing: This is the term for the manufacturing process that produces a *lens blank*, a large round lens (approximately 75 millimeters in diameter) with a specific prescription. The lens surfacing machine polishes both the front and back surfaces of the lens to create the desired lens power.

Edging: Edging is the process of grinding a lens blank to be fit into a frame. The lens blank is placed in the edging machine, or "edger," and aligned according to (1) the lens's optical center, (2) the person's PD, and (3) the size and shape of the frame. The edger follows a specific frame pattern to grind, bevel, and polish the lens edges, so that each one fits exactly into the frame.

Troubleshooting Problems with Your New Glasses

Now, what do all of these factors mean to someone whose new eyeglasses don't work? If your doctor finds that the prescription is correct and that the lenses have been made correctly, then obviously, something else is wrong—and chances are, the culprit is one of these features.

Incorrect PD

If the PD is off, for instance, you might experience blurred vision, aches in the front of your head or in your temples, a pulling or drawing sensation between your eyes, dizziness, reading problems, and possibly double vision. The induced prism (see above) does not allow for your eyes to work together, and your eye muscles will probably ache from trying to compensate for the incorrect eyeglasses.

In a progressive addition lens, an incorrect PD adds another problem. When we read, our eyes need to "converge," or turn in slightly, so that we can focus with both eyes together on the page. When you wear a lined bifocal, you're measured for a *distance PD* and a *near PD*. (The difference between the distance PD and the near PD is called the *inset*.) The near PD takes the needs of reading into account: it allows for the optical centers to be a little closer together, to match how your eyes converge when you read. With a progressive addition lens, the near PD is preset by the manufacturer and is designed so that each eye individually can follow the progressive path down through the lens into the reading area. If a lens is made incorrectly for the distance PD, this could throw off your ability to read: your eye might not fall within the appropriate area of the lens when you look down to read, and the vision will be blurry. When this is the case, you may be able to read with either eye at a time but not with both eyes together, because the image is not clear for both eyes at the same time.

Problems with Frame Adjustments

Occasionally, even with a correct PD you may experience symptoms similar to those of an incorrect PD. If, for instance, your old eyeglasses were made with an incorrect PD and you adjusted to the induced prism (see above), then you might miss that prism when your eyeglasses are made to match your eyes appropriately. The same is true if, because of ill-fitting frames, the optical centers are placed somewhere other than over your pupils.

In either of these scenarios, your symptoms tend to be more vague than when the PD is made incorrectly. Your eyeglasses "just don't feel right," but your vision seems otherwise normal. If the optician hasn't already done so, your doctor needs to determine whether the frame sits unevenly on your face, and he or she should look at you from four different views.

The first is face-on, to see if the frame is tilting and causing one lens to sit higher than the other. (For example, do you have one ear that's higher than the other, making the frame tilt?) If you wear a bifocal, frame tilt might cause the bifocal segment line to cross one pupil and create double vision.

The second view is to look from overhead, to see if one lens sits closer to your face than the other. This pushes one of the lenses farther from your eye, which gives that lens a different vertex distance. One eye's prescription will be less appropriate because the vertex distance will be off, and you'll be uncomfortable seeing with both eyes together. Your vision might be blurry or double.

The third view is your profile for pantoscopic tilt. Too much frame tilt can distort your vision. This extra tilt actually changes your prescription, because the optical centers of the lenses aren't where they're supposed to be.

The fourth view is again from overhead, to determine whether your frame has too much face form tilt and is wrapping around your face excessively. This tends to make the world look bowed in or out.

Generally, if the frame fit is different from the fit of your old eyeglasses, it can affect both your vision and your comfort with the new eyeglasses. *Always take your old eyeglasses with you when you return to your doctor to have the new glasses checked.* This way your doctor can consider how your old eyeglasses fit and try to readjust your new ones to match. Of course, if

your old eyeglasses fit poorly but you adjusted to them, you don't necessarily want to have your new eyeglasses adjusted so that they fit as poorly
as the old ones! However, you might have to compromise the fit of your
new eyeglasses somewhat to improve your comfort. If your doctor is not
comfortable readjusting your frame or doesn't have the equipment to do
so, ask the doctor to write a note for the optician describing specific adjustments that need to be made.

Base-Curve Problems

If the base curve in your new eyeglasses is different from what you're
used to, this can produce symptoms similar to those caused by too much
face form tilt: the world will look curved or bowed. An incorrect base curve
can affect your mobility: your new eyeglasses will make it difficult for you
to negotiate curbs or steps while walking. If this is the problem with your
new glasses, you may feel that the vision "just doesn't seem right" without
being able to pinpoint your specific symptoms.

Like any eyeglass problem, base-curve problems are more common
in higher prescriptions and are usually not experienced when the prescription is mild. If you can't adjust to the new eyeglasses, the optician will have
to remake your lenses to match the base curve of your old pair.

Problems of Having a Different Prescription for Each Eye

When everything has been made correctly with your new eyeglasses
but you still have complaints, the problem might relate to the prescription
itself. That is, a prescription may simply be difficult to get used to with
your eyes *together*, even if it's correct for either eye by itself. If the prescriptions for your two eyes are different, then you have a condition called *anisometropia*. (The symptoms of anisometropia are that one eye's image seems
farther away or a different size than the other eye's image. Someone with
this condition may also see double when viewing with both eyes together.)

When your eyes are different, the placement of the lenses over your
pupils becomes critical for clear and comfortable vision. If, for example,
your eyes sit evenly above the optical centers of the lenses and one lens is
stronger, then that lens will have more induced prism at that eye's pupil
than the other lens. This uneven induced prism will make your vision seem
distorted, create dizziness and discomfort, and create a doubling of the
world so that you see two images, one on top of the other.

A more common problem with each eye having a different prescription is *image jump*. In a lined bifocal, as you move your eyes down to the line, the image will appear to "jump." When both eyes have the same prescription, the jump isn't really noticeable once you adapt to your eyeglasses. But when your eyes have *different* prescriptions, the jump is often greater in one eye than in the other, and thus more conspicuous. If your visual system isn't able to recover from this difference in jump, you may experience double vision when you read. Otherwise, you might describe your problem by saying that "the print swims, moves, or dances" on the page, or that you don't feel like your eyes are "working together for reading."

For these reasons, if you have a different prescription in each eye, you may not be able to wear a bifocal. If having two pairs of eyeglasses—one for distance and one for reading—is too inconvenient, a progressive addition lens might alleviate the symptoms of image jump that you had with a lined bifocal. Occasionally, symptoms of image jump can be relieved with a special type of prism called *slab-off prism*. This is incorporated into one lens of a lined bifocal to counteract the difference in image jump created by different prescriptions. Contact lenses are another solution: they greatly reduce the effects of different prescriptions and offer an excellent alternative for your vision (see chapter 5).

Problems with Materials

Eyeglasses that have been measured and made correctly with an appropriate prescription *still* may not provide you with the vision that you were expecting. Keep in mind that there are many different materials and lens qualities available on the market today. Not all plastic lenses are created equal, and some lenses are clearer than others.

Plastic lenses are made of a material known as CR-39, which is exceptional for transmitting light without distortion and provides an excellent optical-quality image. The Food and Drug Administration (FDA) requires that a lens manufacturer needs to use *at least* 50 percent of this material in a lens in order for that lens to be considered a "CR-39 lens." Different manufacturers use different proportions of the material in their lenses. The finest plastic lenses are 100 percent CR-39; however, they also tend to be more expensive. If you're looking for the least expensive prices, you may inadvertently be buying an inferior lens. The problem is that you never really know what you're getting. In general, if the optician orders a stock lens from a major lens manufacturer rather than manufacturing lenses on site, there is less likely to be a problem. (Keep in mind that *manufacturing* lenses and *edging* lenses to be fit into a frame are two different processes.)

Lenses are also made of many materials other than CR-39. Newer plastic lens materials that look much thinner and feel much lighter can be used to make your eyeglasses look and feel better. Many advertisements for these lenses have made eyeglass wearers aware of their availability. As always, some of these materials work better than others. The first such material to become available was polycarbonate. Originally these lenses were designed to be used in safety eyewear that required a high-impact-resistant lens. Because these lenses were so much lighter in weight than the high-index glass lenses in use at the time, they gained in popularity very quickly. Early on, however, it was discovered that these lenses didn't provide the same quality of image as did standard CR-39 lenses; to make matters worse, this shortcoming was much more noticeable when the prescription was stronger. So people who needed stronger prescriptions were more likely to spend more money for these lenses, only to be disappointed by their vision with the new eyeglasses. Newer polycarbonate materials apparently do not have this problem, but as with CR-39, not all optical laboratories use the same quality lenses. Over the past few years high-index lenses that are made of plastic materials other than polycarbonate have become available. While these materials are not totally free of problems, in general they provide better vision than polycarbonate.

Lens coatings are sometimes the source of complaints with a new pair of eyeglasses. The most common lens coating used today is an "antireflective" coating, which reduces the amount of light reflecting off the lens surface and thus decreases glare. When properly applied, an antireflective coating can improve vision. But a poor-quality antireflective coating will leave noticeable ripples in the lenses and thus distort vision.

Other Things That Can Go Wrong

Finally, some things that go wrong with eyeglasses revolve around the wearer. Here are three things you can do to help avoid these problems.

First, be careful when you choose a new frame. The optician should be skilled at helping you to find the best fit for your face and prescription, but sometimes—how can we put this diplomatically?—a sale becomes more important than offering the best advice. If your frame is too large, it may create a distorted view of the world and affect your ability to navigate while wearing your eyeglasses. If the frame extends past the side of your face on either side, it can create glare from light reflecting off the back surface of the lenses.

Second, be careful to describe your vision needs to your doctor. This is of utmost importance. Your doctor can prescribe eyeglasses based on the average person's needs but can tailor your prescription to fit how *you* use your eyes during the day. The biggest problem with bifocal prescriptions, in particular, is determining a reading correction that allows you to read at the distance that *you* require. Every reading lens power focuses light at a given distance, and as the reading power increases, the reading distance gets shorter. We don't all necessarily have the same reading distance. Our reading distances either come from habit or are specific to a job or hobby. For example, if you sit all day with a computer monitor twenty-four inches away from you, and your doctor assumes that you like to read at sixteen inches, then your eyeglasses won't be very helpful for the computer unless you move much closer to it.

The final thing you need to look at requires some introspection. We've all bought things—clothes, jewelry, and the like—that have gone over like a lead balloon with our friends and family. Many of us respond to this decided lack of enthusiasm by declining to wear that particular thing again. If for some reason you come to hate your new frames, then subconsciously you might not feel as if you see well. You may secretly be hoping that the eyeglasses can be returned. Try to be honest with yourself, the optician, and the doctor—because all of you will spend a lot of time trying to find out the source of your symptoms.

AS A LAST WORD OF ADVICE, always have your doctor write a note for you to take back to the optician describing exactly what's wrong with your new eyeglasses. This helps you to communicate the problem to the optician effectively; it also adds more credence to the problem at hand. Without a note, the optician might just dismiss the problem and tell you that you don't really understand enough about eyeglasses to know what you're talking about.

Some Questions You May Have about Eyeglasses

Does it matter where I get my new glasses?

In a perfect world, every optical shop, optician, optometrist, and ophthalmologist would treat you the same, radiating infinite concern that your new eyeglasses provide ideal vision, comfort, and looks—all, of course, at a reasonable price. Unfortunately, as in any profession, there are some among the spectacle purveyors who can be considered unscrupulous. Some chain stores are the epitome of professionalism; others illustrate in the worst possible way the principle of "caveat emptor" (let the buyer beware). The same can be said for some professional opticians. So the first thing to know is that the individuals you'll be dealing with—their knowledge and their ethics—matter much more than the location. In this regard, word of mouth can be very helpful. Most likely, human nature being what it is, someone who has gotten lousy service will be more than happy to tell you all about it, and someone who has received excellent care from a particular eye doctor or optician will enjoy spreading that word as well.

There are several advantages to buying your eyeglasses at your doctor's office—if, of course, the price is fair. For one thing, you have the advantage of having your doctor available to recheck your prescription if something doesn't seem right. Also, if the new prescription needs to be changed, your doctor will probably not charge you for the second set of lenses. While some doctors tell their patients "old wives' tales" about "getting used to your new glasses" just to avoid remaking them, most doctors feel responsible for any lab work produced by their office. For them, this craftsmanship reflects the values of the office as a whole, and they'll do anything to make sure their patients are happy with their new eyeglasses.

Eyeglasses bought elsewhere might be more convenient for you if the optician's shop is located where you can easily stop by for frame adjustments. However, if there's a problem, you'll find yourself traveling between the optician's and the doctor's offices, probably several times, until the problem is resolved. The "one-hour" opticians can be a lifesaver if you really have an emergency need for new eyeglasses. However, some of these establishments manufacture their own lenses, and the quality of materials may not provide you with the best vision possible.

Ultimately, you need to shop where you're comfortable or have had good references. If you know and trust your doctor, and the doctor's eyeglass prices are pretty much in line with prices elsewhere, it's probably worth getting your glasses made there for the service and quality of the eyeglasses. Remember, most people wear the same pair of glasses every day, usually for two years or more. No other piece of your wardrobe receives as much wear. It's probably worth a little more of your time, and sometimes your money, to make sure that you have the best in vision, comfort, and looks with your eyeglasses. (In other words, it takes a reasonable length of time to make your glasses right the first time, and the people crafting your glasses should be watching the quality, not the clock.)

If I wear my glasses all the time, will I become dependent on them?

No. Remember, your eyes are in a constant state of flux your whole life (see chapter 2). No matter what you do, you can't stop this process; your eyes are going to change anyway, with or without corrective lenses. All eyeglasses do is help us see better *through* these various unavoidable vision changes.

If you're just starting to need a reading prescription or bifocals and you try to put off getting eyeglasses "so that your eyes won't weaken further," you won't be doing yourself any favors—and you certainly won't be toughening up your eyes by straining them, as if they were stomach muscles you could whip into shape if only you did enough sit-ups. Instead, you'll find yourself putting up unnecessarily with blurred vision and headaches. As we age, our reading vision, in particular, falters; this trend increases with each passing year. So even if you don't wear your eyeglasses, your reading vision isn't going to get any better, and anyway, you'll still have more of a "dependency" on eyeglasses in the future. Everybody does. Why should you be blurry and uncomfortable in the meantime?

Conversely, if you don't wear your eyeglasses, your vision won't necessarily get *worse* because of eyestrain. After about the first ten years of life, the critical years for the development of our vision, *not* wearing your eyeglasses has no effect on the outcome of your prescription. (During those first ten years, however, it's very important to provide the retina with the best possible image for vision development, and wearing eyeglasses, if they are needed, is an absolute must.)

There's nothing wrong with being clear and comfortable; you're not giving in to weakness by seeing better. If it means wearing some form of corrective lens to achieve better vision, don't feel that you're harming yourself in doing so.

What does my prescription mean?

Your prescription is written in units called *diopters*. A "one-diopter lens" focuses light at one meter, or approximately forty inches. The diopter designation on your prescription does not indicate what your visual acuity is. (For more on this, see chapter 3.) If, for example, you have a prescription for one diopter of nearsightedness, then you really don't see very well past the length of your arm; but the one-diopter designation doesn't indicate what your vision is without your eyeglasses. Eyeglass prescriptions change by a quarter of a diopter at a time. On average, your vision changes one line on the eye chart for every quarter-diopter of prescription that you need. For someone with one diopter of nearsightedness, vision without eyeglasses is generally about four lines higher on an eye chart than the 20/20 line, or 20/50 vision.

Your prescription will sometimes include a designation for *axis*. The axis is the specific direction in which the correction for astigmatism is placed. Because astigmatism is an optical distortion that is caused by the eye having more curvature in one direction than in the other (see chapter 2), corrections for astigmatism always have a particular orientation.

If you are someone who needs to wear a bifocal, then your prescription will have a designation for *add* (see chapter 2). Your distance prescription will allow your eyes to focus appropriately on objects that are usually twenty feet away and beyond. The "add" describes the amount of reading correction that is added to the distance prescription in order to allow your eyes to focus at a reading (or near-working) distance.

How should I clean my new lenses?

Always begin by rinsing your lenses thoroughly with tap water. (Between cleanings, dust and debris settle on the lenses. Rubbing a lens with a cloth—your shirttail, for instance—actually grinds the dust and debris into the surface of the lens, creating fine scratches.)

After rinsing, spray them with a cleaner designed *especially for eyeglass lenses*—window cleaners often contain ammonia, which can damage lens coatings—or apply a small drop of a mild liquid dish detergent to each lens. Gently rub the cleaner into the lens with your thumb and forefinger and then rinse thoroughly with hot water. Hot water evaporates from the lens surface faster than cold water, making it easier to dry the lens. Finally, always use a soft paper towel or lint-free tissue to dry your glasses. Tissues with skin softeners and perfumes may smudge your freshly washed lenses, and cloth towels can scratch.

What is a "no-line" bifocal?

Actually, it's a little more complicated than it sounds. As discussed in this chapter, a bifocal is an eyeglass that does two jobs: the top part corrects your distance vision, and the bottom is used for reading. Traditionally, these two portions have been separated by a distinct line.

"No-line" bifocals come in two basic varieties. In the first, called a *blended bifocal*, the line is blended out, leaving a thin blurred zone between the distance- and near-lens portions. In the second and more popular kind, called a *progressive no-line bifocal*, there's a gradual progression between the distance and near prescriptions. The big advantage here is that instead of the wasted blurry space, there's a bonus zone for *intermediate vision* ("arm's-length" vision, such as the distance between you and a computer screen or a shelf at the grocery store).

I just bought new glasses. Can I still get some use out of my old pair?

Sure. People do it all the time. Most of our patients keep at least one old pair of eyeglasses around the house as a spare, or to wear when doing yard work or any other potentially lens-scratching activity. Some people have their old eyeglasses darkened with a tint by an optician and made into prescription sunglasses. There are many ways to give new life to an old frame. One of the best is to donate them to a "recycling" agency so that someone else can use them (see below).

Can I recycle my old eyeglasses?

Absolutely—and someone will bless you for it! Eyeglasses, both frames and lenses, are processed at regional centers, categorized by their lens prescription and style, then sent to underprivileged areas in the United States and to underdeveloped countries and dispensed to those in need. Ask your eye doctor, local hospital, or community organizations (in our area, the Lions Club has been particularly involved with this recycling project).

Can I do anything to alleviate computer-related eye problems?

If your long hours in front of the computer are hurting your eyes, you're certainly not alone. An estimated sixty-six million people in this country have computer-related vision problems: eyestrain, irritated eyes, blurred vision, even headaches.

But there are some things you can do. The easiest and most low-tech solution is simply to give those accommodation muscles (see chapter 2) a break every so often by looking across the room or out the window. Administering teardrops several times a day may help. Progressive or "no-line" bifocals, or "computer lenses" (with an intermediate-distance prescription), may help ease the strain on your eyes. You might also ask your eye doctor about getting antireflective coatings or tints on your eyeglasses; these can break up the reflection of overhead lights and improve contrast of the screen. Also, many computer stores sell glare-cutting filters that sit over your screen or monitor. (Speaking of glare, if your computer sits directly in front of a bright window, you'll notice a big improvement if you either move it or keep the curtains drawn.) Finally, positioning your monitor slightly below eye level makes it easier for your eyes to converge (see chapter 2) on the screen.

My daughter sits too close to the television and my husband stares at his computer screen for hours. Will this damage their eyes?

This falls under the "reading in dim light" category of eye worries, and fortunately the answer is the same: no. No research has ever proven that TV screens or computer monitors harm the eye. However, watching any kind of screen, TV or computer, from the same vantage point for prolonged periods can cause eye fatigue and discomfort. (For tips on alleviating computer eyestrain, see the previous question.) As with any prolonged activity involving the eyes, take frequent breaks; look around the room every fifteen to thirty minutes, to give your accommodation muscles a rest. Also, to avoid dry eyes, remember to blink frequently, and use supplemental teardrops if needed. (For more on these, see chapter 13.)

What about those "dime-store" reading glasses? Are they any good?

Over-the-counter, or "dime-store," reading glasses are sold in many drug stores and grocery stores as well as in specialty stores. These glasses come in varying strengths and are usually labeled with the same power system as prescribed reading glasses. Because they are inexpensive, many people who enjoy using them will purchase multiple pairs so that they can leave one at work, one by their favorite reading chair, and one on their nightstand, and never have to worry about where they left their glasses.

Dime-store reading glasses can be an excellent alternative for someone with presbyopia who has little or no need for a distance prescription, or for someone who requires an additional reading prescription while wearing contact lenses. However, because both lenses in these types of glasses have the same effective power, they might not work well if one of your eyes needs a significantly different prescription from the other.

Additionally, these types of glasses are set up with optical centers that provide for an average pupillary distance, one that won't necessarily match your eyes. If you experience headaches, discomfort, print that swims or moves while you read, or double vision with your over-the-counter readers, then the optical centers are probably off with respect to your eyes.

Even if you do get symptoms from wearing these glasses due to inappropriate power or pupillary distance, they will not harm your eyes. The symptoms will almost certainly go away when you stop wearing the glasses.

5

Contact Lenses
Everything You Need to Know

For some people, glasses are a plain old nuisance. They slip down on your nose, get smudged—or worse, misplaced (for folks who rely on more than one pair of glasses, this seems to happen several times a day!).

Thank goodness, then, for contact lenses. For the millions of people who wear them, contacts are the lenses of choice for several reasons. Many find contacts to be much simpler than glasses; once they're in for the day, it's easy to forget about them (except for adding the occasional rewetting drop). Also, they provide much better peripheral vision than glasses. Is this important? Absolutely. Better peripheral vision can help keep your eyes more relaxed when you're reading and focusing—and this, in turn, helps reduce fatigue and eyestrain. For sports and recreational activities, better peripheral vision can even boost your performance.

Also, a contact lens *moves with your eye*, so you're always looking through the *center* of the lens, the part of the lens that provides the best vision. In contrast, when you're wearing glasses and you glance to the side, sometimes your vision seems distorted. (This is because, due to the nature of many eyeglasses, the lens doesn't provide the same quality at its edges as it does in the center.)

If your prescription is strong, your glasses will actually change your perception of the size or relative distance of whatever you're seeing. Once you get used to your glasses, of course, you tend not to notice these things. But contacts give the world a more natural appearance. Putting the lens correction *on the eye itself* minimizes these size differences and often provides better visual acuity, which means you can read smaller letters on the eye chart. (For more on visual acuity, see chapter 3.)

Still, despite these and other advantages, contact lenses aren't ideal for everybody. Are they for you? This chapter may help you decide.

HOW CONTACTS CAME ABOUT: FROM LEONARDO TO TODAY

The notion of putting a corrective lens on the eye to achieve better vision is certainly nothing new. In fact, Leonardo da Vinci came up with this brilliant idea some 450 years ago. (Although no lenses were manufactured at that time, detailed drawings and descriptions were made.) A. E. Fick, a scientist in Zurich, manufactured the first contact lens in 1887 but soon found out that the human eye didn't like wearing lenses made of actual glass. It took a major innovation, in the 1940s, to produce the ancestors of the contact lenses we wear today: plastics. Those original lenses were made of a material called PMMA, which in fact was so well tolerated by the human eye that it's still used for hard contact lenses, for intraocular lens implants, and for orthopedic purposes.

Soft contact lenses didn't become available in this country until 1972, when Bausch and Lomb first introduced them to the American market. The original soft lenses tended to be more comfortable than the hard lenses available at the time, but because they were limited to just a few sizes, these lenses didn't fit many people. The big difference between hard and soft contact lenses was that the new soft lenses allowed oxygen to pass *through* them—not just *around* the lens, as with hard contacts. This made for a much healthier lens environment, because it enabled the eye to "breathe" with a lens in place. Lack of oxygen to the cornea can lead to decreased vision from corneal swelling and epithelial cell damage.

Since 1972, contact lenses have changed and improved considerably. Now, lenses are designed to correct almost any vision problem and are available in special designs for extended wear, cosmetic changes (like eye color), and disposability.

TYPES OF LENSES

Hard versus Soft

Contact lenses come in an impressive variety of materials, sizes, shapes, thicknesses, and colors. In general, they're divided into two major categories: hard and soft.

Hard contacts have evolved significantly since their introduction in the 1940s. Initially their design improved as manufacturing techniques improved, but in the late 1970s came a major breakthrough: the development of hard contacts that "breathed" like soft lenses. We call these lenses *rigid gas-permeable contacts*, or RGPs.

The RGP lenses are more flexible and fit better than earlier hard lenses, and they last longer (with respect to "wear and tear") and sometimes provide better vision than soft lenses. They're manufactured by computer-controlled lathes that can create any kind of surface needed to correct someone's vision. For example, if you have a high degree of astigmatism, an RGP lens can be ground with a curvature to match your cornea perfectly—providing a healthier, more comfortable fit, and vision that's usually superior to that offered by your glasses.

RGP lens materials also allow for bifocal segments to be added. In this sophisticated manufacturing process, a bifocal segment is fused into the lens; the result is similar to bifocal glasses that have a line (except this line is tiny, and it's within a lens placed on your eye; for more on this, read on). Because RGP lenses move significantly on the eye with a blink, these lenses can be fit to *translate* or move the bifocal segment up so that it sits in front of the pupil while you're looking down to read. (Because soft lenses don't move quite as much, translating bifocal soft lenses don't work very well.)

Another significant advantage to RGP lenses is that they can provide, in effect, a new cornea for people with a corneal problem that distorts vision. Because this lens maintains its shape on the eye—as opposed to molding itself to the eye, the way a soft lens does—it masks a corneal irregularity, helps correct the optical surface, and improves vision.

Soft contacts are referred to as *hydrogels*, because they're made of a plastic material that holds water. By varying the amount of water that a lens holds, manufacturers can provide a broad assortment of materials for fitting. Water contents range from 38 percent to 79 percent. (There is no single material that's absolutely best for everyone; by varying the water content, lenses can be custom-designed to fit specific needs.)

Soft contacts are available to correct myopia (nearsightedness), hyperopia (farsightedness), astigmatism, and even presbyopia (that unfortunate loss of ability to focus at near distances that gets worse after our mid-thirties). For years patients with unusual prescriptions, astigmatism, or reading problems were told that they couldn't wear soft contact lenses. But now innovations in lens manufacturing allow for almost any prescription to be made into a soft lens. Computerization and automation of lathing and molding soft contact lenses have made for extremely accurate lens prescriptions.

Daily-Wear versus Extended-Wear

Daily-wear lenses are designed to be put in when you wake up and taken out before you go to sleep. This is very important. All daily-wear lenses are made to provide enough oxygen to the cornea for the eye to breathe while it's open. *No daily-wear lenses are appropriate for overnight wear.*

Extended wear refers to any lens worn longer than twenty-four hours. (*Note:* Some people need extended-wear lenses for daily use, because their eyes require a higher level of oxygen.) These lenses are made to provide enough oxygen so that the eye can breathe even while you're sleeping.

When they were first introduced in the late 1970s, extended-wear soft contacts were advertised as "thirty-day lenses." They're not called that anymore. Research in the early 1980s quickly discovered that very few people could tolerate keeping lenses in their eyes for a whole month at a time, and those hardy souls who tried wearing them that long often ended up with big problems—corneal edema (excess fluid and swelling in the cornea), corneal abrasions, and infections. Subsequent research found that after even one week of continuous wear, there was a significant buildup of bacteria on and in the lenses—so much so, actually, that it's been determined that contact lenses shouldn't be worn for more than one week at a stretch. (However, it wasn't until recently that the Food and Drug Administration forced contact lens manufacturers to change their packaging for these lenses, limiting use to seven days.)

RGP extended wear didn't become available until the mid-1980s. These lenses were approved for only seven-day wear, but they generally provided more oxygen than their soft-lens counterparts and were less prone to the nasty bacterial buildup.

More current thinking with regard to extended-wear lenses centers around the phrase *flexible wear*—which isn't a particular type of contact lens but instead a concept of how these lenses should be worn. *Flexible wear* simply means that a lens material is fine for occasional overnight wear, and that you have the option of keeping your lenses in all night or taking them out before you go to sleep.

Disposable and Frequent-Replacement Lenses

Like everything else, as technology has improved, soft contacts have also gotten more complicated. Now, in addition to the original lens packaging—where you bought a single pair of lenses, built to last from about twelve to eighteen months—there are soft contacts that are packaged as disposable or frequent-replacement lenses.

Disposable extended-wear lenses, available since the late 1980s, are meant to be worn once—kept in your eyes for a week at a time—and then thrown away. Clinical studies in the 1980s found that many extended-wear lenses were more fragile than other kinds of contacts, more prone to wearing out or to being torn, which made this prospect too expensive for many people. In response to this, some lens manufacturers created entirely new production techniques and facilities to make lenses so reproducible, with so few defects, that large quantities of lenses could safely be dispensed at a very low cost per lens. Other manufacturers simply repackaged existing lens designs into lens "multipacks." The safety and efficacy of this method can be called into question because some of the manufacturing techniques for these older designs don't allow for the same lens reproducibility, and some of these older lenses provide less oxygen than the newer ones. Most recently, in 1995, came the first lens designed to be *disposed of daily*. If you have sensitivities to contact lens solutions or are prone to allergic reactions and infections due to contact lens coatings, or simply don't have time to clean your contacts, then daily-wear disposables might be the healthiest choice for your eyes.

Frequent-replacement lenses are designed to be removed, cleaned, and then worn again—but replaced often, at two-week, one-month, or three-month intervals, depending on the brand and the individual wearer. These lenses are made for either daily use or extended wear. (However, any disposable, extended-wear lens can also be used as a daily-wear, frequent-replacement lens.) An important thing to remember is that although these lenses are replaced often, they must be cleaned and disinfected every time they are removed, if you intend to wear them again. Otherwise there is a significant risk of an eye infection.

GETTING YOUR CONTACT LENSES

Which Lenses Are Right for You?

Your first step in deciding which lenses are right for you is a comprehensive eye exam, to determine what your prescription is and also to make sure that your eyes are healthy.

One of the most important parts of this evaluation is your health history. (For more on eye exams, see chapter 3.) Have you had any eye disease—such as dryness, chronic infections, or corneal dystrophy—that may interfere with contact lens wear? Do you have any functional problems with your eyes—a muscle imbalance, perhaps, or any trouble focusing? Do you have any general health problems? (Even though the problem may not be in your eye itself, some conditions may make wearing contact lenses more difficult, so be sure to tell your eye doctor *everything*, even if it doesn't seem important to you right now.) Are you taking any medications? (Some medications can dry out your eyes or otherwise interfere with contact lens wear.) Do you have any environmental allergies or sensitivities to preservatives? (These too may affect your comfort in contacts or your ability to use certain contact lens solutions.)

Another aspect of this evaluation is to determine whether your lifestyle—your work, habits, and hobbies—lends itself to contact lens wear. For example, are you active in sports? Do you work in a dry or dusty environment? Do you stare at a computer for a large portion of your day? Are you routinely exposed to any chemical fumes that may be absorbed into a contact lens? While none of these might absolutely preclude your wearing contacts—many of us who stare at computers all day do just fine with our contacts, for instance—it's certainly smart to consider everything *before* you make this investment, not after the fact.

Finally, it's a good idea to clarify your goals and expectations with contact lenses. For example, if your goal is to wear contacts for competitive swimming, this may not be realistic, because of the chemicals and bacteria found in swimming pools. If your goal is to use extended-wear soft contacts because you travel extensively on your job and don't want the hassle of taking contact lens solutions with you, this may be a fine idea, so long as your eyes can tolerate this type of lens. (The dehydrating environment in airplanes may complicate your plans.)

Getting the Right Fit

Contacts that don't fit right are about as useful as glasses that constantly slip down your nose; in other words, they're not much help. Good fit is essential, because it lets the contacts do what they're designed to do: give you the best vision possible.

To ensure good fit, your eye doctor will begin by measuring the corneal curvature and diameter for each eye. This curvature measurement, taken with an instrument called a *keratometer*, helps determine the right curvature of the back surface of a contact lens, so that it can be custom-made to match your eye. The diameter of your cornea—important in determining what size lens to use—can be measured with a ruler, but often it's best to try on a *diagnostic contact lens* (a nonprescription sample) of a known size; then the doctor can see how that lens fits by viewing it on your eye with something called a *biomicroscope.*

Your doctor will also take into account any surface irregularities on your eye that might hamper a good fit. Do you have any bumps or elevations on your conjunctiva (that clear layer over the "white" of your eye)? These may affect how your lenses move when you blink or may cause the edge of a lens to lift off a little. Is there any corneal disease? This too may affect how a contact lens would fit. And most important, might a contact lens aggravate any of these conditions?

When you blink, your contact lens should move up and down to circulate your tears on both sides of the lens. Good lubrication is very important; it helps keep your eyes and lenses from drying out. It also helps wash any debris, such as dust or even stray mascara, from your lenses and generally keeps the lens surface cleaner.

With this in mind, your eye doctor will also examine your eyelids. If you have a very large *interpalpebral aperture* (or "wide eyes," a large distance between your upper and lower lids), it may be difficult to fit you with RGP lenses, and you may need soft lenses, which are larger. If your lashes tend to turn inward and rub on the lens, this can affect both your vision and comfort. Lids that don't move smoothly across an eye can affect lens movement and lead to discomfort, dryness, and blurred vision. Similarly, eyelids that are very tight may move a lens *too much*, while lids that sag or are loose may not move a lens enough.

Next, your tears—their quantity and quality—will be inspected. Your "tear profile" also helps determine the kind of lens material you'll need. Some people are more comfortable with soft contacts that hold high amounts of water; others don't make enough tears to maintain a soft lens and would do better with an RGP lens that doesn't absorb tears.

Next, the Test Drive

Once you've been examined for your prescription, measurements have been taken, and it's been determined that your eyes are indeed healthy enough to tolerate contact lenses, your eye doctor will probably place "trial contact lenses" in your eyes—choosing lenses that best match your specific needs—to make sure all these measurements and assessments have been made correctly. What will they feel like? If you are trial-fit with a soft lens, you'll probably have some awareness that there is a lens in your eye, but it should be fairly comfortable within a few minutes. RGP lenses at first usually feel much more like a foreign body in your eye, but they typically settle down within about fifteen to twenty minutes. *Note:* If either type of lens feels painful—like you have several eyelashes in your eye—then there's something wrong, and the lens should be removed, rinsed, and tried again.

Some lens designs take longer to settle on the eye than others. For instance, lenses that are designed to correct astigmatism and bifocal contact lenses usually need to sit on your eye for fifteen to twenty minutes before the fit can be assessed. Some soft-lens materials are more volatile than others; they dry more easily on the eye. These lenses should also be allowed a longer settling time, so that the doctor can see whether this material is likely to tighten on your eye as it dries.

Once the trial lens has had time to settle on your eye, the doctor can often double-check your prescription using hand-held lenses. This generally gives you a sense of how well you should see with your "real" contacts (actually, having your full prescription in a well-fitting contact lens should provide even *better* vision than what you'll see with the trial contact demonstration).

Where to Purchase Your Lenses

Now it's time to get your "real" contacts. After all the fitting determinations have been made, your new lenses will be ordered (or set aside, if the doctor already has them in stock). If you're being fitted for contacts for the first time, or being refitted because of problems with a previous lens design, then you should buy your new lenses from your doctor or "lens fitter" (some states allow opticians to fit contact lenses).

Contact lens prescriptions are much more complex than glasses prescriptions. Glasses prescriptions just specify the power of the lens. Contact lens prescriptions specify a power, curvature, diameter, thickness, material, tint, and edge configuration. And we can't stress this point enough: because contacts are worn *on the eye*, they automatically become a health consideration for your eye. If you choose to shop elsewhere for your lenses, careful fitting and follow-up care must be done before your doctor can give you a written prescription and the go-ahead. Think about it: You can't reasonably expect your doctor to see you for an initial contact lens fitting and then write a prescription for you to get your first lenses elsewhere, because if that prescription is not correct, there can be serious complications for your eyes. Sometimes it takes a follow-up visit for the doctor to ascertain that a lens needs to be modified to improve your vision or comfort.

Wearing Your New Contact Lenses

Once you have your contacts, either the doctor or a trained contact lens technician will show you what to do: how to put the lenses in and take them out, plus how to clean and care for them. You'll also be given a wearing schedule—a plan that tells you how many hours at a time to leave your lenses in your eyes—so that you can get used to them gradually. (It's like starting an exercise program: you can't just start out at full throttle, you have to build up to it.)

Contacts do take a little getting used to. The cornea has to adjust to receiving slightly less oxygen from outside air (this doesn't harm your cornea in any way). Your tear-making system has to gear up production so that it can maintain a contact lens as well as your eye. *Therefore, follow the schedule faithfully.* If you try to wear your lenses all day right away, you'll likely find yourself right back in the doctor's office the next day with painful red eyes. (It won't make you feel any better to recognize that you should have known better.)

Before you leave the office with new lenses, your doctor will probably want to check the fit and also make sure that your vision is what it should be. (*Note:* Your vision may be slightly blurry at first; this is perfectly normal, because your eyes are adapting.) If it's determined that the fit looks healthy and that your vision is adequate, then you'll be set up for your first follow-up visit. (Depending on your specific needs, that visit may be scheduled from twenty-four hours to two weeks after this one.)

The follow-up visit is very important, so don't cancel yours! It means far more than just seeing that you're comfortable and making sure that your vision is okay. The big reason to go is this: *contact lens complications, if caught early, are always reversible.*

The doctor needs to check the integrity and health of your eye at every follow-up visit. A typical follow-up schedule for a first-time daily-lens wearer might be visits at one week, one month, and six months, and then a full examination at a year. Someone with extended-wear contacts might return within twenty-four to forty-eight hours, at one week, one month, three months, and six months, and then at a year for a full examination. If you seem particularly likely to develop complications with extended-wear lenses, your doctor may want to see you every three months—or more often, if necessary—even if you've been wearing lenses for years.

TAKING CARE OF YOUR CONTACT LENSES

Solutions

To help launch you into the new world of contact lenses, your doctor or lens technician will probably give you a "starter kit": various bottles of solutions, or "lens care systems." These have been fully tested, under the watchful control of the FDA, to make sure that the solutions work well with each other and that they'll both clean and disinfect your lenses.

Whether you wear soft, hard, or RGP lenses, the basic steps are the same, and they're fairly simple: when you take the lens out of your eye overnight, it needs to be cleaned, rinsed, and stored in a disinfecting solution. Some of the soft-lens solution terms that you need to be familiar with are *saline, daily or surfactant cleaners, weekly or enzyme cleaners,* and *disinfection.*

Saline is a rinsing solution, made up of water and 0.9 percent salt—much like your tears. *Note:* If you use tap water instead of saline, you will contaminate your lenses with bacteria and other microorganisms that can cause severe corneal infection. Saline can be preserved with a chemical to keep it sterile for a longer shelf life. (Some people are sensitive to these preservatives, however, and need to use an unpreserved solution.) *Any time you need to rinse a lens, or temporarily store a lens in a case, use saline.* Homemade saline, made with salt tablets and distilled water, carries a high risk of infection because of the potential for growth of microorganisms in the water. One particularly dangerous microorganism, acanthamoeba, can cause a potentially incurable infection.

Daily cleaners are to be used whenever a lens is left out overnight. (If you take your contacts out every day, you'll need to clean them every day.) If you have extended- or flexible-wear contacts, you'll need to use the daily cleaner whenever you choose not to sleep with your lenses in. This cleaner is a *surfactant,* or soap, that cleans debris and other filmy coatings off the lenses. Daily cleaners help disinfect by killing any bacteria that stick to the surface of your lens, and this in turn helps your overnight storage solution do a better job of killing the remaining bacteria.

Protein coatings that also accumulate on the lenses cling so tenaciously that a daily cleaner just isn't powerful enough to get rid of them. *Weekly cleaners* contain enzymes that "eat away" the proteins without damaging the lenses. (For some people, protein builds up so heavily that it's necessary to clean the lenses with enzymes several times a week.) This usually involves either soaking the lenses separately, in a solution of saline mixed with an enzyme tablet—which fizzes like a tiny Alka-Seltzer—or adding the enzyme tablet to the disinfection cycle.

Disinfection is the process of killing bacteria on the lens surface and within the lens itself. Wearing a sterile lens reduces your risk of developing an eye infection. (Because soft lenses are porous enough to allow water to pass through, bacteria can infiltrate them as well.) Disinfection systems are described below.

Caring for Soft Lenses

You should always wash your hands before caring for your contact lenses. Before you remove each lens, put "contact lens rewetting drops" in your eye to soften and loosen the lens. (This makes removing your lens a lot easier; it also decreases the risk of either tearing your lens or scratching your eye in the process.)

Cleaning and Rinsing

Once you've removed the lens, place it in the palm of your hand concave side up—so that the lens forms a small bowl—and rinse with saline to keep it from drying out. Add several drops of cleaner and *gently* scrub the lens in your palm by rubbing your finger back and forth over it. (This way you'll be washing both sides of the lens at once; the outside of the lens will be cleaned as it rubs against your palm.) Alternatively, you can clean one side and then flip the lens over to clean the other. After scrubbing the lens, move it to your other palm and rinse it thoroughly with saline. If you don't rinse thoroughly, the soap and coatings will reattach themselves to the lens surface, just as food does on dishes that are scrubbed but not rinsed. If you have a "multipurpose" lens solution, in which the cleaner is mixed with the rinsing solution (see below), you can scrub and rinse in the same palm. You should always clean your lenses before disinfecting them.

Disinfecting

There are three basic systems for disinfecting your soft lenses: heat, chemical, and peroxide oxidative.

Heat systems are designed to warm your contact lenses to a temperature hot enough to kill bacteria that would otherwise grow on the lenses overnight. After each lens is cleaned and rinsed, it is placed in the heat unit. The unit heats the lenses for approximately thirty minutes and then has a fifteen- to thirty-minute cool-down cycle.

Heat systems are quicker than most other methods of disinfection. Another advantage is that the lenses can be heated in saline that is "unpreserved" (a good option for people sensitive to solutions that contain preservatives and chemicals). There are several disadvantages, though. Heating a lens often makes lens coatings, particularly protein coatings, worse. If your lens is not thoroughly cleaned before you put it in the unit, protein coatings will be denatured (broken down) by the heat and will bind more tenaciously than ever to the lens surface (the "baked-on, caked-on" effect). Excessive protein buildup can not only make your contacts seem constantly cloudy; it may even lead to a particular allergic reaction to your lenses. (For more on this, see below.)

Another disadvantage is that heat units are compatible with only certain kinds of soft lenses. If your lenses are composed of more than 50 percent water, they can't be heated safely without distorting the lens. (Therefore, check with your doctor before using this kind of system!)

Heat units also have a practical disadvantage: they don't travel well. Wherever you go, you'll need to be sure there's someplace to plug in your heat unit. (This isn't always as easy as it sounds, especially for people who like to camp.)

Chemical disinfectants: If you don't heat your lenses, you'll need to soak them in a chemical bath to kill bacteria. With most of these systems, you place your (freshly cleaned) lenses in a case with a solution. This saline-based solution is mixed with a chemical preservative strong enough to kill specified bacteria in about four to six hours. (The solution has to work within a reasonably short time so that you'll be able to use the lens the next day.)

The advantage to these chemical baths is that unlike the heat system, they don't make lens coatings worse. However, the big disadvantage is that many people are sensitive to the bacteria-killing chemicals in the disinfectant; some soft-lens disinfection preservatives produce reactions in as many as 40 percent of the people who use them. For many people these reactions are fairly minor: just a little stinging and redness. But for some the effects can be much more serious: a full-blown allergic reaction, with significant swelling of the eyelids and conjunctiva, as well as toxic reactions that leave deposits in the cornea. (For more on this, see below.)

Peroxide oxidative disinfectants: The most significant advance in chemical disinfectants came in the early 1980s, with the development of peroxide oxidative solutions. These are based on a 3 percent hydrogen peroxide solution—the same strength as the hydrogen peroxide you can buy in the drugstore. Hydrogen peroxide is a great disinfectant, but it's acidic; if you accidentally got some in your eyes, it would burn, leave your eyes red, and possibly cloud your vision.

To avoid this, peroxide oxidative disinfection systems have a built-in "neutralization mechanism" that oxidizes hydrogen peroxide, breaking it down to its basic components, oxygen and water. The specifics vary, depending on your particular system. One company, for example, uses a catalytic disk, made of plastic that's been coated with a very thin coating of platinum. This disk is left overnight in the lens case, where it takes about six hours to break down the hydrogen peroxide. Another company's solution uses a tablet that contains catalase, an enzyme that also occurs naturally in the body, and that breaks down hydrogen peroxide completely. This system has appeared in several different formats over the years, but the most recent version has a time-release tablet that neutralizes in a two-hour cycle.

These peroxide oxidative solutions have the advantage of combining the best of the two previous concepts. That is, the lenses are not heated, there are no residual chemicals to cause irritation, and these solutions disinfect better than multipurpose solutions (see below). Even when—as inevitably happens in bathrooms full of similar-looking bottles of solutions—people put the disinfectant directly into their eye, there's no harm done beyond some temporary stinging and redness. (If this should happen to you, immediately wash your eye with copious amounts of saline and call your doctor.)

Multipurpose Solutions

In the 1990s, multipurpose solutions, featuring chemical disinfectants plus a cleaner, came on the market. The chemicals are designed to be mild enough to be tolerated directly in the eye, so the solution can be used for rinsing the lenses as well as disinfecting them. These solutions are convenient, which is their best selling point. But any cleaner—no matter how mild—has the potential to cause eye irritation, and the more chemicals, the greater this potential. These systems, however, seem to cause problems only for about 5 to 15 percent of the people who use them, depending on the brand of solution.

Multipurpose solutions don't always make the most effective cleaners or disinfectants. Because the ingredients have to be mild enough to be tolerated by the eye, they don't always do as thorough a job maintaining a contact lens over the long run as other solutions. However, they are an excellent means of lens care when lenses are made for frequent replacement, especially if you replace your lenses at least once a month. Often a frequent-replacement lens can be fully maintained with multipurpose solutions—which means you won't have to bother with weekly enzyme cleaners. (Because everyone's tear composition, environment, and wearing habits are unique, there are some people who can successfully maintain a pair of contacts for its typical twelve- to eighteen-month life with *only* a multipurpose solution.)

What's Next?

In the future you might see some new advances in soft-lens disinfection. Several research groups have tried using a microwave oven as the disinfection unit, and others have experimented with a disinfection unit based on ultraviolet light. Either of these methods would completely sterilize the lenses in approximately five minutes. The significance of this? When a lens is merely *disinfected*, only certain microorganisms are killed (the ones that cause problems, we hope). A *sterilized* lens, on the other hand, is utterly free of all living organisms. These ideas are still experimental and must be further tested to ensure that the lenses aren't somehow damaged during the disinfection process. However, if the soft-lens industry continues in its trend of disposability, *all* disinfection systems may become obsolete in the future.

Caring for Hard and RGP Lenses

The concepts in cleaning hard and RGP lenses are the same as for soft lenses, but the solutions used are very different.

The first step after removing your lenses is to clean each one thoroughly, on both sides, with an RGP cleaner in the palm of your hand. Use a finger that's softer than the index finger on the tip, such as your ring finger or pinkie, to reduce the risk of scratching your lens. If you try to clean an RGP lens between your thumb and forefinger, the lens will be more likely to warp because of the extreme pressure from your finger.

After thoroughly scrubbing your lens, rinse it with tap water. Be sure that the water is not too cold (it might shatter the lens) or too hot (it might warp the lens) and—this is essential—*be sure to close the drain!* You can use tap water instead of saline to rinse the cleaner off your RGP lenses, because the lens isn't porous enough to absorb the water. However, you should never use tap water to insert a lens into your eye, because of the risk of infection.

After cleaning and rinsing your lenses, soak them in a case filled with an RGP soaking solution. This solution has preservatives to disinfect the surface of your lenses and make them safe to wear the next day. In fact, you'll probably use the same bottle of soaking solution to wet your lenses when you insert them the next day. The solution refreshes the lens surface to make it more "wettable" with your tears; with every blink, your tears should coat the lens surface smoothly. When a lens is not "wettable," your tears will bead up on the lens surface, just like rainwater on a freshly waxed car. *Note:* Always clean your lenses at night. If you clean a lens in the morning after a night of soaking, you'll undo all the good that the soaking did. Your lens will lose its surface "wettability" until it's soaked again for a few more hours. (If you happen to be wearing your lens at the time, this means that the soaking will take place *in your eye* for the first few hours. As a result, until the lens is properly wettable again, it will feel very dry or seem foggy.)

In general, for any type of contact lens, always use fresh solutions for cleaning and disinfection. Empty out your lens case after you insert your lenses. Rinse the case, if necessary, and let it air-dry to kill any bacteria remaining in the case. Bacteria need moisture to survive, so air-drying the case will ensure that you're placing your lenses in a sterile environment the next time you clean them. A solution that is reused will not be as effective and can possibly lead to an eye infection.

REPLACING YOUR CONTACT LENSES

Maybe your prescription changed. Or you lost or tore a lens, or your lenses just wore out. Maybe you want to keep a spare pair of lenses handy, in case of an emergency. Maybe you wear tinted lenses, and you want several different colors. Whatever the reason, it's inevitable: at some point, you will need to replace one or both lenses.

So, where will you go to do this? There used to be just one choice: your eye doctor. But these days there are so many alternatives that you can actually shop around. (Believe us, your doctor is well aware of this and as a result will probably offer competitive prices.) Although most doctors don't have the buying power of a major lens retailer or discount mail-order business, they can usually come close to the best prices you can find elsewhere.

Why should you buy from your doctor if you can save a few dollars and get the exact same lens from someplace else? With soft contacts the reason is simply that no contact lens manufacturer ever produces lenses with a zero defect rate, for either a doctor or a major retailer. Your doctor, however, will be better equipped to troubleshoot a contact lens problem than the retail outlet or mail-order house, as well as make sure that the problem is with the lens and not with your eye. It's not uncommon, for instance, to receive a lens that's marked correctly on the bottle but doesn't perform as it should. It might not be clear for your vision or fit like your old lens. Occasionally lenses are received with a small defect in the material itself that affects how you see or how the lens feels.

Some RGP lenses as well turn out not to have been made to your doctor's specifications and must be returned to the lab. Also, every lab has its own manufacturing technique; these may vary slightly, and this could alter the fit of even a "brand-name" lens. Say your doctor orders your first lens from one lab, and you replace it with a lens from another lab. Although the lens material and specifications may be exactly the same, the lens still may not fit or perform exactly as your original lens did. Not only can this affect your vision and comfort, it can also harm your eye. If you do shop around for your RGP lenses, make sure that your new lens supplier gets in touch with your doctor's lab for your exact specifications and tolerances.

The mail-order contact business is booming. You've probably seen the commercials and read the ads, in which a spokesmodel suggests that you can now buy lenses using a convenient toll-free number for up to "60 percent less." Just have your credit card ready! Such ads may be misleading. To start with, no lens manufacturer has ever set a "manufacturer's suggested retail price" for contacts. If you look hard enough, you'll probably come across a greedy doctor somewhere who overcharges for lenses so exorbitantly that the mail-order company's price is indeed 60 percent less. But this is not the norm. And it's not the whole story, either. Most mail-order companies want to sell you a "membership fee," which adds to the cost of each "discount" lens; they also charge a pretty penny for shipping and handling, and these hidden costs often make the lens price *equal to or more than* the price your doctor charges. Mail-order companies are in the business to sell lenses and make a profit. Most doctors, in contrast, sell lenses to their patients as a service and charge only a nominal markup to cover any office expenses associated with ordering lenses. Reputable eye doctors make their living caring for eyes, not selling lenses.

So, if you do buy from mail order, be careful. There have been many cases in which mail-order companies haven't called the doctor to verify the prescription before sending the lenses. Also, mail-order phone representatives often try to sell you other products and services—including lens solutions, or even suggesting their own network of doctors. In some cases phone clerks, dispensing "expert" advice without the benefit of examining the person's eyes or seeing his or her patient records—or, for that matter, having the medical education to make their opinions valid—have even suggested that a patient wear his or her lenses differently from the way the doctor prescribed. And this, frankly, is reprehensible. Your doctor has carefully selected a lens care system that's appropriate for *your* lenses and *your* eyes in particular. Such careless advice could potentially cause damage. Also, your doctor has prescribed a personalized schedule for you so that you can wear your contacts safely. If you've been told by your doctor, for example, to dispose of your extended-wear disposable lenses every week, don't try to wear them for two weeks just because Joe at the mail-order house said you could. (One of the ways mail-order companies promise "big savings" on disposable lenses is by telling you to wear them twice as long— advice that might be easy on your wallet, but tough on your eyes.) Finally, if you like and trust your doctor—and you should, or else you should find another doctor—why change?

COMPLICATIONS: WHEN SOMETHING'S NOT RIGHT WITH YOUR CONTACTS

Dry Eyes

This is an extremely common problem; in fact, dry eyes are probably the largest impediment to successful contact lens wear. Unfortunately, as the eye gets older, it makes fewer tears. In addition, medications such as hormonal supplements, diuretics, antidepressants, and Accutane can make the eyes dry. Many people who have worn contact lenses for years, with no problems at all, suddenly find themselves unable to tolerate their lenses.

However, the key may simply be finding the right lens material for your eyes. It may take trying several different lens designs and materials before you and your doctor can find the least-drying contact lens for your eyes.

Tears are more complicated than you might imagine (see chapter 13). They've got three major layers, for one thing. The innermost, called the *mucin layer*, is produced by goblet cells on the conjunctiva. (For more on the eye's anatomy, see chapter 1.) Mucin is viscous; it enables tears to cover the eye more evenly. The huge middle layer (which takes up about 90 percent of each tear), mostly water, is produced by the lacrimal glands that sit just above and outside your eyes. Outermost is an oily layer, produced by a row of Meibomian glands along the margin of each eyelid; the coat of oil helps keep tears from evaporating too quickly.

A soft contact lens contains water, and so soft contact lenses must absorb tears in order to stay soft. After the lenses have been in your eyes for about fifteen minutes, their water content is actually made up of your tears. If your eyes are dry because of poor tear *quality*—that is, if you have plenty of tears, but they lack mucins or oils—then a *higher-water-containing* lens will probably keep more tears on your eyes and, as a result, be less drying. If, however, your eyes are dry because of poor tear *quantity*—if, in other words, your tears are perfectly fine, but there just aren't enough of them to go around—then a *lower-water-containing* lens will usually cause less dryness, because it won't have to absorb as much tear volume to maintain itself. Finally, if you have both poor-quality and poor-quantity tears, you'll most likely have problems wearing soft contacts at all—but RGP materials may work well for you.

Corneal Edema

As we've discussed in previous chapters, we see because light passes through the "window" of the cornea and focuses on the retina. The innermost portion of the cornea is constantly in contact with the aqueous humor, the fluid within the eye, but this fluid is never allowed to build up. Tiny efficient "pumps" continuously force it out, to keep the cornea clear (see chapter 11). These pumps run on oxygen; most of it comes from the environment, but extra oxygen also comes from blood vessels around the cornea and under the eyelid.

A contact lens has the potential to decrease the supply of oxygen to the cornea, and this can cause the pump mechanism to slow down. In turn, fluid begins to seep into the cornea—a swelling called *edema*—causing it to become cloudy. This can happen if a lens is too tight, if it's too thick, or if it's worn too long.

Signs of trouble: You'll probably notice symptoms first when you take out your contacts and put on your glasses: your vision will look hazy. If this haziness disappears within the first ten to fifteen minutes, the edema is probably not very significant. However, the haziness can persist for days or even months, depending upon how much edema was present. If the edema is left untreated, small water bubbles will eventually form in the cornea. Your cornea is like skin, in that the surface layer constantly replenishes itself; cells formed below the surface rise and eventually slough off. When edema is present, these bubbles float along with the rest of the cells right to the top. When they reach the surface of the cornea, they burst, leaving tiny abrasions. If you accumulate enough of these abrasions, in addition to the hazy vision you will have red and painful eyes.

Treatment: Your doctor can prescribe drops or ointments to reduce the edema and heal the abrasions. Corneal edema almost always resolves with treatment and discontinuing wear of the lens that's causing the trouble.

Corneal Neovascularization

Neovascularization is the growth of new blood vessels. As discussed above, the cornea needs oxygen to maintain its clarity; oxygen also supports a protective barrier that keeps blood vessels out of the cornea. If the cornea is oxygen-starved, blood vessels invite themselves in, taking upon themselves the matter of "turning up" the oxygen flow. Unfortunately, these vessels also scar the cornea.

Treatment: If this condition is caught early, neovascularization can be reversed simply by removing the offending contacts and either switching to a better-fitting, more oxygen-permeable lens or discontinuing lens wear for a time. But when these blood vessels spread unchecked like ivy, right into the center of the cornea, they can cause big trouble: a significant loss in vision that can be treated only by corneal transplant.

Because there really aren't any early warning signs or symptoms of corneal neovascularization—that is, until it's too late to reverse—routine examinations with your doctor are essential, so that your doctor can make sure your cornea is as healthy as it should be.

Giant Papillary Conjunctivitis

Giant papillary conjunctivitis, or GPC, is an allergy that's caused by an autoimmune reaction to your own protein coatings, the ones that build up on poorly cleaned contact lenses. Who's at risk? You are, if you don't use a weekly protein cleaner with your soft lenses, or if you don't do a very good job cleaning any type of contact lens.

On any typical day of wearing your contacts, your upper lid travels about three hundred yards—the equivalent of three football fields—over the surface of your lens. The upper lid therefore has the most interaction with protein coatings and is the best indicator of GPC: its inside surface becomes swollen and red and produces large amounts of mucins that coat your contact lens with a film that clouds your vision when the contacts are worn.

Signs of trouble: One common early symptom is an itch that gets worse when you remove the lens (when your upper lid comes in direct contact with your cornea). Also, as more mucins are produced, the lenses begin to appear foggy while you're wearing them. Sometimes—because with each blink your swollen upper lids grab the sticky, coated contact lenses more vigorously than usual—they even slide off the center of your cornea. Lenses also tend to wear out much more quickly than normal with GPC. Many lenses designed to last a year will wear out in as little as one to two months. Often someone with this problem will replace many lenses in a short period of time before finally going to the eye doctor and having the problem checked out.

Treatment for GPC has varied over the years, but a common remedy is to stop wearing contacts for at least two weeks, to give the lids a chance to recover. (Often this alone is enough to treat the problem, without the need for any additional medications.) If your GPC is severe, or if you still have symptoms after you stop wearing your lens, your doctor may prescribe antiallergy and/or anti-inflammatory eye drops. Over-the-counter artificial tear supplements can also help.

Because GPC is an allergy, if you start using the same contact lenses after this two-week breather your symptoms will probably come back; the proteins will accumulate again and produce a new allergic reaction. Therefore, if you want to keep wearing contacts once the GPC has resolved, you'll need to switch to another kind of lens. In the past, someone with GPC either moved to a more "deposit-resistant" soft contact lens—and a much more rigorous cleaning regimen, including more frequent enzyme cleaning—or switched to a gas-permeable lens. But in recent years it's been found that wearing disposable or frequent-replacement contact lenses also reduces the problem dramatically. Because there's so little buildup of protein on a new contact lens, replacing your lenses every day to every two weeks keeps the lenses free enough of proteins that GPC usually doesn't return.

Infections and Corneal Ulcers

Everybody gets eye infections, whether we wear contacts or not. We all have bacteria around our eyes; most of the time our tears keep them in check, but occasionally those bacteria can take over. A well-fitting, well-tended contact lens does not cause eye infections, but it can make any infection worse; the warm, moist space between the lens and your cornea can act as an incubator for bacteria and allow them to flourish.

A corneal ulcer is a severe eye infection. It can be extremely painful—and potentially disastrous when it comes to your sight. An ulcer can permanently scar your cornea and cloud your vision if that scar is inside your pupil.

Who's at risk? Mostly it's people who often sleep with their contacts in. A common scenario is this: Say you have a small corneal abrasion, from debris that got trapped under your lens. If you take out your lens for the night, the abrasion will have a chance to heal, and you'll wake up with no ill effects. But if you sleep with the contact lens in, the bacteria that grow between the lens and your eye can work their way into the abrasion and cause a corneal infection.

If you suspect that you have an infection—your eye is red, with a discharge, or is uncomfortable in any way or is sensitive to light—remove your lens immediately and call your eye doctor. Getting medical attention in time usually means that your eye will heal completely and that you can start wearing your contacts again as soon as your eye recovers.

If your infection turns out to be bacterial (caused by bacteria), then your usual methods of cleaning and disinfecting your contacts will probably be enough to save your lenses and enable you to wear them again. But if your infection was caused by a virus, disinfection alone may not be enough to remove the contamination, and the lens may need to be replaced.

Tight-Lens Syndrome

Tight shoes can cause debilitating foot problems. A too-tight shirt collar can hamper your breathing and produce symptoms that mimic a heart attack. Well, your eye doesn't respond well to tight-fitting garments, either. When a soft contact lens is too tight, it can cause problems ranging from mild discomfort to serious, vision-threatening complications. The trouble is that a tight lens doesn't make room for your tears to flow underneath the lens and refresh the cornea. Instead, tears tend to pool under the lens and stagnate—like a fetid pond, a perfect breeding ground for nasty bacteria. As the bacteria proliferate, they ooze toxins that create cloudy patches in your cornea, called *corneal infiltrates*, and cause infections.

A soft lens that's too tight also smothers the cornea, leaving it constantly oxygen-starved. The chronic lack of oxygen (as discussed above) in turn makes the cornea more susceptible to edema (swelling) and neovascularization (the growth of new blood vessels within the cornea).

Tight-lens syndrome can happen with any kind of soft contact lens—even disposable lenses that are thrown away every day. If the lenses don't fit properly, it doesn't matter how long you leave them in or whether you take them out every night; you're still harming your eye.

Signs of trouble: Warning symptoms include foggy vision, fluctuating vision (your vision gets better or worse with a blink), dryness, irritation, and redness. Often, redness is noticeable around the entire cornea, but it can appear in isolated patches as well. If the edges of your lens bear down on blood vessels running through your conjunctiva, this can cause tiny hemorrhages to appear around the edges of your contacts. Also, you can almost always see a distinct stamp of the lens left on the eye after you take out the lens, just as you can trace the outline of painful shoes after you take them off your feet. (However, some people can see such an impression even if their lenses fit appropriately.)

An RGP lens that's too tight can cause similar symptoms, but because it doesn't cover the entire cornea, as a soft lens does, the symptoms can take longer to express themselves. A tight RGP lens can actually stick to your cornea, making it difficult to remove, and will probably leave a contact-shaped indentation in the cornea afterward. If, after you remove your RGP lens, your vision is foggy and distorted with your glasses—and it doesn't return to normal within ten to fifteen minutes after you take out your contacts—your lens may be too tight.

A tight-fitting lens doesn't necessarily mean that your lens fitter did a poor job of fitting your eye. Contact lenses can tighten on their own after they're worn for a few hours, especially if your eyes are dry. Thus, it's important that you have your lenses in for a few hours before you return for any follow-up visit, so that your eye doctor can get an accurate idea of how your contact lenses really fit. (Of course, if your lenses are too uncomfortable to wear for even a few hours, then don't harm yourself just to demonstrate your level of discomfort!)

Reactions to Contact Lens Solutions

First, read the label. No matter how a solution is packaged, before you buy it, make sure it doesn't contain any chemical or preservative that you've reacted to before. Many manufacturers label their solutions as being "for sensitive eyes," but even some of these contain preservatives— milder, less sensitizing ones, but preservatives all the same—and you may still react to them. Thus, if you need an "unpreserved" solution, make sure the bottle is labeled that way.

Signs of trouble: Sensitivities to preservatives can range from stinging, burning, and redness to full-blown allergic reactions that can cause tremendous itching and swelling and may even harm the cornea. These reactions occasionally require treatment but almost always go away when use of that preservative is discontinued.

Two preservatives known to cause problems for many people are thimerosal and chlorhexidene. Thimerosal produces allergic reactions in more than 40 percent of the people who use it; these reactions can develop even after years of use. Chlorhexidene can be toxic to the cornea and can cause significant redness, burning, and irritation. Polyaminopropyl biquanide (also known as Dymed), a newer, milder, version of chlorhexidene introduced in the early 1990s, has decreased this problem tremendously. Still, some people have reactions to this chemical as well (symptoms are similar to those caused by chlorhexidene).

You can avoid some major eye reactions simply by making sure you're putting the right solution in your eye. Mistakes happen more often than you might think, and it's no laughing matter. Accidentally putting in contact lens cleaner instead of the rewetting drops you thought you had picked up can cause severe chemical burns, painful red eyes, and cloudy vision that lasts for days or even weeks. Some cleaners contain abrasives that will scratch your cornea; others contain alcohol, which can strip off the surface of your cornea. Occasionally someone mistakes disinfectant for saline, rinses a lens with a disinfectant, and inserts it. This too can cause a significant chemical burn.

Treatment for all of these reactions always starts with removing the offending chemical or preservative. You'll have to stop wearing your lenses until your eye heals completely, rid your old lenses of every last trace of the chemicals, or replace your lenses altogether. If your symptoms are severe enough, you may also be prescribed a medication. Because your symptoms can be vague, when you seek treatment make a list of every solution you've been using, or take your solutions along with you, to help your doctor or lens fitter pinpoint the problem.

Of course, one big remedy for solution sensitivities is disposable contact lenses. If you throw them away after every use, you'll never have to worry about reactions caused by cleaners and disinfectants.

Torn or Damaged Contacts

A torn or damaged lens can irritate your eye, causing symptoms of redness, pain, discharge, watering, and blurred or distorted vision that may not clear up right away when you take out your lens. It may also injure your cornea—in which case you might still feel like the lens is in your eye even when it's not—or even lead to infection. So if you have persistent redness, pain, or discharge, see your doctor and get your eyes (and contacts) checked.

No matter whether your lens is hard or soft, if it's torn, warped, broken, or simply worn out, it will have to be replaced. Once they're damaged, lenses can't be fixed.

Itching, Burning, and Redness

It's simple: itching, burning, and redness all indicate that there is something wrong with either your contact lenses or your eyes. If the symptoms go away when you take out your lens, this could indicate a problem with the fit of the lens, the lens itself, or the solutions that you're using, and your doctor or lens fitter should scrutinize your lens-wearing and lens-cleaning habits to figure out what needs to be changed. If your symptoms persist after you remove your lenses, this could suggest an infection, allergic reaction, or abrasion. In any event, you should seek medical attention.

Problems with Extended-Wear Lenses

Extended wear of a contact lens magnifies the risk of any of the complications we've discussed above. Think about it: The lens is in your eye twenty-four hours a day. Your eye never gets a break; there's no downtime.

This can cause serious eye infections and complications from lack of oxygen to the cornea.

We're not all cut out for extended-wear contacts. Some of us require more oxygen in our eyes, just as some of us need more sleep to refresh us or more heat to feel comfortable in the winter. Maybe you can do well with extended wear. Or maybe your eyes have such a high demand for oxygen that you need an extended-wear lens just for daily wear.

In any event, you can dramatically reduce your risk of extended-wear complications by just using a little common sense. The most important thing to do, before you decide to sleep with your contacts in, is to take a good look at your eyes. If they're red, irritated, or significantly dry before bedtime, then the answer should be pretty obvious: Don't sleep with your lenses. Take them out. Give your eyes a breather.

If you wake up with any symptoms of redness, persistent blurred vision, discomfort, discharge, or pain, the answer should be equally clear: Take out your lenses immediately. If the symptoms go away, see your eye doctor or lens fitter to make sure the lens fits properly. If your symptoms don't go away, again, seek medical attention promptly. Don't wait for a problem to become serious. When in doubt, find out what the problem is; some problems are serious, and some aren't, but you won't know unless you find out.

Some Questions You May Have about Contact Lenses

Can I wear contact lenses if I have astigmatism?

Sure. Statistically, about 40 percent of potential contact lens wearers could benefit from correcting astigmatism with contact lenses. If you've read chapter 2, you know that astigmatism is considered a "refractive error," like nearsightedness or farsightedness. In a perfect eye, light enters through the cornea at the front of the eye and is focused to a precise point on the retina at the back of the eye. But with astigmatism, this focusing is skewed. Instead of being focused to a sharp *point* of light onto the retina, the light gets stretched out almost into a *line;* as a result, your view of the world is stretched in one direction and blurred. Eye doctors compensate for your astigmatism by prescribing lenses that have the *opposite* curvature of your eye; these lenses even out, or counterbalance, the way your eyes focus light. *Note:* Astigmatism does not reflect the health of your eye and should not be considered an impediment to contact lens wear.

The original hard lenses could correct mild to moderate degrees of astigmatism, but they weren't too helpful for people with more significant astigmatism. What a difference a few years makes! Today highly precise RGP lenses, made by computer-driven lathes, can correct any degree of astigmatism.

The early soft contacts couldn't do much to correct astigmatism. By 1980, as technology improved, several soft-lens designs incorporated corrections for astigmatism. And today many lens designs do a fine job of correcting astigmatism. However, there are still some practitioners out there who tell patients that they can't wear contact lenses because they have astigmatism. This is not true. If you've been told that astigmatism prevents you from wearing contact lenses, take your business to a more enlightened establishment.

Am I too old to wear contact lenses?

Not unless you think you are. There's no age limit on wearing contacts; plenty of patients enjoy their contact lenses well into their nineties. Actually, the only real limiting factor is the state of your general health. Arthritis can make it more difficult to insert and remove lenses, for instance. Dry eyes are more prevalent as we get older and can make lens wearing difficult—but certainly not impossible. Certain diseases (thyroid disease, collagen vascular disease, corneal dystrophies) and some medications (hormone replacement therapy and diuretics, for example) can cause problems for contact lens wear. But by all means, if you're interested in contacts, talk to your eye doctor!

How can I see to clean my lenses more easily, once they're removed?

Place your lenses in a temporary case, put on your glasses, and then clean your contacts.

What happens if I leave my contacts out of their case and they dry out?

A soft contact lens will shrink considerably when it gets dry; it will also become brittle and fragile. But if you place the lens—gently—in a case with some saline, the lens will immediately start soaking up moisture like a sponge. It will probably take a good soak of at least thirty to sixty minutes before the lens is fully hydrated. Then, just clean and disinfect the lens again before you put it in.

With RGP contacts, drying causes no damage to the lens itself.

However, these lenses have a surface treatment to make the lens surface more "wettable" (which helps your tears coat the lens surface evenly every time you blink). When an RGP lens gets dried out, this temporarily interferes with the "wettability," and you'll need to soak the lens for about four hours to replenish it. If you try to insert the dried-out lens right away, before it's had time to recover, it will "soak" anyway—in your eye—and will feel dry and uncomfortable for those four hours until it's finally refreshed.

How long do lenses last?

Generally, soft contacts that are neither disposable nor frequent-replacement lenses last from a year to eighteen months. This is based on an average wearing day of about twelve to fourteen hours, seven days a week. But if you wear your lenses longer—eighteen hours a day, for example—they might wear out sooner, in as little as nine months to a year. Even if you take the most meticulous care imaginable—if you're an eye doctor's dream, in fact—the material will still wear out. Several things contribute to this. Just rubbing your lenses, the act itself, tends to break down the lens surface over time. (However, if you *don't* scrub your lenses they'll wear out even sooner, because the coatings that accumulate will eventually form permanent, impossible-to-clean deposits on the lenses.) Every time you blink, you wear down the lens a little. Eventually the surface of the lens begins to erode and become dimpled, like the surface of a golf ball. Deposits start to form in those dimples, and they bind to the lens so tenaciously that they can't be cleaned off.

The life span of disposable lenses is based on your wearing schedule; they should be replaced every one to fourteen days. By the end of their cycle, nearly all of these lenses show signs of wear, so even if your lenses *feel* fine, they should be replaced. If you wait until the lenses hurt before replacing them, you may wind up with one or more of the problems these types of lenses were designed to avoid (such as giant papillary conjunctivitis and corneal oxygen deprivation).

Frequent-replacement lenses are generally meant to last two weeks to three months, depending on your particular schedule and the lens material.

For RGP lenses, the life span of the lens depends very much on how you take care of them. If, with all good intentions, you rigorously clean your lenses between your thumb and forefinger, your lenses may actually warp within a few cleanings. If you're a careful cleaner (see above for tips on cleaning), these lenses can last for years. Your doctor or lens technician can even prolong the life of your lenses by polishing them to remove any fine surface scratches that may accumulate over time. Polishing can also remove any rough spots on the lens edge, which can cause irritation.

There has been some research to support the theory that RGP lenses eventually wear out like a soft lens; electron micrograph photos have shown tiny surface disruptions on aging RGP lenses. However, because these photos show a lens magnified up to one million times, there's some dispute as to whether these irregularities are clinically significant, and whether they actually reduce the life of your lenses.

What are those white bumps that I see on my soft contact lenses?

They're the deposits that inevitably form on a worn-out lens, a conglomeration of mucins, oils, debris, and protein. Every time you blink, you contribute a thin layer to these evolving deposits, like an oyster working on a pearl. Eventually the deposits get larger and larger, resulting in the sizable white bump you're seeing. And this means it's time to replace the lens.

How do I care for my lenses if I don't wear them every day?

If you use a chemical disinfection system with your soft lenses, such solutions can usually maintain a lens for long-term storage of up to two weeks, depending on the product. If you use a heat system, you'll need to find a saline solution with sufficient preservative potential to keep your lens sterile after it has been heated. The problem here is that most saline solutions lack adequate preservatives to keep a lens sterile for long-term storage—which opens the door for potential bacterial and fungal growth on the lenses and in the lens case. Thus, heat disinfection is not terribly practical for the occasional lens wearer. Hydrogen peroxide solutions can maintain your soft contacts for much longer storage periods—so long as there is nothing to neutralize the hydrogen peroxide. (Which means that you'd need to remove the neutralization mechanism before storing your lenses.)

For soft-lens wearers, one-day disposable lenses address this dilemma nicely. You can wear the lens once and throw it away, and store the rest of your lenses in a cool, dry place until you're ready for them.

With RGP lenses, most soaking solutions are fine for storage of up to one to two weeks. If you're storing an old pair to keep as an emergency backup for your current lenses, you'll want to store the lenses dry after a thorough cleaning, to ensure that the lenses don't get contaminated by sitting around in old solution. Be sure to soak your lenses for at least four hours before again trying to wear them.

If I wear bifocal glasses, can I still wear contacts?

Absolutely. The primary problem here is that you're dealing with at least two different glasses prescriptions: your distance prescription doesn't work for reading, and you can't see far away with your reading prescription. Also, some people who wear bifocals need intermediate-distance vision (generally from two to four feet) prescriptions. (In glasses, this is handled either with progressive addition lenses or with trifocals. For more on this, see chapter 4.)

Any decision that you and your doctor or lens specialist make together will be a compromise; what you need to decide is whether that compromise is more suitable to your needs than the compromise of wearing glasses alone.

A good option—the one that probably provides the best vision—is to use contact lenses for your distance vision and to wear reading glasses over the contact lenses. If you have demanding visual needs, or if your work requires some eye protection at a close distance—if you're a dentist or auto mechanic, for instance—then this can be an excellent way to go. If you need trifocals, you can have your reading glasses made in a format that addresses both intermediate and close-up visual needs. (Of course the compromise here is that you'll still need to put on glasses for part of the day.)

Another option sounds like a special effect in the movies. It's called *monovision:* using one eye for distance vision and the other for seeing close up (generally, the distance contact goes in your dominant eye). This is not as taxing as it sounds, and it can be achieved with any kind of contact lens. Even if, for instance, you need custom-made lenses to correct an unusual astigmatism, the lenses can still be modified so that one eye sees distance and the other reads. (A prerequisite for monovision is that both of your eyes must have excellent vision, and each must work properly by itself.)

Since its inception more than thirty years ago, monovision has been a controversial idea. However, recent studies have shown that it's safe, in that it doesn't affect how you use your eyes together. Even people who have worn monovision contacts for years still have good *binocular* vision (using both eyes together) when they wear glasses.

Of concern to many patients who wear monovision contacts is a loss of depth perception. At a long distance, you perceive depth based on information that can be provided to either eye and is not dependent on how you use your eyes together. For example, when you see a car parked in front of a building, you know that the building is farther away than the car. You can see this with either eye by itself, just the same as you would with both eyes together; you don't see the car as being *in* the building when you close one eye. Other clues to depth are relative differences in shadowing, shading, coloring, and contrast.

Recently, researchers at the University of California School of Optometry in Berkeley studied how well contact lens wearers who need bifocals functioned with various types of lenses, in terms of hand-eye coordination and depth perception. The study found that patients who wore contacts with reading glasses could perform up-close tasks best, and that patients who wore monovision contacts did exceptionally well and better than those who wore soft bifocal contacts (another option; see below).

A major advantage to monovision is that you can view up-close objects from any angle. Say you go to the grocery store and you're wearing bifocal glasses. You want to read a product label that's at or above eye level. Well, you probably can't without first taking the product off the shelf and holding it at the appropriate angle. With monovision, though, you just look up and read the label, just as you did before you had bifocals.

The compromise with monovision is that your vision is generally not as sharp as it is with your glasses. You lose what's referred to as *binocular enhancement*, the enhanced visual image you see when both eyes work together. For the most part this is a concern only under specific circumstances, such as driving at night—in which case you can resolve the problem by using driving glasses. (You wear them over your monovision contacts to offset the near-vision contact lens and bring that eye back to a distance prescription. The other side is a nonprescription lens.)

Also, with monovision there can be a compromise to intermediate vision, if you're accustomed to wearing trifocals or progressive addition bifocals. Some people resolve this by replacing the near contact lens with a progressive addition bifocal contact lens that will provide good vision close up but will extend your working distance to allow for good intermediate vision.

The last option is bifocal contact lenses. These are designed either as simultaneous-vision or translating-vision lenses. A *simultaneous-vision lens* has both distance and near optics that focus light into the eye at the

same time: when you're looking at a distance, your brain learns to ignore visual information from the up-close part of the contact lens, and
vice versa. Simultaneous-vision designs are accomplished either by creating different distance and near zones within the lens or by varying the
power of the lens from the center to the edge. (This is akin to the way
progressive bifocal eyeglasses vary the power from top to bottom.)
Many of these lens designs provide 20/20 vision, but the *quality* of that
vision may be reduced from the loss of contrast, and the things you see
might not seem sharp or well defined. One advantage, as with monovision contacts, is that you can read up-close objects at any angle. The
compromise is that although you use both eyes together, the vision is
still not always as good as it is with your glasses.

A *translating bifocal contact lens* works like traditional bifocal glasses:
there's a tiny line that separates the distance prescription at the top from
the reading segment at the bottom. (A built-in stabilization system
makes sure that the lens always sits the right way in your eye so that the
distance part is always at the top.) When you glance down, the lens
should move, or "translate," up, placing the reading area in front of your
pupil so that you can see up close. Soft translating bifocal contact lenses
tend not to work well, because these lenses generally can't move enough
to bring the near optics where you want them, in front of your pupil.

The best of these designs are made in RGP materials; they can provide excellent vision that can match or even surpass your glasses. However, they also have the same limitations as standard bifocal glasses.
When you glance down at the floor, it's blurry; to see anything clearly
up close, you have to hold the object down at a certain angle, just as you
would with glasses. So if you work at a computer and your monitor sits
at eye level, for example, you won't be able to use the near optics of your
contact lens to see the computer monitor. If you can't adjust your work
area, then this lens design might prove more of a hassle than a help.

Why does my lens just stick to my finger whenever I try to put it in? Why won't it stay on my eye?

No matter what kind of contact lens you have, when you insert it, the
inside surface—the side that rests on your eye—is wet enough to "pull"
the lens onto your eye. This works because fluid is naturally drawn to
fluid; a wet lens naturally wants to stick to your wet eye. But if your finger is too wet, there's too much "fluid attraction," and the lens sticks to
your finger instead of your eye.

When you're putting in soft contacts, make sure that only the *bottom* of the lens (not the edge) is resting on your finger. Next, open your eyelids wide enough to provide a clear shot at your eye, so that the lens won't be waylaid by your lashes. Don't poke your eye, and don't press so hard that you just push the lens back onto your finger. Simply get the lens within striking distance—close enough that it can "work off" of your finger and onto your eye. If you can't get the hang of it, go back to your eye doctor or lens fitter for a refresher lesson. After all, the contact can't help you much if it stays on your finger!

How can I tell if my contact lens is inside out?

It's *almost* impossible to turn an RGP lens inside out. However, it can be done. You'll know something's not right, because your lens will look almost flat, and if you can put it on your eye, it probably won't stay on. If you manage to turn the lens right side out again, it will most likely be too warped to wear, and you'll need to get a new one.

If you have soft contacts and aren't sure if a lens is inside out, look at the lens, invert it, and look at it again. (Often it's difficult to tell by just looking at the lens one way; by comparing both views, you'll have a more accurate assessment.) If the lens is as it should be, right side out, the edges will point up and the lens will form a bowl. If it's inside out, the edges will point more out to the sides than up to the skies, and the lens will appear "flared," like a champagne glass.

A second way to tell is to place the lens in the crease of your palm and gently cup your hand so that it starts to fold the lens. If the edges roll into each other, like a taco shell or clam shell, the lens is right side out. If the edges start to fold *back*, away from the center, the lens is inside out.

If you place an inside-out soft contact lens on your eye, your vision might still be clear. However, you will feel uncomfortable, and you'll probably feel that the lens is going to fall out. If you have this sensation, try removing the lens, inverting it, rinsing with saline, and reinserting it. If the lens feels fine, you've solved the problem. If it feels worse, it's likely that you had inserted the lens right side out the first time, and that either you had some debris on the lens that altered the fit or there's a nick or tear in the lens. If you can't get it to fit so that it feels right, let your eye doctor or lens fitter take a look at it.

Can I wear my contacts if I have hay fever? Can I use allergy eye drops with my contacts?

It depends on your symptoms. If hay fever for you means irritated, dry, and itchy eyes, then you might not be able to wear contact lenses during allergy season; the lenses might make your eyes feel drier and increase your itching. Also, some allergy medications can make the problem worse by drying out your eyes even more, making contact lenses uncomfortable.

However, if you get relief from one of the many allergy eye drops available, you might still be able to wear your contact lenses during allergy season. *Note:* These drops should not be inserted while your contact lenses are in your eyes. Soft contacts, especially, will soak up the drops and keep the medication and preservatives concentrated on your eye much longer than is safe, and this may harm the cornea. If you use the drops ten to fifteen minutes before inserting your contacts, the drop should have provided its relief and dissipated, and your lenses should be safe to insert.

How can I tell if my lens is worn out?

It depends on how bad the lens is. The most common symptom is that your lenses will feel drier than usual, and you may not be able to wear them comfortably for as long as you used to. Often the dryness is so significant that there's no relief, even with rewetting drops.

Quantity of vision—how many letters you can read on a chart—is occasionally poorer with a worn-out lens, but usually it's the *quality* of vision that people notice first. Worn-out lenses provide less contrast; nothing looks crisp.

Many people find that they need to increase their use of cleaners when the lenses are wearing out. For instance, you might need to remove the lens in the middle of the day and clean it with your daily cleaner. Weekly enzyme cleaning won't seem to have the same benefit when a lens is worn out, and you might need to increase the frequency of this cleaning regimen as well.

For RGP lenses the symptoms may be similar, but often the lens can be polished and effectively refurbished. A soft contact lens that is worn out should be replaced.

If you're not sure whether your lens is worn out, see your doctor or lens fitter. Unfortunately, many people simply replace their lenses without having anyone take a look at their eyes—which is fine, unless there's another problem that needs to be addressed. Say, for example, you have a contact lens allergy (not hay fever, but a reaction to your contacts; see above). Your symptoms may be similar to those you'll have with a worn-out lens, and not treating the symptoms may be harmful.

Why do I have a red streak on my cheek after I insert my lenses?

Most likely you're sensitive to the preservative sorbic acid (also called potassium sorbate). This is the preservative that has traditionally been used in solutions labeled "for sensitive eyes," and while it *is* much less sensitizing than any of its predecessors, sorbic acid still causes reactions in as many as 5 percent of those who use it. But even if you are sensitive to this preservative, you still may not have any symptoms in your eyes, or you may experience only mild stinging. You can test yourself by placing several drops of a contact lens solution containing sorbic acid on the back of your hand and checking for any skin redness.

Why have my soft contact lenses discolored?

Soft contacts can discolor when they wear out. However, the culprit is usually a preservative in your contact lens solution. If you tend not to stick with one particular brand but buy "whatever's on special," and as a consequence mix various solutions containing different preservatives, these preservatives can interact. This can discolor your lenses, usually turning them yellow, red, brown, green, or gray. Also, if you use heat disinfection, check your saline solution: a saline that's not recommended for heat disinfection may contain preservatives that will discolor contact lenses when heated.

Can hairspray "gunk up" my contact lenses?

Yes. Over time the sticky protein in hairspray can indeed build up on contact lenses and shorten their life span. So try not to use hairspray after inserting your contacts (or even to insert them in the same room after using hairspray, because the stuff can linger in the air for several minutes). Similarly, it's a good idea to use water-based mascara (such as Almay, Lancôme, or Borghese), hypoallergenic or "sensitive-eye" makeup remover, oil-free moisturizers, and soaps that aren't lanolin-based (such as Neutrogena in the bar form).

Can my contact lens get lost behind my eye?

No. Your eye is very well sealed off by several safeguards, including your sclera (the "white" of your eye), conjunctiva (the clear layer over the sclera), and eyelids. There is one, smooth, continuous flow of tissue from the margin of your lower eyelid, across the eye, and to the margin of the upper eyelid (see chapter 1). If your contact lens goes where it's not supposed to in your eye—above your cornea, for instance—it will just stay there, under your eyelid, until you get it out.

What is orthokeratology?

This is a method of fitting a rigid contact lens to the eye that is flatter than the curvature of your cornea. The lens effectively flattens the eye while you wear it; then, when the lens is removed, the cornea remains flattened. (Because the lens is curved less than the cornea, it won't be too tight.) If someone is nearsighted, flattening the cornea reduces the degree of myopia, or nearsightedness. In theory this means that after you remove the lens, you'll be able to see without *any* correction. (However, the flattening may not be even on the cornea, in which case your vision can appear distorted when you remove the lens.) Once the desired effect has been achieved, contact lenses must be worn for at least a few hours every day, or worn overnight while sleeping, to maintain a flattened cornea. If you stop wearing the lenses, the cornea should simply return to its original shape without damage to the eye, and you won't be any worse off than you were before.

This method of vision correction, said to lie somewhere between contact lenses and refractive surgery (see chapter 6), varies in effectiveness, and often the results are only short-lived. The safety and efficacy of molding the cornea remain controversial.

6

Refractive Surgery
Don't Discard Those Spectacles Just Yet

Life without glasses—wouldn't it be wonderful? If only there were some way to correct vision permanently, to fix the problem that made us need glasses or contacts in the first place. An intriguing thought, one that has fascinated doctors and patients alike for years. Is it possible? Yes, it's called *refractive surgery.* Is it perfect? No. Is it for you? Maybe.

If you decide to undergo refractive surgery, it's imperative that you go into it—pardon the pun—with your eyes wide open. Refractive surgery will most likely reduce your prescription, yes. But there's absolutely no way to guarantee that it will provide you with even the same quality of vision that you had before surgery with your glasses or contact lenses. You may wind up needing something—glasses or contacts—afterward, to fine-tune your vision, and you'll still face presbyopia later in life. If you wear bifocals, you'll still need glasses or contacts to help you see up-close. If your potential surgeon leads you to believe otherwise, find another doctor.

A LITTLE BACKGROUND

The idea behind refractive surgery is, as its name suggests, to adjust the way your eyes refract, or bend, light, by changing the shape of the cornea (the front surface of your eye; for more on refraction and how the cornea works, see chapter 2). This was first attempted in 1885, by a Norwegian surgeon named Dr. H. Schiötz, in a procedure we now call *astigmatic keratotomy,* or *AK.* The patient's trouble was severe astigmatism (a focusing problem, in which the eye doesn't refract light evenly; see chapter 2), a result of previous cataract surgery. Dr. Schiötz decided to make an incision in the patient's cornea to flatten it and thus counterbalance the astigmatism. The operation was successful, and refractive surgery was born.

It wasn't until the 1940s, however, that refractive surgery expanded beyond astigmatism. The first procedures to reduce myopia, or nearsightedness, were done by a Tokyo eye surgeon named Tsutomu Sato. He found that if incisions were placed radially—like the numbers on a clock face—around the corneal surface, the cornea would flatten uniformly, and as a result nearsightedness would improve. Unfortunately Dr. Sato took a good idea and went too far with it, trying to do too much at once. He attempted to reshape the cornea from both the front and the back, and instead of seeing better, his patients actually wound up with worse vision than they'd had before.

Dr. Sato's theories were put aside until the early 1970s, when Dr. S. N. Fyodorov, of the Soviet Union, evolved a more prudent approach that improved myopia with significantly less harm to the cornea. A few years later Dr. Fyodorov's procedure, called *radial keratotomy,* or *RK,* found its way to the United States. At first there was a flurry of interest. But many patients who underwent this procedure found that not only was their vision *not* fully corrected, sometimes it wound up being so distorted that even glasses couldn't help! For some of these people, hard contact lenses saved the day, providing a smooth optical surface on the cornea and making adequate vision possible again. RK had other limitations as well, in that it couldn't fully correct severe cases of myopia (and thus help the patients who needed the procedure most). As a result of these drawbacks, RK's popularity faded in the 1980s. But the procedure was given new life in the early 1990s, as equipment and surgical techniques improved dramatically.

Although these cornea-shaping operations themselves were less than flawless, doctors knew that the basic ideas behind them were sound, and they kept exploring new techniques and refining procedures. One of these new techniques, developed in the 1980s, was called *epikeratophakia.* Epikeratophakia involved removing a section of cornea, freezing it, lathing it into a new shape, and then reinserting the newly curved section back into the cornea. Because of the complexity of this procedure, there were too many things that could (and did) go wrong, and it was considered too risky for elective surgery. (Actually, this technique proved most successful as a means of correcting vision in babies after the removal of congenital cataracts.)

By the late 1980s, lasers had come on the scene, designed for *photoablation:* selectively vaporizing the tissue at the center of the cornea, thereby sculpting the eye into a new shape. This technology gave rise to several other surgical procedures. The first, *photorefractive keratectomy,* or *excimer PRK,* is performed by a highly sophisticated computer-driven piece of machinery called an *excimer laser.* The computer, reading a topographical map of the cornea, selectively reshapes the cornea by telling the laser precisely which bits of tissue to remove. Like radial keratotomy, PRK can't fix all vision problems; currently it's limited to correcting myopia and some astigmatism. *Laser-assisted in-situ keratomileusis*, or *LASIK* (also known as *laser automated lamellar keratoplasty*, or *laser ALK*) also uses an excimer laser to vaporize tissue in the cornea. But this technique can correct more severe cases of myopia than PRK; it can also correct some astigmatism and moderate cases of farsightedness. *Holmium laser thermokeratoplasty*, or *holmium LTK*, uses a different laser, called the holmium:YAG. This exquisitely precise laser heats (instead of vaporizes) individual collagen fibers within the cornea, causing them to shrink permanently. As the collagen contracts, the central corneal curvature increases and adds more refractive power to the eye. This technique is used to treat patients who have hyperopia, or farsightedness. (People who are nearsighted already have too much refractive power.)

MAKING THE DECISION TO HAVE REFRACTIVE SURGERY

Realistic Expectations

So, today it's surgically possible to correct myopia, astigmatism, and, to a lesser degree, hyperopia. But don't be dazzled by hype or unrealistic expectations: *none of these techniques is guaranteed to provide perfect vision or to prevent you from ever needing glasses or contacts again.* You're still going to get older, and so are your eyes; nothing can change that. And because presbyopia—the trouble focusing close up that sneaks up on all of us eventually—is inevitable, *and because it's a problem with the lens and ciliary muscles, not the cornea,* refractive surgery on the cornea won't do anything to prevent it, and you may still wind up needing a reading prescription. If you're moderately nearsighted and wear glasses for distance vision only, you'll have a trade-off: instead of needing glasses to see across the street, you'll need them for reading. And if you spend your days in front of a computer, you'll end up wearing glasses *more* than you did before surgery.

Aiming for Undercorrection

If you decide to have refractive surgery, your doctor will evaluate you to determine which technique (if any) is appropriate. (Sometimes, to correct more than one problem, more than one technique is used.) Most refractive surgeons err on the conservative side, aiming for undercorrection of your refractive error. Why? Because if your eyes are targeted for the ideal correction and the surgery works too well, you'll end up with the opposite problem. In other words, if a surgeon "overshoots," or overcorrects your nearsightedness, you'll wind up being farsighted. Undercorrecting the problem leaves a margin for future action; you and your surgeon can decide together whether to try to enhance the surgery with a second procedure (which effectively doubles the risks involved in having had surgery to start with). But undercorrection also means that you'll *still* have to wear glasses or contacts (although sometimes contact lenses aren't possible if the cornea is considered too delicate after the surgery).

HOW THE PROCEDURES ARE PERFORMED

RK

In RK, the surgeon first anesthetizes the eye and then uses a diamond-bladed knife calibrated to reach a certain depth (about 90 percent of the thickness of the cornea) to make uniform incisions, or cuts (usually about four to eight in all), around the cornea. The more incisions, the flatter the cornea becomes; with milder cases of myopia, fewer incisions are needed. The length of the incisions also makes a difference: the longer the incision, the greater the correction. The patient's age is still another factor: the older the patient, the greater the potential for refractive change with a given size and number of incisions. If a patient has astigmatism, AK is performed as well (see above), with incisions made to compensate for the cornea having more curvature in one direction than another. And that's about it.

Recovery: Afterward, there's no patching or bandaging. You'll probably be given a combination of antibiotic and anti-inflammatory drops to help your eyes heal without infection or scarring—other than the scarring deliberately caused by the incisions—and to reduce pain from the nerves being exposed. It usually takes three months for your eyes to become fully comfortable and your vision to stabilize.

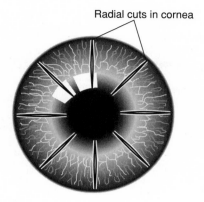

Radial cuts in cornea

Fig. 6.1.   Radial cuts in cornea for a radial keratotomy

Excimer PRK

Before the excimer laser can be used to reshape or "sculpt" the cornea, the front surface of the cornea, the epithelium, must be removed. This is done either manually, by scraping the cornea (while it is anesthetized), or with the laser itself—or in a combination of both. The laser is then used to change the cornea's curvature by vaporizing the tissue deep inside it.

Recovery: Because the corneal surface has been removed, you'll probably be fitted with a protective clear "bandage" contact lens until the epithelium has time to regenerate, a process that takes about four days. You'll be given antibiotic and anti-inflammatory drops to help your eyes heal. You'll probably need some form of oral painkiller as well; stripping the epithelial surface exposes certain sensitive nerves, and the resulting pain can be severe until the epithelium regenerates to cover these nerves again. Because PRK alters the cornea more than RK does, recovery time is longer—generally about six months.

LASIK, or Laser ALK

LASIK evolved from a procedure called *automated lamellar keratoplasty,* or *ALK,* in which tissue from the central cornea was removed to reduce myopia. In ALK, the surgeon creates a flap in the epithelium (the top layer of the cornea) and carefully lifts it to the side. Then the surgeon re-

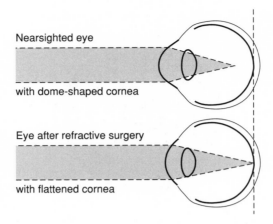

Nearsighted eye

with dome-shaped cornea

Eye after refractive surgery

with flattened cornea

Fig. 6.2.   Nearsighted eye before and after radial keratotomy

moves a section of stroma (the tissue just beneath the epithelium) to re-shape the cornea. The flap is then replaced and allowed to heal.

Although the idea behind ALK seems sound, in practice the operation's success rate has proved disappointing; because it is so complex, there is much room for error. In recent years surgeons have sought to improve the technique with high-precision lasers, which brings us to LASIK (laser-assisted in-situ keratomileusis), or laser ALK.

The laser procedure is basically the same as ALK, except that tissue is vaporized, or photoablated, instead of cut out. It's much less painful than RK or PRK, because corneal nerves are not left exposed, and the original corneal epithelium is preserved—so you don't need to grow a new layer of cells over your cornea. Thus, it takes less time for your eyes to heal.

Recovery: You'll still need to use antibiotic and anti-inflammatory eye drops, but for a shorter time than with RK or PRK. Recovery time is about three months.

Holmium LTK

The big difference with holmium LTK is that tissue is merely heated, not vaporized. First, you'll be given eye drops to constrict the pupil and drops to anesthetize your eyes. Now for the procedure, which is fairly simple: The surgeon marks the cornea with an instrument to pinpoint precisely where to aim the laser probe. The laser then heats *only* those selected portions of the cornea, to shrink the collagen fibers around the cornea's edges.

Recovery: You'll be given antibiotic drops for the next two to three days while your eyes are healing. With this procedure, unlike the others, there's little injury (or, as surgeons say, "insult") to the corneal epithelium, and so most patients experience no pain, or only minor discomfort.

HOW WELL DO THESE PROCEDURES WORK?

An easy question, but a complicated answer—mainly because most of these procedures are still too new and still evolving. The largest follow-up studies to monitor the results of refractive surgery have been done on patients who have received RK. One reason for this is simply the comparative volume of patients. Before 1995, RK was the refractive surgery of choice (actually, it was the *only* approved refractive surgery in the United States). The laser techniques have been "under investigation," and have been done on limited numbers of patients in research centers, but they were not widely available until 1995. PRK was approved by the Food and Drug Administration only in 1996. Therefore, the total number of patients undergoing laser procedures is still small when compared with the many patients in this country who have had RK.

What's Considered Effective?

A successful result for most studies is *uncorrected vision of 20/40 or better.* This is the minimal level of vision required by most states in granting a driver's license without a restriction for glasses or contact lenses. So basically, with 20/40 vision you could see well enough to drive a car. However, for most of us, seeing at a level less than 20/20 is not ideal; we don't feel that our vision is as clear as it should be. And many RK patients, even those with results considered to be "successful," still need glasses at least part-time. (Most of these people, however, feel that this is less of a compromise than wearing glasses full-time.)

The most widely publicized study on refractive surgery so far is the PERK (Prospective Evaluation of Radial Keratotomy) study, sponsored by the National Eye Institute at the National Institutes of Health; it was started in the late 1970s and has been updated as surgical techniques have changed. Because it's been around the longest, the PERK study's findings give a better sense of what happens to an RK patient's vision over time. The most recent findings show that results of RK surgeries are still very dependent on the amount of myopia that someone has before surgery. The more myopia, the less likely for uncorrected vision after surgery to be better than 20/40. For patients with mild myopia, 92 percent maintained 20/40 vision or better at five years after the surgery. For those with moderate myopia, the number drops to 86 percent, and for those with high myopia, 72 percent had 20/40 vision or better. And 64 percent of all RK patients with any degree of myopia wore neither glasses nor contacts five years after surgery. Some people with RK required eyeglass prescriptions because their corneas continued to flatten after the surgery and they became much more farsighted over time.

Early studies on the laser procedures show slightly better results. However, the patients these studies represent—those who enrolled in research programs—were carefully screened to meet certain criteria, so they may not be representative of the general population; therefore, the results may be slightly skewed.

Surgical Complications

Your doctor has probably told you this, but it's worth repeating: *with any type of eye surgery, there is a risk of loss of vision.* With RK, the main complication is perforation of the cornea by the knife used to make the incisions. While vision loss from a small perforation is rare, it can happen. Perforations of the cornea can lead to endophthalmitis (an infection of the entire inside of the eye), a breakdown of the cornea, corneal infections, and traumatic cataracts. The second major complication happens when the incisions aren't placed accurately; this can result in irregular, and sometimes uncorrectable, astigmatism.

One way to measure a procedure's safety and efficacy is to compare patients' best "corrected" level of vision (with glasses or contacts, if needed) after surgery with their best corrected level before surgery. After RK, 98 percent of patients have been reported to maintain the best level of corrected vision they had before surgery. This still leaves 2 percent of patients with potentially worse corrected vision after surgery (even though they are very likely to have better "uncorrected" vision—that is, to see better *without* glasses or contacts—than they did before surgery).

Other postoperative complications from RK include pain, glare, and vision fluctuations. There is also an increased risk of corneal damage from trauma due to a structurally weakened cornea. While all are fairly common, these complications usually resolve over the first few days to months as the eye heals. However, occasionally the glare from corneal scarring and vision fluctuations can persist for years. Vision can fluctuate because the cornea has been effectively weakened by the surgery (with less tissue to support it, it's not as sturdy as it used to be). For someone who has undergone RK, a closed eyelid during sleep tends to flatten the cornea slightly. Upon waking, there is less myopia. By the end of the day, as some of this flattening goes away, the myopia tends to get worse.

Laser procedures seem to have fewer complications than RK, but there are a few. The primary symptoms are pain, hazy vision, halos around lights, and glare. As with RK, these symptoms usually go away within a few days to months; however, haze, halos, and glare can persist beyond the usual six months after surgery. PRK and LASIK both alter tissue in the central cornea (as compared with RK, which leaves the center of the cornea alone). It has been reported that, for between 1 percent and nearly 9 percent of PRK patients, scarring may persist in the central cornea indefinitely. With LASIK surgeries, corneas have been shown to stabilize in as little as one month with less risk of scarring than with PRK.

REFRACTIVE SURGERY, WHEN IT'S MOST SUCCESSFUL, will give you the best vision soon after the surgery is performed, but whether or not you have the surgery, the vision you have today is not the vision you'll have ten years from now. Surgery to your cornea won't affect what happens to the *rest* of your eye (the lens in particular), which will keep right on changing over your lifetime—and therefore, so will your vision.

PART III

The
Big Problems
for Aging Eyes

7

Cataracts

It's probably cataracts. My friend's aunt had cataracts, and so did her husband. I'm the right age for it, and I'm having problems with my eyes—cataracts, that's it. I bet I need surgery.

Well, you may. Then again, you may not—depending on whether you do indeed have cataracts. Although cataracts are probably the most talked-about eye problem today and a major reason for visits to an eye doctor as we get older, they're also—right up there with astigmatism—among the most misunderstood disorders of the eye.

Difficulty reading for prolonged periods of time, excessive tearing, occasional feelings of having something in your eye, double vision in both eyes, pain in or around the eye—these are *not* typical symptoms of cataract development. (Of course, if you're having *any* troublesome eye symptoms —whether you think the diagnosis is cataracts or not—you should seek medical attention.)

Instead, cataracts more commonly cause problems with distance vision, blurred vision, frequent changes in eyeglass prescriptions, and poor night vision; they can also cause glare, make it appear that there's a halo around lights, and make it necessary for the person to use ever-brighter lights to see to read. Our goal with this chapter is to help you understand about cataracts, their development, symptoms, and treatment, and to help give you realistic expectations about what their surgical removal *can* and *cannot* achieve.

The first thing you need to know is that if you have developed cataracts, you couldn't have picked a better time to do it. Not long ago cataracts were removed through large incisions in the eye. These surgical wounds were closed with thick sutures that caused a lot of pain and swelling. Also, *intraocular implant lenses* were in their infancy just twenty to thirty years ago; before this, cataract patients had to wear thick cataract

What Are the Symptoms of Cataracts?

Symptoms associated with cataracts include:

- Impaired distance vision
- Blurred vision
- Frequent changes in eyeglass prescriptions
- Poor night vision
- Glare
- Appearance of a halo around lights
- Need for ever-brighter lights for reading
- Double vision in one eye

glasses or extended-wear contact lenses. Today, thanks to great surgical advances, things are dramatically different. Most people with cataracts who need surgery undergo the modern *phacoemulsification* procedure, which enables surgeons to remove the cataract through a tiny incision in the eye. Complications are fewer, and recovery time is quicker. Now more than 99 percent of patients who undergo cataract surgery receive a permanent implant lens for better focusing power and sight.

WHAT IS A CATARACT?

A *cataract* is an opacity or haziness that develops in the eye's lens. For most people a cataract simply develops as part of the normal aging process. *All* people over age sixty-five have at least some degree of cataract development; although this aging process usually affects both eyes at the same time, it can progress at different rates. Just because you've never been told that you have a cataract doesn't mean that you *don't* have some degree of cataract development in your eyes. Cataracts are somewhat like gray hair and wrinkled skin in this regard: everyone eventually gets some of these changes, but we really don't take notice or make mention of them until someone has a lot of gray hair or wrinkled skin (and ideally even then we'd hold back, just to be polite!). Similarly, most eye doctors feel that cataracts are hardly worth mentioning at the beginning. However, rest assured that we become acutely interested in them as they progress and begin to affect vision.

Many people ask if a cataract is actually a film, like the skim on fresh milk, or maybe a sheet of algae on a pond, growing on the eye's surface.

Actually, no. A cataract occurs in the *lens*, which is deeper within the eye. (The cornea is the clear outer surface of the eye, the "window" through which light must pass. Although there are conditions that cause whitening or clouding of the cornea, these aren't cataracts.) The lens is located inside the eyeball, within a membranous "bag." (Because it sits behind the iris, it's not easily seen without special instruments, and without first dilating the pupil.) So even if your eye *looks* clear in the mirror, this doesn't necessarily mean that you don't have a cataract.

Types of Cataracts and Their Symptoms

The typical cataract that occurs with age is called a *nuclear sclerotic cataract*. The name refers to the center, or nucleus, of the lens. As the normal lens ages, the nucleus enlarges, and its protein structure starts to change. The lens gradually loses its clear appearance and becomes a yellowish or greenish color. Over time, as the nuclear cataract progresses, the lens can actually turn brown. (This is what eye doctors mean when we use words like *clouding* or *haziness* to describe cataracts.) People with nuclear sclerotic cataracts typically have trouble seeing at a distance. Many stop driving at night because of poor vision and because car headlights appear blurred. They also find that the quality and brightness of light becomes very important for seeing. They have trouble in dim light and must increase the wattage of light bulbs at home to help them read and get around

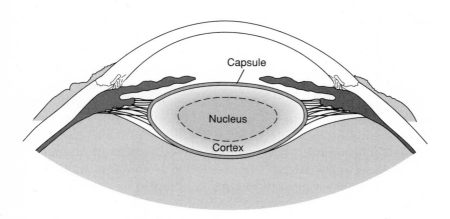

Fig. 7.1. The parts of the lens

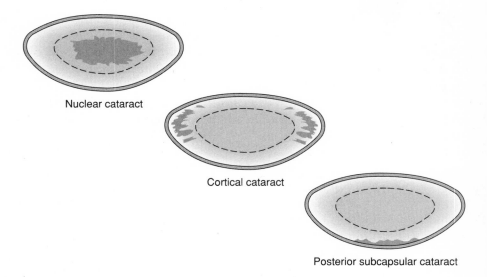

Fig. 7.2.   Types of cataracts

the house better at night. They often read best in bright sunlight, unless glare becomes a problem; then, hazy days may bring more comfort and better vision.

Other developments also seen with cataracts may include cortical changes and posterior subcapsular lens changes. *Cortical changes* occur in the outer layer, or lens cortex; they're the result of chemical imbalances that cause water to be drawn into the outer cortex. This excess water has an adverse effect on lens fibers—think of waterlogged carpet strands—causing a decrease in the clarity of the lens. (Interestingly, one of the dictionary's definitions of *cataract* is "a waterfall or great downpour.") Whitish, irregular lens areas and streaks caused by this flooding create problems with diffraction (how light is bent and focused; see chapter 4). People with cortical lens changes that fall within their visual axis often complain of *monocular double vision* (double vision or a "ghost" image seen when looking through only one eye). When double vision occurs with both eyes open, but not in either eye alone, it's very rarely due to cataracts. (Double vision with both eyes open needs to be carefully evaluated by an eye doctor for eye muscle imbalances or other problems.)

These nuclear and cortical lens changes usually happen slowly, and at a different pace in each eye. *Posterior subcapsular lens changes*, on the other hand, can progress rapidly and tend to be much more advanced in one eye than the other. These are often known as *fast cataracts*. People with posterior subcapsular cataracts form an opaque, plaquelike cell growth on the back surface of the lens. This is different from the diffuse haziness of nuclear sclerotic cataracts or the focusing problems and distortion of cortical lens changes. This growth often occurs dead center in the lens, right in the path of central light rays that pass to the macula for reading vision. It can cause people to have more problems seeing close up than at a distance, and to experience a lot of discomfort from glare. People with diabetes, people taking oral steroids, and people who have suffered eye trauma or undergone previous eye surgery are more prone to develop these cataracts. But posterior subcapsular cataracts can also occur in young, healthy people who don't have any of these risk factors. Because of their rapid onset and marked impairment of reading vision, these cataracts are often tremendously debilitating.

There are many other, rarer types of lens changes including cholesterol cataracts, "sunflower" cataracts, phenothiazine cataracts, and congenital lens changes. But nuclear sclerotic lens changes—alone or in combination with other lens changes—are overwhelmingly the most common.

Symptoms Not Typical of Cataracts

A hazard of automatically blaming cataracts for many eye problems is that making this assumption—without the medical diagnosis to back it up

What Symptoms Are Not Typical of Cataracts?

Symptoms unlikely to be associated with cataracts include:

- Eye discomfort
- Pain
- Redness
- Discharge
- Excess mucus
- Tearing
- Itching
- Irritation
- Aching in the eyeball

—often delays the diagnosis of other eye diseases until it's too late for treatment. As mentioned above, cataracts usually cause problems with vision; on the other hand, they do *not* typically cause eye discomfort or pain, or any change in the appearance of the eye or the production of tears.

Cataracts are also not a major cause of eye fatigue or tired eyes; as we get older, these symptoms are usually due to dry eyes or the need for new glasses or contacts. Also, a rapid deterioration in vision is usually not due to a cataract. (However, as always, there are a few exceptions to this rule, and a careful examination by an eye doctor is necessary to determine the true cause of deteriorating eyesight.) Likewise, cataracts usually aren't to blame for a sudden loss of reading vision or lost side vision (two symptoms, by the way, that call for immediate professional attention!).

WHO'S AT RISK?

Among the risk factors associated with developing cataracts, age is by far the biggest. It's important to note here that most cataract lens changes are simply part of the *normal* aging process; theoretically, all of us will eventually experience some degree of cataract if we live long enough. And again, although everybody has at least some cataract lens changes by age sixty-five, these usually aren't commented upon by eye care specialists unless they appear to be affecting a patient's vision or unless they can help explain symptoms such as glare, foggy vision, or difficulty with night driving. Many people, however, live their whole lives without ever having cataract problems that need treatment.

Cataracts have been found to be more common in women than men, in blacks than whites, and in people living in developing countries near the tropical belt than people living in the United States and Europe. Having diabetes, a strong family history of visually significant cataracts, or taking certain medications (in particular, corticosteroids) have also been shown to increase someone's likelihood of developing cataracts. Smoking has also been shown to increase a person's risk of developing nuclear, but not cortical, cataracts. The role of nutrition in cataract formation is not clear.

Do sunglasses help? Advertisements for sunglasses have popularized the notion that sunlight and its associated ultraviolet rays can increase someone's risk of developing cataracts. Several epidemiological studies appear to support this claim; in particular, a study from the Johns Hopkins Hospital in the 1980s found that watermen on the Chesapeake Bay, who, by reason of their occupation, had increased exposure to the ultraviolet-B

(UV-B) radiation in sunlight, were found to have over a threefold risk of developing cortical cataracts compared with those with much lower exposure. The exact role of sunlight and UV rays in lens changes and cataract development needs further study. However, because there's good evidence that the two are indeed linked, we recommend sunglasses for all our patients—especially those at risk for cataract development (including people with diabetes as well as people on certain medications that make them more sensitive to the effects of light exposure).

Although most sunglasses provide adequate protection from UV radiation, you should look for labeling claiming "100 percent UV-A and UV-B filtering." The color of the sunglasses has little effect on their ability to protect your eyes. The tint should simply tone down the sun's brightness to a level that's comfortable for you. (The embedded chromophores in the lens that provide UV protection have little effect on the color or darkness of the sunglass.) Very dark gray lenses can decrease contrast, but gray is an acceptable color at lighter shades, as well. Amber and brown lenses are popular because people find that they alter natural colors minimally. Green lenses, on the other hand, cause the most color distortion. Yellow lenses have been touted on midnight television commercials as great improvers of vision, especially outdoors. There is little scientific support for these claims, but hunters and other people who spend a lot of time outdoors have found them particularly comfortable. Polarized lenses have little effect on ultraviolet light, but they do cut glare substantially. Glare is a frequent complaint before and after cataract surgery, and polarized lenses may provide considerable comfort, especially for people who are exposed to a lot of reflected light (fishermen, boaters, and those who spend a lot of time driving on highways). Mirrored lenses, on the other hand, are purely cosmetic (especially if your goal is to look like a state trooper), have no true protective or comfort value, and may reflect unwanted UV rays onto the surrounding skin, causing sunburn.

VISUAL IMPAIRMENT, AND PARADOXICAL IMPROVEMENT, FROM CATARACTS

Like the lens in a camera that focuses light rays onto the film inside, the lens in the eye focuses light rays onto the retina. As cataracts develop over time, the lens becomes cloudy or hazy, allowing less light to reach the retina. The rays that do penetrate the lens can become distorted and scattered, accounting for such symptoms as blurred vision and halos around lights at night. Eventually this dimming of the lens reaches the point where stronger eyeglasses can no longer improve vision. This is because cataracts are not a *refractive* problem (one that can be corrected simply by changing your prescription). Rather, cataracts are a problem *inside* the eye. The lens becomes cloudy, like a dirty window. No matter what kind of glasses you put up *outside* the eye, they can't focus light rays adequately through this hazy or dirty cataract window inside the eye. For your vision to get any better, the window will eventually need to be cleaned—or, as in the case of cataracts, removed.

One of the earliest signs of cataract development is called *second sight*. It's an amazing phenomenon. Some people actually stop needing their glasses as they get older (see chapter 2). Even though they may once have needed glasses for distance, now they can see just fine without them. Others who were always dependent on reading glasses may slowly discover that they read just as well without any glasses. So how, you may be wondering, if a cataract is a clouding of the lens in the eye, can this cause better vision? The answer is that in its earliest stages, the clouding is minimal and has little effect on decreasing light and distorting vision. But at this early stage, as the cataract begins to form, the change in the consistency of the lens can have an effect on someone's eyeglass prescription. These changes can alter the focus of light rays by the lens, so that people who were farsighted may gradually become nearsighted, and vice versa (though more often the former). This tendency toward nearsightedness as a cataract develops is called a *myopic shift*. Myopic shifts can have many other causes, such as certain medications (sulfa antibiotics, miotic eye drops), systemic disorders (diabetes), and other ocular conditions (ciliary muscle spasm). Nevertheless, people with large changes in their eyeglass prescription over one or two years, especially if there's a big difference between the two eyes, should be checked for cataract development. This change is occasionally the first clue that a cataract is developing despite only minimal changes in the lens visible during an examination.

CAN CATARACTS BE PREVENTED?

Vitamins

As we discussed above, age is the big cause of most cataracts—and as we all know only too well, there's not much we can do to stop or turn back the clock. However, it has been suggested by several investigators that nutrition plays a role in cataract development, and changes in nutrition and vitamin supplementation have been tried to slow cataract development. Specifically, antioxidants such as riboflavin, vitamins C and E, and carotenoids, as well as niacin, thiamine, and iron, may alter cataract development.

The effect of nutrition, specifically antioxidants, on cataract development is currently being investigated by the National Institutes of Health (NIH) in a large clinical trial. This study, known as the Age-Related Eye Disease Study (AREDS), has enrolled some forty-five hundred people nationwide with various stages of cataracts and macular degeneration. These people have been randomly assigned to groups. Some groups take vitamin supplements containing copper, zinc, and an assortment of antioxidants, and other groups take placebos. Study participants will be carefully followed for ten years to determine the effects of dietary supplementation on these age-related eye conditions. Because nobody knows if these vitamins will have any effect at all—the only suggestions that they might help have come from a limited number of studies—at present we urge you to use caution here. Don't rush right out and raid the health-food store. Vitamins aren't candy, and you may risk your health if you take high-powered nutritional supplements without medical supervision. If you want to take something, a multivitamin with zinc, copper, and antioxidants can't hurt.

Sunglasses

It has also been suggested, as discussed above, that wearing sunglasses with UV filters may slow cataract development. Ultraviolet rays penetrate the cornea and are absorbed by the human lens; laboratory animal and epidemiological studies suggest that exposure to sunlight and ultraviolet light may have an effect on cataract development. But whether (and how much) *ordinary* exposure to sunlight accelerates cataract development is uncertain. If you decide to use sunglasses—and this is probably a good idea—to cut down on light exposure when you're outside, you should purchase the darkest-tinted lenses you can tolerate, and look for UV coating that specifies that it blocks wavelengths below 400 nanometers.

Medications

Various medications, including aspirin, have been studied for their effect on cataract development. Aspirin appears to have a minimal effect, if any, on inhibiting cataract lens changes. However, there are several medications that have been specifically designed and marketed as "anticataract drugs." These are much more popular outside the United States and include catalin, phacolysin (Lutrax, Quinax), bendazac, and phaka. However, spend the money at your own risk. The usefulness of these drugs in retarding or reversing cataract development is not widely accepted, especially in light of today's excellent surgical results. That is, cataract surgery usually has such a good outcome that using unproven drug remedies seems not the best approach.

WHAT ARE MY TREATMENT OPTIONS?

At first, the best treatment is education: having a good understanding of this problem and its effect on vision, and getting the most accurate eyeglass prescription possible, can help you cope with the often annoying consequences of cataract development. Improving the lighting at home with more and brighter lights (halogen lights, or 100-watt to 150-watt incandescent bulbs), positioning reading lamps over your shoulder for maximum illumination of the printed page, wearing sunglasses on bright sunny days to reduce glare, and limiting your night driving—all of these can be very helpful steps for people with early cataracts.

But also know that cataracts, like all age-related changes, will progress. There will come a point when stronger eyeglasses will no longer do the job, when the lens changes will impair your vision to a degree you find unacceptable, when you're no longer comfortable performing daily activities such as driving, reading, or even walking around in varied lighting conditions. At this point, cataract surgery becomes a treatment option that you need to consider.

MAKING THE DECISION TO HAVE
CATARACT SURGERY

As we've said before, the lens (and the cataract in it) sits in a "bag" inside the front part of your eye. When the lens becomes so hazy or opaque that a cataract operation is necessary, we must remove the lens from this bag. This is true for all kinds of cataracts, including the three most common types: nuclear, cortical, and posterior subcapsular (see figure 7.2).

Cataract surgery usually involves opening the front of the bag, removing the lens, and leaving the back of the bag in place. An intraocular ("within the eye") implant lens is then inserted in place of the old lens, inside the old lens bag.

Who Needs Surgery?

Do you need surgery? A big part of the answer is that it's up to you; it depends on what you can tolerate and the degree of vision you consider necessary for a normal life. Surgical removal of cataract lenses is considered when people find that the visual impairment has progressed to the point where their normal activities are curtailed and stronger glasses aren't an option. An older person who doesn't move around very much has fewer visual needs and can better tolerate a more advanced cataract than can a more active person, who may not be able to tolerate even an early cataract.

So, how active are you? This is an important question. And in answering it, by the way, don't sell yourself short—or let your doctor or well-meaning relatives talk you out of surgery—with a rationale such as "Well, I'm in my seventies, I guess I should slow down anyway." Poppycock! It's your life, and the decision to undergo cataract surgery is an *individual* one; there are no strict rules to be applied here. There's also no age cutoff. Is the visual impairment interfering with your job, special interest, or hobby? Is it affecting your level of independence, as driving becomes a problem or you become afraid to leave the house because of trouble seeing?

Cataract surgery may also be performed for other reasons besides improving your vision. A dense cataract will obscure an eye doctor's view of the retina. This will make it difficult to follow conditions in the back of the eye such as glaucoma, diabetic retinopathy, and macular degeneration. Laser treatment of the retina is also difficult when there is a dense cataract. Very mature cataracts can lead to glaucoma or inflammation in the eye and should probably be removed.

Consideration must also be given to what you expect to achieve with the surgery. In most instances, cataract surgery is done to improve vision; in other words, you expect that after the surgery, your vision will be better than it was before, whether you need to wear glasses or not. *You should not undergo cataract surgery with the idea that you won't need to wear glasses anymore.* (Or because you hope cataract surgery will improve your golf game. It's the old story: "Doctor, will I be able to play the piano after the operation?" "Yes," replies the doctor. "Great! I never knew how to play it before.")

When Should Surgery Be Performed?

When surgery should be performed is another difficult question. Visual acuity, as measured with eye charts, varies from office to office and from one tester to another. The most common acuity measurements used today in the United States are the familiar "Snellen acuity" measurements of 20/20, 20/40, and so on. In general, someone whose visual acuity cannot be brought to better than 20/50 with eyeglasses should consider surgery. This visual impairment must also be judged to be consistent with the degree of cataract observed clinically and the health of the eye. Also, a careful eye examination must be performed to make sure that this visual impairment isn't due to other problems, such as corneal or retinal disease. Fortunately, modern microsurgical techniques make it no longer necessary to wait until cataracts are "ripe" before they can be removed.

When discussing such concepts as visual acuity and the level of impairment due to cataracts, it may be helpful to think of your vision in terms of a scale from 1 to 10. On this scale, 1 is the best vision you can have (about 20/20) and 10 is the worst. Right in the middle, at level 5, is 20/50 vision; at this point, cataracts are usually significantly affecting a person's activities. *Cataract surgery in most people can be expected to improve vision, with or without glasses after the operation, to a level below 5, and preferably to a 1, or approximately 20/20.*

Although 20/50 is generally the accepted level at which many eye surgeons feel comfortable recommending cataract surgery in an otherwise healthy eye, sometimes cataract surgery may be warranted in patients at lower levels on this scale. Cataracts causing severe impairment in someone's occupation or lifestyle due to reduced acuity, monocular double vision, distortion, or glare can prompt a surgeon and patient to decide to proceed with surgery in an eye at levels of 4 (20/40), 3 (20/30), or better.

Note: Before undergoing any surgery it's a good idea to *get a second opinion.* (In fact, some insurance plans require patients to get two opinions before undergoing any surgery for which the insurer will be asked to pay.) This is especially important if there's a possibility of insincere motives on the doctor's part or unrealistic expectations on yours.

Will the Surgery Actually Help?

This should go without saying, but cataract surgery shouldn't be performed unless your eye doctor believes there's a good chance that your vision will be improved by it. If the retina or the optic nerve isn't healthy, then rarely will the removal of a cataract improve someone's visual acuity. (Imagine trying to focus light rays in a camera onto bad or exposed film. The lens can be as clear as possible, with the best focusing ability, but none of that will matter if the film is simply bad.)

Before performing cataract surgery, it's essential for the doctor to assess the health of the rest of your eye behind the cataract. This requires carefully going over your medical history, asking many questions about past vision problems, eye trauma, and eye disease. Your doctor may use instruments such as a potential acuity meter (PAM) to test the health of your eye behind the cataract. In this test, a visual acuity chart—similar to the classic ones you see in an eye doctor's office—is projected *through the cataract* and focused onto the retina in the back of the eye, using two pencil-thin beams of light. If someone can see the chart *better* this way, then the retina is usually judged as healthy. If, on the other hand, the person can't see the PAM test chart on the retina, this implies that the retina or the optic nerve may not be healthy, and it's doubtful whether removing the cataract would improve vision. (*Note:* Sometimes the PAM test can provide misleading results. Therefore, it should be done by doctors who have a great deal of experience using these instruments and interpreting their results.)

What about the Risks?

We've talked about the benefits of cataract surgery (improved vision); we also need to consider the risks. Many people hear from their friends how easy it was to have cataract surgery, and because the surgery is relatively safe these days, fewer people have heard about those who had complications. *But cataract surgery is an operation.* As with any operation, there are risks, and there is a recovery period.

One risk of cataract surgery is an eye infection. Many surgeons give their patients antibiotics around the time of surgery, in theory to help lower this risk—although studies have yet to prove this rationale. (Some patients may be given antibiotics *before* surgery.) Another big concern is retinal detachment, during and after cataract surgery. The retina is like wallpaper lining the back of the eye. If there's any weakness in the retina at the time of surgery, it can become detached, like peeling wallpaper, from the back of the eye. This is why people are examined frequently after the operation. If a retinal detachment occurs, it is repaired right away. (We have also seen patients sneeze their implants out of place, rub open their cataract wounds, and even fall on their eyes soon after cataract surgery.)

Many other complications are also possible, either during or after cataract surgery. Any surgeon who performs cataract surgery sees these complications; fortunately, they're infrequent—on the order of 5 to 10 percent—but they do happen. This is where the experience and competence of your surgeon can make all the difference in the world. *Usually, if complications are recognized and treated early, the eye can still heal well after surgery and achieve improved vision—even if this requires a second surgery soon afterward.* If an infection gets out of control or a retina becomes very badly detached, however, there's a chance that the vision in the eye could end up worse than it was before the operation. In rare cases, people have lost an eye from cataract surgery. In extremely rare cases, people have had unforeseen reactions to anesthesia and have even died from it. *Fortunately, complications of all kinds are unusual, and most cataract surgery goes very well.* But it's worth repeating that cataract surgery, no matter what you've heard from friends, is not without some discomfort, and a good outcome is certainly not guaranteed.

How's Your Health in General?

Your overall health is another important consideration. Although today, with modern microsurgical techniques, cataract surgery is relatively safe, with few complications, there are still risks. People taking Coumadin, aspirin, and other blood-thinning medications are at risk for excessive bleeding during the operation. Because it's necessary to lie flat during the operation for a period of time ranging from as little as fifteen minutes to greater than an hour, someone with severe scoliosis, debilitating arthritis (especially in the cervical spine), or chronic obstructive pulmonary disease may have difficulty.

Also, a certain level of patient cooperation is necessary for cataract surgery. Today it has become standard to perform cataract surgery under local and not general anesthesia (in which the patient is "asleep"). Local anesthesia is safer and avoids the potential complications associated with general anesthesia; patients also recuperate faster after the operation and can go home the same day, with little drowsiness and few residual effects. At the start of most cataract operations, people are given an intravenous injection of a Valium-like drug to induce a "twilight sleep." While they're in this relaxed state, most patients also receive injections of local anesthesia around the eye, to keep them from closing their eye or blinking during the procedure. These injections also block sight in the operated eye. Patients are awake during the operation but are so relaxed that they hardly notice what is going on around them; in fact, many people doze during cataract surgery. *But patients must make an effort to lie still; sudden movements can have devastating visual consequences.* This is especially true for patients of doctors who choose to perform cataract surgery with only topical and intraocular anesthesia, without a retrobulbar block (see below). Combative patients, people with dementia, or others who are likely to have trouble keeping still for sustained periods may not be good candidates for cataract surgery.

Other Concerns You May Have

It's perfectly normal to be concerned before any surgery. You'll probably have a lot of questions, such as, How much better will my vision be after the operation? What if something goes wrong? Could I be blinded? How long will it take after the operation for me to drive, get back to work, read, and resume my other normal activities? Will the other eye need cataract surgery in the near future?

The stakes are much higher for people who have only one working eye, since for them an unsuccessful operation can have a much graver outcome; the risks of surgery for these individuals become magnified and potentially devastating.

There's no master list of answers to these questions, because everybody's situation differs slightly; in fact, there are as many sets of pre- and postoperative cataract surgery instructions as there are eye surgeons. But one standard applies in every case: You should feel free to raise your concerns and questions with your cataract surgeon and his or her staff before surgery, not only to ease your worries but to establish realistic expectations regarding this procedure. If your surgeon flunked the bedside-manner course in medical school, and either doesn't fully answer your questions or concerns or doesn't seem inclined to take the time to listen to you, you may want to seek a second opinion or consider going to a different surgeon altogether. You should also be comfortable with your surgeon's arrangements for your postoperative care. Today not all cataract surgeons follow their patients after surgery, instead sending patients back to their ophthalmologist or optometrist for postoperative management.

CATARACT SURGERY

Cataract surgery has progressed remarkably over the last thirty years. Not too long ago people routinely spent a week or two in the hospital recuperating from a cataract operation. At that time the hazy cataract lens was removed using mainly manual techniques. Sandbags—how primitive it seems now!—were placed around the patient's head in an attempt to prevent movement while the wound healed. The results of these procedures varied, and there were much higher rates of infection and inflammation following surgery than we see today. Furthermore, after cataract surgery many people had to wear thick cataract glasses that overmagnified and distorted their vision.

Welcome to the microsurgery revolution. Special microscopes, designed to give ophthalmologists a better view of the cataract and other eye structures during surgery, have enabled us to refine our surgical incisions and other delicate procedures performed inside the eye. As microsurgery has evolved, surgeons have developed many new instruments for use within the eye. And new sutures, finer than human hair, and smaller cataract incisions have allowed for better wound closure following cataract surgery. This advance too has speeded the patient's recovery, and it's also helped us maximize the chances for achieving good vision after the procedure.

Intraocular Lens Implants

The lens provides focusing power for the eye. When it's removed, as it is during cataract surgery, the eye loses its ability to focus properly. So, the dilemma: how to fix one problem (getting rid of the hazy lens) without creating an even bigger one (removing someone's ability to focus incoming light rays, and therefore see in that eye, altogether).

Years ago the most widely accepted options for correcting this lack of focusing power in the eye after cataract surgery were the thick cataract glasses or contact lenses mentioned above—inadequate solutions, both of them. Many people found it difficult, if not impossible, to adjust to the distortion and magnification created by the thick glasses. And contacts weren't an ideal option because they were difficult to handle, especially for people with arthritis or a mild tremor; they also increased the risk of developing an eye infection.

Eye surgeons continued to search for a more acceptable option for returning focusing power to the eye, eventually developing an artificial lens, or intraocular lens implant. This implant, which can be placed in the eye during cataract surgery, restores some of the eye's ability to focus after the old lens has been removed. In addition to the lens implant, you may also need a pair of normal reading glasses to provide more focusing power for close work, or a bifocal prescription that will also fine-tune your distance vision. Although they don't create perfect vision, intraocular implants have eliminated the magnification problems created by those thick cataract glasses and have helped many people avoid the difficulties associated with the use of contact lenses. After cataract surgery, you can still wear contacts if you want to.

A Bit of Background

A complete history of intraocular implant lenses is beyond the scope of this text (and is in fact the subject of several books). But the story of their development is an interesting one. Dr. Harold Ridley, an English ophthalmologist working during World War II, is credited by most people as the person responsible for originating the idea of implant lenses in cataract surgery. During the war he treated many Royal Air Force pilots who had been injured when their planes' cockpits shattered. In a number of these pilots, cockpit fragments had penetrated the cornea and lodged in the anterior chamber of the eye. But surprisingly, Dr. Ridley noticed, these fragments were actually well tolerated by the eye! This gave him the idea that a prosthetic lens could be developed of similar material and placed in the eye after removal of a cataract.

As you might expect, early attempts to create implant lenses met with many problems and complications, since manufacturing techniques and materials were limited. Glass implants were too heavy and would not remain properly fixed in the eye. But over the years technology finally caught up with the idea, and newer implant designs were of plastic—which, as with contact lenses, eventually became the material of choice. Surgeons tried various methods of getting these implants to stay put inside the eye; all met with varied success. After many years of study we have found that it's best to place intraocular implant lenses *behind the iris* inside the old cataract bag, where they're better ensconced and in a better position for the restoration of eyesight.

Just like transistor radios, implants have gotten smaller over the years as our technology and surgeons themselves have become more sophisticated. Now, thanks to better surgical instruments, it's possible to remove a cataract through narrower incisions—and the finer the incision, the more rapidly someone will heal after cataract surgery. Also, these smaller wounds are less likely to induce unwanted astigmatism in the eye, a common problem after cataract surgery. We continue to strive for ever-tinier incisions and implant lenses. Currently the trend is to make a 3-millimeter incision and use foldable implant lenses. But who knows what the future holds—perhaps a needle-sized incision and an injectable implant?

Advances in Anesthesia

The major surgical advances, the new, highly sophisticated equipment, plus an expanded spectrum of medications to decrease infection and inflammation after the operation have helped make cataract surgery a much safer and more effective procedure. Because of improved techniques, cataract surgery today is usually done under local anesthesia (instead of general anesthesia, which carries more risks). As noted earlier, you'll probably receive a relaxing medication, given by intravenous injection, before the procedure to make you sleepy. Then you may be given injections of a local anesthetic around the eye to decrease sensation and movement (similar to the injections the dentist uses when working on your teeth). Patients are usually in a "twilight sleep" during surgery, aware but not caring; these injections also block your vision in that eye during cataract surgery. Some doctors today even choose to perform cataract surgery using only topical anesthetic eye drops. This may be supplemented with an intraocular anesthetic, but either way requires a very cooperative patient to keep the eye from moving during surgery.

Improved techniques of closing the incision and new ways of controlling inflammation have done away with those prolonged stays in the hospital patients used to endure (remember the sandbags!). In fact, most cataract surgery today is done on an outpatient basis: patients have their surgery and then go home the same day.

BEFORE SURGERY

The A-Scan Measurement

The A-scan measurement, an ultrasound measurement of the length of the eyeball, is an important calculation that must be performed before surgery to help determine—along with other measurements such as your eyeglass prescription in each eye, corneal curvature readings, and the intraocular lens constant—the appropriate power of the lens implant you'll be getting. Unfortunately this calculation is not always as accurate as we would like, especially in very nearsighted or farsighted people. Because the intraocular implant lens is a *gross* estimation of the power the eye needs to focus correctly, glasses are often necessary after a cataract operation to fine-tune vision.

Presurgical Testing

Even though cataract surgery is performed under local anesthesia, it's usually advisable to undergo presurgical tests to check for any medical conditions that might cause problems during surgery. Presurgical testing usually includes a history and physical, an EKG, a chest X-ray, blood work, and a urinanalysis. If you have multiple medical problems, it's probably a good idea to have these tests performed by your internist, family practitioner, or other specialist familiar with your medical history. (Otherwise, the testing can be done at the hospital or surgical center prior to the operation.)

Scheduling

Surgery dates are scheduled in coordination with the A-scan measurement and presurgical testing. Typically surgeons begin working very early in the morning and continue doing operations until midafternoon; your surgery will probably be scheduled sometime between 7:30 A.M. and 3:00 P.M.

Preoperative Instructions

Preoperative instructions vary from surgeon to surgeon. Patients are generally asked not to eat or drink anything the night before surgery, from midnight onward. (This is a routine precaution before any type of anesthesia is given; it can vary greatly depending on the surgeon, the surgical center, and the specific anesthesia that will be used.) You'll probably be told to continue taking any medicines you normally take on a daily basis (but on the day of surgery to swallow them with only small sips of water). *Note:* Bring a list of your medications, and when you last took them, to the surgical center before the operation. Your surgeon may also want you to take antibiotic eye drops before the procedure.

If you take insulin, be sure to check with your internist, family doctor, or endocrinologist about the doses you'll need on the morning of surgery. If you usually take prophylactic doses of oral antibiotics—to protect a damaged heart valve, for instance—before dental procedures, it's a good idea to check with your medical doctor about taking these antibiotics before cataract surgery.

Aspirin and Coumadin are both known to interfere with blood clotting. Therefore, most doctors recommend that *all aspirin use be stopped at least two weeks before cataract surgery* because of the risk of intraocular bleeding or hemorrhage during retrobulbar anesthesia (see below). However, this should be done only with the consent of the internist, family doctor, or specialist who put you on aspirin in the first place. Stopping Coumadin before cataract surgery is a trickier prospect, because interrupting it for even a short period of time can put some patients at serious risk for a stroke. (In this case you and your eye surgeon, after a thorough discussion of the risks of being anticoagulated at the time of cataract surgery, may decide to continue the Coumadin and go ahead with the operation.)

THE PROCEDURE ITSELF

Your surgery may be performed at a hospital, at an outpatient surgicenter, or in a surgical facility connected to your doctor's office. Wherever it is, you'll probably be asked to arrive early, sometimes as much as an hour and a half before the actual scheduled time of the operation, to allow plenty of time for preoperative preparation. (This usually includes a review of the presurgical testing results, interviews by nursing and anesthesia staff, and eye drops.) The regimen of preoperative eye drops varies, but it usually includes dilating drops (such as Mydriacyl and NeoSynephrine) and may also include an antibiotic and a corticosteroid or nonsteroidal anti-inflammatory medication such as flurbiprofen (Ocufen). Anesthetic eye drops are usually applied to *both* eyes—to numb the eye that will be operated on, and to make the other eye more comfortable during surgery.

Patients often ask if they'll need to remove their clothes for the procedure. A reasonable question; the answer varies depending on the surgical facility. Even if you do get to keep your own clothes on, you'll wear a surgical gown or covering during the procedure. Human nature being what it is, it's a good idea to keep such personal articles as watches, rings, money, and wallets to a minimum (and preferably to leave them locked up at home).

Note: A quick trip to the bathroom before surgery can be very important and help avoid an embarrassing situation. (But even if you take this precaution and still have to go, don't worry: if necessary, you can use a urinal or bedpan during the surgery.)

In the operating room, your eye and the region around it will be cleaned with an antibacterial and antiseptic solution. Sterile drapes and sheets will also be laid over and around the eye to lower the risk of infection. Oxygen is usually provided to the patient through a nose tube because it can be hard to breathe under the drapes. At most centers, patients' blood pressure, blood-oxygen levels, and cardiac rhythm are also monitored throughout the procedure.

We should note again that there is considerable variability among surgeons and centers regarding the procedures on the day of cataract surgery. But in general, all patients receive some degree of sedation, followed by injections of local anesthesia around and behind the eye. A local injection to prevent the eye from closing may also be given. As mentioned previously, some patients may receive only topical anesthesia. *Note:* The medication used is usually lidocaine or something similar—just like the lidocaine your dentist uses. So if you've ever had any problems with local anesthesia in the dentist's chair, be sure to tell your surgeon!

Retrobulbar anesthesia, a local injection of anesthetic behind the eyeball, works by blocking the nerves leading to the muscles that control the movement of the eyeball and eyelid. This injection is performed with a long, thin needle that is usually inserted through the lower eyelid to a point behind the eyeball where the ocular nerves and muscles nestle closely together. A retrobulbar injection is not without risk. Your doctor guides the needle without being able to see the structures behind the eye such as blood vessels, nerves, muscles, and—most important—the eyeball itself. Although eye surgeons and anesthesiologists perform this injection with great care and complications are rare, they do occur and can include nicking a blood vessel (causing a retrobulbar hemorrhage), perforating the eyeball, or injuring the optic nerve. These complications can occur in even the most experienced hands and usually require postponing the planned cataract surgery until a later date. But the vast majority of these injections are performed each year without any complications at all. (However, because the risk of these complications, small though it may be, is present, some surgeons advocate other anesthesia and surgical techniques that are associated with less risk. The indications, safety, and effectiveness of these newer techniques are currently being assessed.)

After retrobulbar anesthesia, pressure is applied to the eyeball, either manually, by the doctor's finger, or using a special device or weight over the

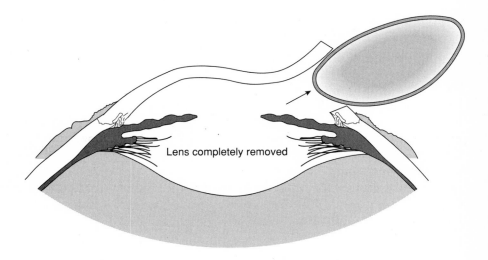

Fig. 7.3. Intracapsular extraction

eyeball. This pressure on the eyeball serves two purposes. First, it encourages any bleeding—if a blood vessel was nicked or severed during the retrobulbar injection, for instance—to stop, and it maximizes clotting. Second, pressure on the eyeball decreases the pressure within the eye by displacing fluid from the eyeball into the systemic circulation. (And lower intraocular pressure decreases the risk of surgical complications.)

The atmosphere in the operating room probably won't be nearly as intense as it's usually portrayed in the movies and on TV; many patients are pleasantly surprised to find that the staff is congenial, with a warm, comforting attitude. Many patients worry that they won't be able to keep their eye open throughout the whole operation—that they'll accidentally blink and derail the procedure. As the old slogan goes, "Leave the driving to us." We'll keep your eyelids open, using a lid speculum or specially designed retraction device.

Now it's time to remove that cataract. First, an incision must be made into the eyeball. Most incisions are placed somewhere in the upper half of the eyeball, relatively near where the cornea meets the sclera (the "white" of the eye); this area is known as the *limbus* of the eye. The length and specific placement of the incision depend on which technique the surgeon will be using to remove your cataract. Smaller surgical incisions speed up recovery time; they're also less likely to cause postoperative astigmatism, an

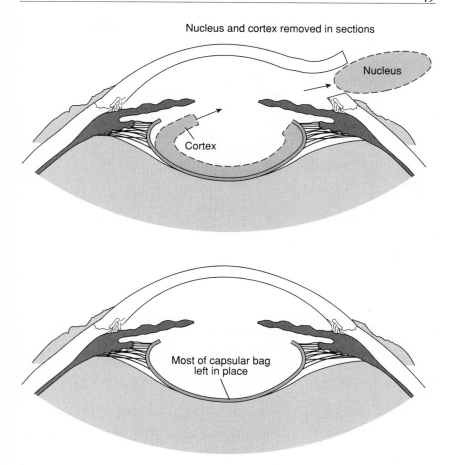

Nucleus and cortex removed in sections

Nucleus

Cortex

Most of capsular bag
left in place

Fig. 7.4. Extracapsular extraction

abnormal curvature of the corneal surface that is created as the wound heals. But in intracapsular and extracapsular cataract surgery, where the lens of the eye is removed in one piece, the surgical incision must be large, as long as 10 to 12 millimeters, or about half an inch.

Intracapsular cataract extraction (ICCE), very popular many years ago before modern microsurgical techniques were developed, is rarely performed these days. In an ICCE the lens is removed intact, complete with the surrounding capsular lens bag. *Extracapsular cataract extractions* (ECCE) involve opening the capsular lens bag and removing the lens located within

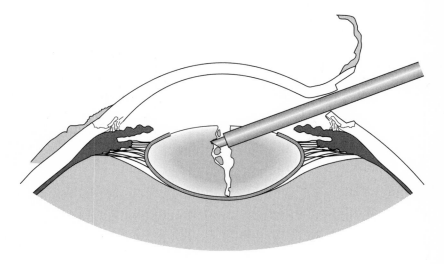

Fig. 7.5. Phacoemulsification

it. The inner lens is extracted from the eye in one piece. A surgeon may choose this technique if he or she is more skilled in this procedure than in other methods of cataract surgery. Also, this technique is often reserved for very dense and firm cataracts that would be difficult to break up with phacoemulsification.

In *phacoemulsification cataract extraction*, incisions can be much smaller—approximately 3 millimeters, or one-eighth of an inch. In this very popular form of cataract surgery, the cataractous lens is broken up inside the eye with ultrasound waves emanating from a specially designed surgical instrument inserted through the incision. This instrument then vacuums up these small lens fragments as they're broken up. (The use of lasers for cataract surgery will be discussed later. At this point, lasers are *not* used to remove cataracts from the eye. Since a cataract is a solid structure, it must be removed, either in one piece or in fragments. None of the above techniques involves the use of a laser, which burns or cuts through an object or tissue.)

With extracapsular extraction and phacoemulsification, after the cataract is removed from the eye, it's often necessary to use an irrigation and aspiration technique to clean up any leftover fragments of the cataract. Although this technique can be performed manually, most surgeons prefer to use an automated system.

10 mm incision

3-5 mm incision

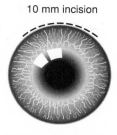
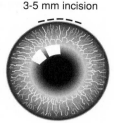

Extracapsular extraction

Phacoemulsification

Fig. 7.6. Incisions for extracapsular extraction and phacoemulsification

Now it's time to insert the intraocular implant lens. At this point the incision is either large (approximately 10 millimeters) or small. Different implant lenses require different-sized incisions to be made in the eye, ranging from approximately 3 millimeters for foldable lenses to 7 millimeters for larger-diameter solid plastic polymer implants. Depending on the surgeon's choice of implant lens, then, the opening may need to be enlarged for its insertion. (Once again, the style and size of the implant lens chosen for each patient vary, depending on a multitude of factors.)

Closure of the opening, or wound, has become a highly publicized issue in cataract surgery advertisements. Advertisements for "one-stitch" or "no-stitch" surgery, popularized by surgeons as the most modern, state-of-the-art approach to cataract surgery, imply that the eye surgeons who use these techniques are a cut above all the rest. The truth is that the *majority* of eye surgeons today perform phacoemulsification and one-stitch or no-stitch surgery. What's the difference between one-stitch and no-stitch? Well, think about why most men wear belts: they probably don't actually need a belt to keep their pants up, but they feel more secure knowing it's there. Most small incision wounds don't need to be sutured, but many surgeons put one suture in anyway just to help them sleep better at night. Smaller incisions with no sutures (or one suture) really help patients recover faster. There's also less chance for unwanted postoperative astigmatism due to sutures being too tight or too loose. On the other hand, procedures involving a larger surgical incision must be closed using many more sutures. Recuperation from these procedures is usually longer, with a greater chance for astigmatism.

At the end of surgery, you'll probably receive an antibiotic medication in the eye; then a light eye patch and shield will be placed over it.

You'll be taken to a recovery area where—finally—you can break your surgical fast. Eat, drink, and be merry, for the operation is over!

AFTER SURGERY

You'll be able to go home shortly after the operation, but somebody else must drive you, because you'll still be drowsy. (Even if you think you're fully alert, have someone drive you anyway.) You'll probably need someone to drive you again for your first follow-up appointment, the next day. Overall, most people don't find the surgery difficult; many patients report that it was painless and not nearly as taxing as they had expected.

You'll go back to your eye surgeon and/or your referring eye care provider for several postoperative visits. These are generally scheduled as follows: the day after surgery, and then at one week, three weeks, and six to eight weeks afterward. You may need to be seen more frequently if you have any complications or an unusual postoperative course.

Rest and relaxation are the marching orders during the first twenty-four hours after cataract surgery. For most patients the evening of the operation usually includes some mild eye discomfort and headache, which can be treated with over-the-counter analgesics. Lingering postoperative drowsiness, an effect of the anesthesia, is not uncommon. (*Note:* Immediately report any severe pain, nausea, vomiting, or other unusual symptom to your eye surgeon.) The next day you'll go back to your surgeon and have the eye patch and shield removed (if you were given them after surgery). Many patients notice an immediate improvement in vision; lights are brighter, colors are more vivid, even objects are better defined. Your vision will continue to improve gradually over the next several weeks.

The old restrictions—in which patients were warned not to lift or bend after cataract surgery—are becoming passé. Stories of patients dislodging implant lenses or tearing open their cataract wound as they bent over to tie their shoes or brush their teeth now belong to cataract folklore. Today most cataract patients resume their normal activities—including reading, driving, and working—almost immediately after surgery. Recommendations regarding showering, bathing, and visiting the beauty parlor have also been changed. (However, it's a good idea to discuss these activities, as well as the resumption of golf, tennis, swimming, bowling, or gardening, with your doctor beforehand.) Common sense is usually your best guide to resuming normal activities after cataract surgery.

You'll probably need to wear some covering over the operated eye for one to two weeks after surgery, either your old eyeglasses or a lightly tinted pair of sunglasses. This will help protect the eye from an accidental finger (your own or a grandchild's), foreign object, bump on the eye, or other form of trauma. At night you'll probably wear an eye shield to keep you from inadvertently rolling onto the operated eye or rubbing it during sleep. Antibiotic and anti-inflammatory eye drops are commonly prescribed after surgery to prevent eye infections and eliminate swelling and discomfort.

Complications

Complications of cataract surgery are generally mild, but it's important for you to be aware of the warning signs.

Cystoid macular edema, a common problem, is a swelling that occurs in the retina after the surgery. Fluid accumulates in small spaces in the area of the retina responsible for central or straight-ahead vision. This swelling can cause blurred vision during the weeks immediately following the operation. The edema usually goes away in one to two months without causing any damage to the retina or eye, but occasionally it can remain much longer and may require medical treatment.

Postoperative eye infection is another well-recognized complication of cataract surgery. The most severe form, which occurs in the eyeball, is called *endophthalmitis*. It is very difficult to treat, and the earlier it's diagnosed and treated, the better the chances for minimizing the damage from this potentially devastating complication. Endophthalmitis often causes the eye to become very red and painful, with an associated decrease in vision. It usually occurs within the first week after surgery. Although the problem isn't nearly as common today as it once was—thanks to sterile surgical techniques, plus the use of antibiotics—it's definitely something you should be aware of, so that you can seek treatment as soon as possible. Other, less serious postoperative infections such as bacterial conjunctivitis, allergic reactions to topical medications, and suture abscesses also may cause milder degrees of inflammation, discomfort, and alterations in vision.

Retinal detachment is another potentially serious postoperative complication. If there's any weakness in the retina at the time of cataract surgery, the retina can become loosened or detached by the procedure. The tricky thing is that this may not happen immediately after surgery but may occur weeks or even months later. *If you've ever had cataract or any other form of eye surgery, contact your surgeon immediately if you notice the sudden on-set of floaters, flashing lights, or a "curtain" that seems to be blocking part of your vision.* These may be signs of a retinal tear or detachment, and they should be evaluated immediately. The quicker this is discovered and treated, the better the chances for repair and a good visual outcome.

Other problems that may arise after cataract surgery include a marked *change in your eyeglass prescription*, making it difficult for you to ad-just to your new vision after surgery. Healing can also lead to unwanted *astigmatism* in the eye (a complication that, fortunately, is much less com-mon with smaller incisions). *Double vision* is also not uncommon, especially within the first two weeks after surgery. The brain has to get readjusted to the change in vision between the two eyes. When double vision persists or develops several weeks or months after the surgery, this may be due to a problem with someone's ability to turn the images from each eye into a sin-gle picture. (This is best evaluated with special testing and may require a "prism" correction in your eyeglasses to help your eyes work together. For more on this, see chapter 2.) *Corneal damage*—much less common today with microsurgery—is another potential problem. This can lead to pro-longed visual blurring after the surgery and, very rarely, may require a corneal transplant.

Other fairly common complications are *spontaneous anterior chamber bleeding* from the cataract wound and *recurrent postoperative inflammation*—both easily treated if promptly brought to the attention of the eye surgeon. Annoying *floaters* and *intermittent flashing* in the operated eye are also fre-quent postoperative complaints. These are related to a change in the vitre-ous dynamics in the back of the eye after surgery and should be brought to your eye doctor's attention, since they may be the first sign of a retinal tear or detachment (see chapter 15).

Although many patients worry about them, implants rarely slip out of place after surgery, and sutures very seldom come loose. Again, we've come a long way from the days when these were common postoperative problems.

As potentially devastating as these complications can be, if they're caught early and tended properly, in most cases there's still an excellent chance that the eye can heal normally and you can have better vision than you had before surgery—even if you need a second surgery soon after the first to correct a particular postoperative problem. Unfortunately—al-though it doesn't happen often—there is a chance that if an infection gets out of control, a retina becomes badly detached, or a complication does not respond to treatment or management, you may end up with worse vision in the eye than you had before. Some patients have even lost their vision or their eye after cataract surgery. Although the local anesthesia we use today has significantly lower risks than general anesthesia, there have also been extremely rare instances in which patients have died during the procedure.

This is why, even though you may feel fine, your doctor will want to monitor you closely after the operation. It's also why you should call your doctor immediately at the first sign of unusual discomfort or a sudden change in vision. But again, for the vast majority of patients, serious complications are rare, and the benefits of cleared sight often far outweigh the risks of surgery.

How Will This Improve Your Life?
Realistic Expectations

People have different expectations after cataract surgery, some realistic and others not. Most people still need to wear glasses to fine-tune their vision after cataract surgery. Although we've all heard of people who swear they no longer need glasses after cataract surgery, most surgeons would agree that these fortunate souls are the exceptions rather than the rule. Remember, implant lenses are artificial, and they're only so good at replacing the eye's focusing power. The more active you are, and the more you depend on good eyesight for activities such as driving and reading, the more likely you are to need corrective eyeglasses or contact lenses after surgery.

Patients who have had cataracts removed almost universally notice that colors are brighter and more vivid after the surgery. Since the cataract acts like a dirty window, removing it allows more light to pass to the back of the eye. (A particularly happy patient once returned after cataract surgery to tell us that she had been prepared to redo the wallpaper in her dining room. After the surgery she realized that the wallpaper was fine, as bright and colorful as she remembered it being when she bought it; it had only seemed faded because of her cataract.) Night driving is easier and so is reading, especially in dim light. Occasionally the increase in light makes people rely more on sunglasses when they go outside than they did before the operation.

The Second Eye

Now that you have had one cataract removed, what should you do as the cataract in the other eye continues to advance? The criterion for surgery on the second eye is generally the same as that (discussed above) for the first eye—mainly, visual acuity of 20/50 or worse. However, a surgeon may operate on the second eye in other situations—for example, if someone has severe discomfort due to the visual imbalance resulting from the presence of a remaining cataract. This is particularly common when the cataract has been removed from a nondominant eye; suddenly the nondominant eye has better vision than the dominant eye, and the brain becomes "confused." This conflict can cause visual discomfort until the cataract is removed from the dominant eye and binocular vision is restored.

No two operations are ever the same, and so it is with cataract surgery. Many patients feel that the second operation took longer, hurt more, or otherwise did not go as well as the first. Rarely do they report that it was a better experience. But as with childbirth, recollections of the event fade with time, making a comparison very difficult. (*Note:* This applies to listening to friends' experiences, too. When it comes to cataract surgery, improved eyesight often seems to cloud the memory.) Be cautiously optimistic about the surgery, and you'll have a better chance of being pleasantly surprised.

The "Second Cataract" behind the Implant Lens: Lasers in the Management of Cataracts

Lasers—highly sophisticated instruments that harness energy and release it on demand at a specific point—have greatly improved our ability to treat eye disease. A question we're regularly asked by patients contemplating cataract surgery is, Do you do the laser cataract surgery? Well, we all do, yet we all don't. Confused? So are the patients. Much of the bewilderment stems from marketing campaigns by ophthalmologists hoping to convey the idea that they're one step ahead of the competition. The bottom line is that all ophthalmologists basically perform the same cataract extraction operations with implantation of intraocular lenses. So where do lasers come in?

Remember, we treat the cataract surgically by removing the hazy lens, as described in detail above. But lasers don't work that way; we can't simply use a laser to cut a clear zone through the lens.

But we can still use lasers to treat cataracts—kind of. Sometimes, with time, the back portion of the lens bag that was left in the eye, and now is located behind the intraocular implant lens, becomes very cloudy. This "second cataract," or opacified posterior capsule, can cause a gradual decrease in vision *even though the cataract has been removed.* In the past an eye surgeon needed to insert a needle into the eye to open this cloudy membrane. Ophthalmic scientists later developed lasers (YAG lasers) able to open these membranes with less risk than the needle technique. This outpatient procedure is virtually painless and usually provides immediate improvement in a patient's vision.

So this is how we explain it to our patients who ask if we perform laser cataract surgery: Cataract surgery initially requires removing the cataract lens from the eye. A laser can be used later, if necessary, when a cloudiness develops *behind the implant lens.*

Special Eyeglass Considerations after Cataract Surgery

Most people who have had cataract surgery eventually need some form of eyeglasses to maximize their distance or reading vision. As discussed previously, this has a lot to do with a person's own visual demands and level of activity.

No two patients are the same; everyone heals at a different rate, and each surgery may cause a different amount of postoperative swelling. Most patients get their "final" eyeglass prescription about six weeks to three months after surgery. But as your eye continues to heal over the first year, your prescription may change again at six months to a year later; even after this, you may still require slight alterations in your prescription from time to time.

What kind of eyeglasses will you need after cataract surgery? Again, much depends on you. Important considerations include the style of glasses you wore before the operation, your particular visual needs after surgery, and how much you want to spend. Bifocals, trifocals, and no-line progressive lenses are popular options, because these are usually what patients wore before surgery, and they continue to provide corrected vision at various distances after surgery. Occasionally patients require only single-vision distance or reading glasses after cataract surgery. Some patients are even fortunate enough to be able to use inexpensive premade drugstore reading glasses. Contact lenses can even be worn after cataract surgery if you have worn them before or are interested in trying them (see chapter 5).

Similarly, the choice of various lens options is largely up to you. Options include antireflective lenses, polarized lenses, photochromic lenses (which change color when you move from a light area—like outside—to a darker area, and vice versa), and other tinted lenses. Many people experi-

ence visual discomfort from too-bright sunlight and indoor light; antireflective coatings on lenses can reduce the glare and dazzle of lights, especially at night. (These lenses have also been helpful for people who play indoor tennis, where the lighting is often poor.) Ultraviolet protection in the
intraocular implant lens or glasses after cataract surgery is felt to be important to protect the retina once the natural lens has been removed. (For
more on lens options, see chapter 4.)

Some Questions You May Have about Cataracts

Do cataracts need to be "ripe" before they can be removed?

Although many years ago it was necessary for cataracts to mature to
a certain stage before a patient could have cataract surgery, this is not
true today. Modern microsurgical techniques have made it possible to
remove cataracts at earlier stages of development based on the level of
visual problems they are causing, not on their degree of maturity.

What is phacoemulsification cataract surgery?

Phacoemulsification is an advanced cataract-removing technique that
uses ultrasound waves to shatter the cataract in the eye. Suction is then
used to remove the lens fragments, making room for an implant lens.
The tiny incision used in this technique either seals itself closed or requires only one stitch thinner than a strand of human hair. Most people
recuperate quickly from this procedure and are able to resume their
normal activities within a few days.

How can I find a good cataract surgeon?

Perhaps a better thought is "How to find a good doctor," because a
good cataract surgeon will have all the characteristics of a good doctor
plus excellent surgical skills. In this case, *good* implies a skilled medical
and surgical ophthalmologist who is caring and able to communicate
well with patients. Whether you're looking for an internist, dentist, or
ophthalmologist, finding the right doctor for *you* can be the most important step.

Frankly, the ideal way to find the right doctor is probably not the Yellow Pages. Many doctors are also a little suspicious of their colleagues
who promote themselves in newspaper, television, and radio advertisements. On the other hand, relatives and friends who have had cataracts
or cataract surgery are usually excellent sources for referrals. Talk to

your internist or family doctor too about the eye surgeons in your area.

Finally, make an appointment to meet the eye surgeon, to decide for yourself. Ask to speak with some of the surgeon's other patients with cataracts or who have had cataract surgery. Ask how often the doctor performs cataract surgery. *This is extremely important.* You don't want someone who does this procedure only occasionally; you want someone who performs this surgery at least once or twice a week. Specifically, find out if he or she performs phacoemulsification, and if you are a candidate for this technique. Make sure that you're comfortable with the surgeon's postoperative care arrangement.

Remember, you have only one pair of eyes. And although cataract surgery is fairly safe these days, not all cataract surgeons are equal. A poorly performed or complicated surgery can cause you problems for the rest of your life.

I'm in a managed-care program. Will my program cover cataract surgery?

Cataract surgery is one of the most common health insurance services. The bottom line is that it costs insurance companies, and state and national health insurance programs like Medicare, a lot of money each year. As managed health care becomes more popular, there will be increasing pressure on doctors and hospitals to perform fewer cataract surgeries at lower levels of reimbursement. There has even been talk of only covering surgery on one eye! The choice of surgeon, facility, and time of the operation will also change from a patient-doctor decision to a health insurance company–dictated system. It is important to be aware of your health insurance coverage concerning your eye care, especially cataract surgery. Being informed about your options as a patient will help you get the care you desire when it comes time for cataract surgery.

If I have cataract surgery on one eye, how long do I have to wait to have the second eye done? Can't I have both eyes fixed at once?

Anyone who would benefit from cataract surgery on both eyes should have two separate surgery dates. The time between operations usually averages about six weeks. Doctors rarely advise someone to have both cataracts operated on at the same time. For one thing, it's helpful to leave one eye unoperated, to make it easier for you to see to get around after the operation. For another, any complications during or after surgery may change your surgeon's approach when it comes time to operate on the other eye. And finally, depending on your experience with the first operation, you may decide you don't even want to have the other eye done right away, if at all.

Can cataracts grow back after cataract surgery?

No, because the lens has been removed, and an artificial one has been implanted in its place. Occasionally, however, a cloudy film can develop *behind* the implant lens (see above). Ophthalmologists use state-of-the-art laser surgery to remove this cloudy film, thereby restoring the person's vision.

8

Glaucoma,
the "Silent Thief"

It's often called the silent thief of vision.

One of the most troubling conditions to affect the eye, glaucoma indeed sneaks in, with the stealth of a master prowler. It rarely causes warning symptoms and yet is a leading cause of blindness—accounting for 12 percent of new cases of blindness each year in the United States. An estimated two out of every hundred people in the United States over age sixty-five have glaucoma. And it is estimated that half of those with glaucoma don't know that they have it. Understandably, detecting and managing glaucoma is of major concern to eye doctors.

It is not a simple disease. In most cases glaucoma is instead a *collection* of eye problems that elevate pressure within the eye, damaging the optic nerve, and seriously affecting vision. Its onset is furtive, usually very gradual over several years; during this time people seldom have any symptoms to alert them of their elevated eye pressure. Most people who develop glaucoma can't feel it. Even the loss of peripheral vision, one of the first signs of trouble, is so subtle that for many people it's virtually unnoticeable. (Some people even develop optic nerve damage and visual field loss *despite* having normal eye pressures. More on this unusual form of glaucoma, called *normotensive glaucoma*, later in this chapter.)

One form of the disease, called *acute closed-angle glaucoma*, in which the pressure in the eye rises rapidly, does cause acute eye pain. This condition hits suddenly and is *an ophthalmic emergency that requires immediate treatment*. But it's also pretty rare.

The more common form is called *open-angle glaucoma*. This is our old nemesis, the silent thief. Open-angle glaucoma can advance undetected for years; during this time the constantly elevated eye pressure can cause irreversible vision loss by severely damaging the nerve fibers that pass through the optic nerve in the back of the eye. The nerve fibers most frequently damaged by this are those that make peripheral vision possible. Losing enough peripheral vision can, over time, lead to tunnel vision, in which people can see only when they're looking directly ahead. In people with very advanced cases of glaucoma, this loss of vision can deteriorate into total blindness.

What's your best protection against the potentially devastating consequences of glaucoma? Because its onset is so insidious, don't trust yourself to notice early symptoms; chances are, you won't. But your eye doctor will. *This means that regular eye exams are essential! Only by monitoring the eyes regularly can glaucoma be detected early and managed well.*

WHAT HAPPENS TO THE EYES IN GLAUCOMA

Think of the eye as a balloon. Inside the eye there's a fine balance between the outer atmospheric pressure and the eye's own internal pressure. This balance helps maintain the shape of the eye, or the balloon. Too much or too little internal pressure can easily change this balance.

Like a balloon, the eye is basically hollow, but it has an inner core that maintains its shape. This core is made up of two separate compartments, one filled with fluid and another filled with jelly. The front compartment, or cavity, of the eye is filled with a fluid called *aqueous*. Within this watery cavity (the aqueous cavity) are two areas, the *anterior chamber* and the *posterior chamber*, both of which are located in front of the lens. Behind the lens, the rear cavity (the vitreous cavity) holds a jellylike substance called *vitreous*.

Together, the aqueous and vitreous cavities help maintain the eye's shape. While the vitreous, like jelly, is relatively inert and stable, the aqueous has a dynamic turnover with constant production of new fluid entering the eye and drainage of old fluid out—much like what happens in a storm drain. The big problem in glaucoma—the elevated pressure that damages the optic nerve—is caused when there's a problem with the drainage. In keeping with our image of a storm drain, imagine the drain clogged by leaves, and the poor drainage—and water backup—that results.

Now for a little anatomy. The anterior chamber of the eye, which contains most of the aqueous fluid, is bordered by the back surface of the cornea and the front surface of the iris. The posterior chamber, which also contains aqueous fluid, is bordered by the back surface of the iris and the front surface of the lens.

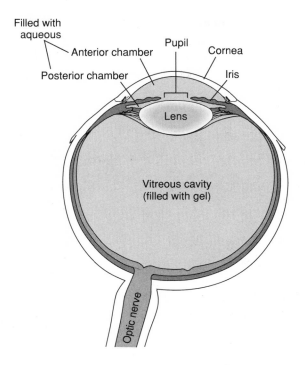

Fig. 8.1. Fluid and gel cavities in the eye: the vitreous cavity is filled with gel, and the anterior and posterior chambers are filled with aqueous (fluid)

The fluid itself is made by the *ciliary body*, eye tissue located near the root of the iris in the posterior chamber. It's then pumped into the posterior chamber, where it circulates through the pupillary space and into the anterior chamber of the eye. The fluid drains out from the anterior chamber—and this is critical—*at an angle*, where the cornea and iris meet. (This is called the *anterior chamber angle*.) As it leaves the eye through this angle, the aqueous fluid passes through a filter of connective tissue called the *trabecular meshwork*.

The trabecular meshwork encircles the eye like a ring on a finger. Normally the anterior chamber angle is wide open, a straight shot to the trabecular meshwork, and the clear aqueous fluid freely exits the eye. It filters out through the trabecular meshwork into an aqueduct called *Schlemm's canal*. Schlemm's canal transports the fluid through a network of aqueous veins. The aqueous is then gradually absorbed into the blood supply by vessels in the conjunctiva.

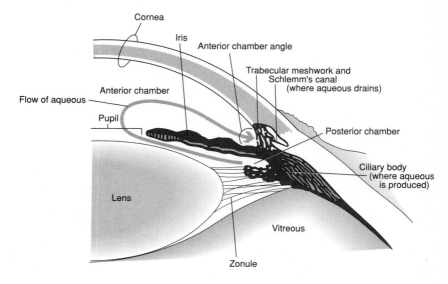

Fig. 8.2. The path of fluid movement in the eye: aqueous flows from the ciliary body to the trabecular meshwork and Schlemm's canal, where it drains from the eye

Not a terribly complicated drainage system, but it's got plenty of places for trouble to occur. When the flow of aqueous is interfered with somewhere along the route—from its beginnings, at the ciliary body, to the trabecular meshwork and Schlemm's canal—the fluid backs up. And pressure within the eye—picture an overfilled water balloon—begins to rise. This, then, is the elevated pressure that can damage the optic nerve, gradually lead to nerve death and loss of peripheral vision—if, that is, the pressure is not lowered by treatment.

TYPES OF GLAUCOMA

The type of glaucoma—there are two basic forms—depends on the specific obstruction that's hampering the aqueous fluid's drainage from the eye. *Closed-angle glaucoma* (also called *narrow-angle glaucoma* or *angle-closure glaucoma*) results when the fluid's access to the trabecular meshwork is physically blocked by the root of the iris. The more common condition, *open-angle glaucoma*, happens when, despite an open drain in the anterior chamber angle, the trabecular meshwork filter itself is somehow clogged. *Note:* Unfortunately, it's possible for someone to develop a combination of both types of glaucoma in the same eye.

Closed-Angle Glaucoma

The problem with closed-angle glaucoma is an obstruction in the drainage of aqueous fluid due to a narrowing in the angle of the anterior chamber. This anatomical defect can best be seen during a comprehensive eye examination with a technique known as *gonioscopy,* using a specially designed contact lens with angled mirrors to observe the anterior chamber angle. In people with a narrowed anterior chamber angle, the iris appears to crowd this area, limiting aqueous access to the trabecular meshwork.

Farsighted people, who have smaller eyeballs to begin with, are more prone to developing closed-angle glaucoma; as you might imagine, in a smaller eye it's easier for the iris to block the anterior chamber angle.

Also, some people were just born with narrow anterior chamber angles; although most of them have normal eye pressures, their risk of acute closed-angle glaucoma is higher. And for these people, even normal activities can bring on an attack—watching a movie in a darkened theater, for

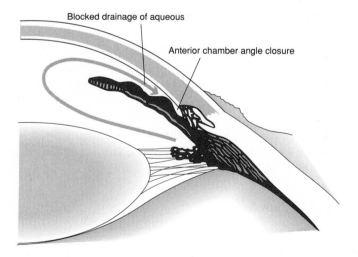

Fig. 8.3. Closed-angle glaucoma: drainage of aqueous is blocked by closure of the anterior chamber angle

example, which causes the pupil to dilate mildly, displacing the iris into the narrow anterior chamber angle. Or trouble can be incited by certain dilating eye drops or oral medications such as antihistamines, which can affect the position of the iris and lead to a precarious further narrowing of this angle. If this narrowing becomes extreme enough to block or close a significant portion of the anterior chamber angle, the eye pressure will rise. This will develop into a harmful cycle of increased angle blockage and higher eye pressure. Eventually, when the eye pressure rises to very high levels, the person will have a painful, red eye. Most people also experience nausea, vomiting, and a severe headache during an attack of acute closed-angle glaucoma. Again, the consequences of an acute angle-closure attack can be devastating. *This is a medical emergency and must be treated immediately and aggressively to preserve vision.*

The primary goal of emergency treatment is to lower the pressure in the eye. This may involve eye drops, pills, and occasionally intravenous or intramuscular injections. In the acute stages of an attack, it may also be necessary to operate if medical treatment fails to lower the eye pressure.

Laser or surgical treatment makes a hole or opening in the iris so that the fluid can escape. This procedure, called a *peripheral iridectomy*, creates an opening for runoff in the periphery of the iris, improving the flow of aqueous fluid from the posterior chamber into the anterior chamber. The iridectomy is, in effect, a short-cut, allowing aqueous fluid to bypass the narrowed approach to the trabecular meshwork.

Peripheral iridectomies are often recommended as a means of prevention against these attacks. For example, the procedure is recommended in the second eye of someone who has suffered through an attack in one eye already. (Preventive, or prophylactic, peripheral iridectomies are discussed later in this chapter.)

Closed-angle glaucoma can also develop more chronically over time. The anterior chamber angle gradually seals closed to a point where the pressure builds up in the eyes. This chronic closure of the angle is less painful than the acute variety, but it can be just as visually devastating.

Open-Angle Glaucoma

In open-angle glaucoma—by far the more common form—the site of trouble is the filter, or trabecular meshwork, leading into Schlemm's canal. There's no single anatomical problem causing the drainage block, as in closed-angle glaucoma. Instead, many conditions can lead to open-angle glaucoma;

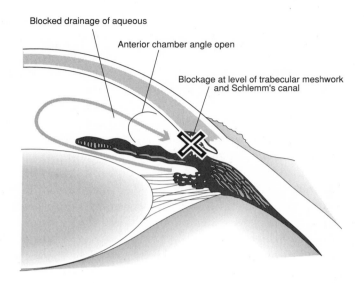

Blocked drainage of aqueous

Anterior chamber angle open

Blockage at level of trabecular meshwork
and Schlemm's canal

Fig. 8.4. Open-angle glaucoma: drainage of aqueous is blocked at level of
trabecular meshwork

but in each of these the trabecular meshwork is clogged or obstructed.

What are some of the things that can go wrong and lead to open-angle glaucoma? For one, inflammation in the anterior portion of the eye, such as *iritis*, can temporarily clog the trabecular meshwork with inflammatory cells. Also, bleeding, or *hyphema*, a separate problem in the anterior chamber, can lead to elevated eye pressure through a similar mechanism. In hyphema, red blood cells collect in and on the trabecular meshwork, impeding the outflow of aqueous fluid.

In *pigment dispersion syndrome*, another form of open-angle glaucoma, pigment granules from the iris spill into the aqueous-filled anterior chamber, especially during exercise or other exertion. These pigment cells are jiggled loose from the surface of the iris and flow with the aqueous to the trabecular meshwork filter in the anterior chamber angle. The trabecular meshwork can eventually become clogged with these cells; this impedes further aqueous drainage and leads to temporary elevations in eye pressure. People with this condition may experience dull pain in their eyes and see halos around lights after exercise or vigorous exertion. Pigmentary glaucoma is more common in men between the ages of thirty-four and forty-six who are mildly to moderately nearsighted.

Pseudoexfoliative glaucoma, yet another form of open-angle glaucoma, happens when the trabecular meshwork becomes clogged with cells that flake off, like dandruff, in the anterior chamber of the eye.

The most common form of open-angle glaucoma is *primary open-angle glaucoma*. In this case the use of the word *primary* means that doctors are not certain what's causing the blockage at the trabecular meshwork. They know it's *not*, however, due to a narrowed anterior chamber angle (thus, by default, it's a form of open-angle glaucoma). Nor is it caused by a recognizable cell or substance clogging the trabecular meshwork, as in the forms of open-angle glaucoma mentioned above. Some researchers believe that the pressure elevation in primary open-angle glaucoma may be due to a change in the structural integrity of the trabecular meshwork that just happens with age. Others have suggested that a problem exists with the drainage through Schlemm's canal.

Whatever the exact mechanism, the changes in the trabecular meshwork seen in this form of glaucoma have also been observed in older people who do *not* have glaucoma. Therefore, these may simply be normal aging changes which for some reason are accelerated or further advanced in people with glaucoma. This is why many ophthalmologists, in moments of frustration when trying to control difficult cases of glaucoma, have declared that this disorder is an aging process that is often as tough to treat as wrinkling skin. *This is not true!* We have many successful ways of controlling glaucoma, as we will soon discuss.

Normotensive (Low-Tension) Glaucoma

Normal eye pressure is usually considered to be 21 millimeters of mercury (mm Hg) or less. Some people have normal pressures within the eye but nevertheless have progressive optic disc and visual field changes similar to those observed in people with primary open-angle glaucoma (which, as noted above, is due to elevated eye pressures). When someone develops glaucoma despite having normal eye pressures, that person is said to have *normotensive glaucoma* or *low-tension glaucoma*. This diagnosis is made only after other ocular or systemic problems that can damage the optic nerve and cause visual field loss are ruled out. These include a period of elevated eye pressure (in this case, even though the ocular pressure has returned to normal, there is residual optic nerve damage); daily fluctuations of eye pressures in and out of the "normal" range; and a past episode of very low blood pressure as the result of severe blood loss or myocardial infarction.

It is believed that many people have *undiagnosed* normotensive glaucoma. Eye doctors often miss diagnosing this disorder because the person has normal intraocular pressure during an eye examination. This is why the doctor must carefully evaluate the eye for other signs of glaucoma, such as significant optic disc changes and visual field loss. Many glaucoma screening programs at health fairs and senior centers also rely heavily on the intraocular pressure readings to screen large numbers of people for glaucoma, so (obviously!) they often miss picking up normotensive glaucoma.

What's causing optic nerve damage in people with normotensive glaucoma despite eye pressures in the normal range? Unfortunately, we don't yet know the answer to this question. Perhaps *normal eye pressure* is a relative term, since some people can tolerate intraocular pressures of 24 mm Hg for years without developing optic nerve damage. For other people an intraocular pressure of even 16 mm Hg may be too high, causing damage to their optic nerve and visual field loss. It has also long been speculated that this increased susceptibility may be related to a poor blood supply to the optic nerve. Or there may be a defect in the support tissues of the optic nerve that makes the nerve more likely to be damaged at lower eye pressures.

The treatment of normotensive glaucoma, as in other forms of glaucoma, is directed at lowering the eye pressure as much as possible, first medically and later surgically, if necessary. Patients are also thoroughly evaluated medically to make sure they do not have an underlying anemia or other condition that can directly or indirectly affect the optic nerve. A brain scan is sometimes part of this workup to evaluate the health of the optic nerve behind the eyeball.

We still know little about what makes one person's optic nerve susceptible and another person's resistant to changes in eye pressure. Normotensive glaucoma underscores this problem as well as the complex nature of glaucoma.

DIAGNOSING GLAUCOMA

Measuring Pressure within the Eye

Although today we recognize that glaucoma can occur in eyes with "normal" eye pressure, the relationship between elevated eye pressure and visual field loss was recognized centuries ago, though at that time physicians were unable to measure eye pressure accurately. For many years the accepted method of estimating the pressure in the eyeball was simply to feel, or "ballot," the eye with one's fingers. Eye doctors of the eighteenth and early nineteenth centuries prided themselves on their ability to judge eye pressure simply "by feel." So confident were they, in fact, that they scoffed at the development of more objective methods to measure pressure.

But eventually eye doctors were won over by the sensitivity of measurements made through *tonometry*, a noninvasive way to measure pressure within the eye. Over the years many tonometry techniques have been developed, all of them measuring how much force is required to indent or flatten the cornea. This measurement, in turn, allows the ophthalmologist to estimate the pressure in the eye.

Many tonometers use weights or specially designed contact tips, which are placed on the eye or cornea. The *Goldmann contact tonometer*, or "blue light" test—many people are familiar with this from eye examinations—is the most accurate method of measuring eye pressure. This is an *applanation tonometry system*, in which a circular tip is placed on an anesthetized cornea. A scale measures the amount of pressure in millimeters of mercury required to cause a specific degree of corneal flattening. Fluorescein (orange) dye and a cobalt blue filtered light are used to help illuminate the tip as it comes in contact with the eye. Many patients are fearful of tonometry, or the "glaucoma test." Most are squeamish about having someone touching their eyes (in applanation tonometry, it's often necessary for the examiner to hold open the patient's eyelids). Others are afraid because they remember some negative past experiences with tonometry techniques, particularly the frightening and sudden loud click associated with some "air-puff" tonometers.

Although it's difficult to define normal eye pressure—since what's "normal" varies from person to person—it is generally accepted that the "average" intraocular pressure of individuals without glaucoma is around 16 millimeters of mercury. In the general population, however, there appear to be more people with pressure readings above 16 than would be expected on a purely statistical basis. Therefore, it is only when someone's pressures reach above 20 or 21 millimeters of mercury that ophthalmologists may consider additional tests to diagnose or rule out a diagnosis of glaucoma.

Anyone with intraocular pressures above 21 millimeters of mercury is considered to have elevated intraocular pressure (or simply "elevated IOP"). Many people with elevated IOP never go on to develop glaucoma, but they must be carefully monitored for early signs of it. Some people have eye pressures of 24 for their entire lives and do not develop any signs of glaucoma, while other people with this pressure develop severe glaucoma. Even more perplexing are those patients with *low* eye pressure (see above) who develop glaucoma, which suggests, again, that glaucoma is caused by other factors besides elevated eye pressure. And although IOP does appear to be the most important factor, intraocular pressure readings by themselves are inadequate predictors of glaucoma.

To make things still more complicated, although intraocular pressures are usually highest in the early morning, they can fluctuate *day to day* and even *hour to hour*. They can be affected by such variables as age, gender, race, the presence of myopia, a family history of glaucoma, medications (for example, steroids and antihistamines), and certain systemic disorders (such as eye disease related to a thyroid disorder). Hypertension, or high blood pressure, has been associated with elevated eye pressure but not with the development of glaucoma.

The Effects of Elevated Eye Pressure in Glaucoma

Let's take a moment to review the machinery of the eye. First, of course, light rays enter the eye. They strike the retina, where they induce chemical reactions in specialized cells called *rods* and *cones*. (For more on the eye's anatomy, see chapter 1.) These cells then send impulses to the brain via nerve fibers—tiny telegraph lines, if you will, conveying essential information. The mass of all of these nerve fibers—approximately one million in all!—forms the *optic nerve*, way at the back of the eye. The optic nerve's job is to transmit all of this information to the brain, where it's translated into images that make sense. The exact area where these fibers come together at the back of the eye, before exiting the eyeball, is called the *optic nerve head*, or *disc*. Within this optic disc, major retinal blood vessels enter and exit the inner part of the eyeball.

What does all this have to do with glaucoma? Intraocular pressure elevations—such as those found in the majority of people with glaucoma—cause structural damage to these nerve fibers at the optic disc. Exactly *why* these fibers are so susceptible to damage here is not well understood. In normal aging, these fibers appear to diminish gradually anyway; but in people with elevated eye pressures and glaucoma, this loss is accelerated.

These million nerve fibers are somewhat loosely organized. The fibers responsible for central vision are generally located on the temporal

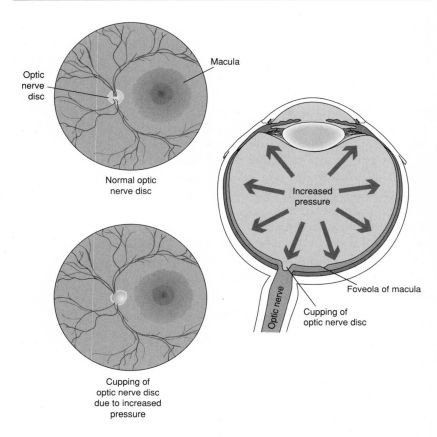

Fig. 8.5. Cupping of optic nerve disc caused by elevated ocular pressure

side of the optic disc (the side nearest the temples). The ones responsible for peripheral vision are mainly found at the top, bottom, and nasal side of the disc, and it is theorized that these are the first to be damaged by elevated eye pressure. Unfortunately, these peripheral fibers can be damaged before any loss in vision can be noticed by the patient or discovered in an eye exam. When this loss of peripheral vision is detectable, the structural change that eye doctors see on the disc looks as if someone has excavated, or scooped out, part of the normally flat optic disc, making it resemble a cup (see figure 8.5).

At first this scooping is subtle and mild; in advanced glaucoma, however, the optic disc can become markedly excavated, as if someone had physically drilled out the center of its tissue. When this happens, as you can imagine, many nerve fibers have been lost and the loss of vision is severe.

Eye doctors often use the term *cupping* to refer to the relationship between the size of this scooping and the overall size of the optic nerve disc. The cup-to-disc ratio—basically, how much of the disc is damaged—is estimated by the eye doctor when he or she directly observes the optic nerve head using one of several techniques during an eye examination. Loss of vision—eye doctors often say "loss of visual field"—is found with increased degrees of cup-to-disc (C:D) ratio. The larger the C:D ratio, the greater the chance of visual field loss. A C:D ratio of .1 implies a relatively healthy optic nerve head with minimal cupping—an optic nerve head usually not associated with glaucoma. A ratio of .9, on the other hand, refers to a major degree of excavation and tissue loss, usually seen in advanced glaucoma. The C:D ratio and its progression over time are important measures for detecting and managing glaucoma.

Note: As always, there are exceptions. Some people have congenital forms of optic disc cupping that can mimic glaucoma. These normal variations, which are present from birth, aren't associated with glaucoma; but they can confuse an untrained observer, leading to misdiagnosis and unnecessary treatment for glaucoma that doesn't exist.

Classically, glaucoma's damage to the optic nerve head leads to peripheral, or side-vision, loss. And unfortunately, as stated before, this can be very difficult to detect in the early stages. Many people try to check this on their own, by placing their fingers far out to the sides of their vision. But this isn't a very precise gauge, and results aren't nearly as accurate as those produced by today's sophisticated tests, performed by specially trained observers.

Many years ago eye doctors relied on manual visual field tests to measure side vision, a process known as *perimetry*. (Testing devices are called *perimeters*.) Early perimetry consisted of holding small test objects to the side of a patient's vision, noting and then mapping what could or could not be seen. In recent years computers have automated perimetry testing, making it much more reliable; these sophisticated "visual field machines" can store vast amounts of information about someone's range of vision, greatly improving our ability to analyze and interpret the test results.

Caution: Because these computerized perimetry machines are so popular, they've also been bought by eye care providers who aren't terribly knowledgeable about how to use them or how to interpret their results—which means, unfortunately, that improper or inappropriate testing is not

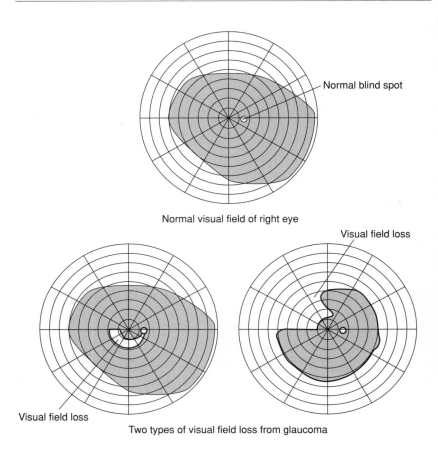

Normal blind spot

Normal visual field of right eye

Visual field loss

Visual field loss

Two types of visual field loss from glaucoma

Fig. 8.6.   Visual field loss from glaucoma

uncommon. Certain things can skew the test results, including testing patients while they are wearing their eyeglasses or checking someone's side vision without placing the person's proper eyeglass prescription in the perimeter of the testing field. Using pilocarpine, a kind of eye drop, can also cause misleading results.

In addition, some eye doctors may perform tests much more often than necessary. How often visual field tests need to be done is a question with no simple answer. In fact, there aren't many simple answers to questions about glaucoma, including the question of deciding whether someone really has it. Although automated visual field testing is reliable for assessing someone's peripheral vision, the value of this testing as a screening

Are You at Higher Risk for Glaucoma?

Risk factors include:

- Being over age fifty-five
- Having a family history of glaucoma
- Being very nearsighted
- Having diabetes
- Being African American
- Being Native American (according to some studies)

technique for glaucoma is debatable. Furthermore, visual field test results *alone* should never be used to diagnose or manage glaucoma.

Similarly, glaucoma screening tests—like those conducted at senior citizens' centers, shopping malls, or health fairs—are of rather limited benefit in detecting glaucoma. (Unfortunately, the old adage "You get what you pay for" is largely true here.) The big problem with such events is that they're often conducted by untrained observers, whose unenviable job is to screen a large number of people in a fixed amount of time, and who often rely on measurements of eye pressures and visual fields that are less accurate than those available in a doctor's office. Therefore, these glaucoma screenings do not replace a comprehensive eye examination for glaucoma performed by a trained eye doctor. This is especially true for people considered to be at higher risk for glaucoma than the general population (see box).

TREATING GLAUCOMA

Because glaucoma is a diverse collection of disorders with a common endpoint—a damaged optic nerve resulting in loss of vision—and because everybody is different, there is no one preferred form of treatment. In general, however, the basic goal of managing glaucoma is to lower someone's intraocular pressure—and keep it lowered—sufficiently to prevent further nerve damage and loss of vision.

Frequent Monitoring

At first, when you're beginning a new antiglaucoma medication or changing to a new regimen, you may require weekly or monthly monitoring of your intraocular pressures. Then, once a particular regimen seems to be doing its job—controlling eye pressure and stabilizing your visual field—your eye doctor will probably lengthen the time between visits to every three to six months or so. (Visual field testing may be performed less often, depending on such factors as your eye health, degree of vision loss, intraocular pressure readings, and the appearance of the optic disc. If you have severe glaucoma, this testing may be done more frequently.)

What's the point of such frequent checkups? Eye pressure is not a constant. Your doctor needs to monitor your intraocular pressure readings while you are on medication and also will occasionally need to take a reading after asking you *not* to take your medication. Another reason for frequent monitoring is that many patients become resistant, over time, to the effects of a particular antiglaucoma medication; despite faithful use of the eye drops, their intraocular pressure gradually sneaks back up to where it was before treatment. For such patients it's clearly important to detect this problem as soon as possible, so that they can be switched to a different type of medication. Also, your eye doctor needs to make sure that your vision isn't deteriorating by using perimetry and by watching for any significant changes in the appearance of the optic disc.

Note: Because eye pressures fluctuate constantly, even from morning to afternoon, it's a good idea to schedule your office visits at different times of the day. *Also, be sure to report any changes in your general health, any other medications you may be taking, or any other visual or medical symptoms that you feel may be important.*

Glaucoma Medications

Now, welcome to the world of eye drops.

There are two basic theories in lowering eye pressure. One is to *reduce the production* of aqueous fluid in the eye; the other is to *improve the drainage* of this fluid from the eye. All forms of antiglaucoma therapy are designed to do at least one of these.

Currently, the first line of treatment is to start glaucoma patients on antiglaucoma eye drops to lower the eye pressure. These drops can be used either alone or in combination with other eye drops. No matter what kind of eye drop you're taking, here's an important point to keep in mind: The eye can hold only about 20 percent of one drop. Therefore, it's customary to place *one drop in an eye at a time*, not two drops. If multiple eye drops are to be given around the same time, then they should be *spaced apart by about three to five minutes*—so that they can be absorbed properly, and to minimize the chances of washing out one drop with the next.

If you're taking a combination of eye drops, it may not matter much in which order you put them in. However, over the years we've found that taking the drops in one order rather than in the reverse order may reduce problems of burning or stinging associated with a particular drop. (This may be because one drop has more of an anesthetic or lubricating quality than the other.)

So, which drops will you take? Here's a brief discussion of some of the more popular "antiglaucomatous" eye drops, their dosages, and potential side effects.

Pilocarpine

Pilocarpine, the first eye drop developed for treating glaucoma (developed nearly 120 years ago), comes from a South American plant and generally produces few allergic or toxic reactions in people who take it. Pilocarpine is commercially available in strengths ranging from 0.5 percent to 10 percent; most glaucoma patients are prescribed strengths of between 1 percent and 6 percent. (Most doctors feel that there's a point of diminishing returns, in that concentrations above 4 percent don't effectively reduce pressure any more significantly than lower concentrations. However, this can vary from patient to patient; patients with dark irises, for instance, often require higher dosages.)

After it's administered, pilocarpine lowers intraocular pressure, or IOP, in about an hour, with its effectiveness peaking after an hour to an hour and a half and lasting about eight hours. It's usually given as one drop four times a day. Pilocarpine is also available in a once-daily gel, and in a slow-release ocular insert that's placed in the eye for a week at a time. You may want to discuss these alternatives with your doctor.

Pilocarpine's most common side effect is miosis, or a small pupil. This can cause diminished vision, because less light will be able to get into the eye. Other important side effects in the eye include browache, induced nearsightedness, and retinal detachments. (For more on warning signs of retinal detachments, see chapter 15.) Systemic, or bodily, side effects are rare but can include increased salivation, sweating, nausea, vomiting, diarrhea, and trouble breathing.

There are many other antiglaucoma drugs that have a pharmacological action similar or related to pilocarpine's. These include carbachol, physostigmine (Eserine), demecarium (Humorsol), isoflurophate (DFP, Floropryl), and echothiophate (Phospholine Iodide).

Epinephrine and Propine

Epinephrine is a hormone that's found naturally in the body; dipivalyl epinephrine (Propine) is a synthetic, inactive derivative of epinephrine that seems to be more effective in the eye. The exact mechanism by which they lower intraocular pressure is poorly understood; however, they seem to have an effect on *both* aqueous production and outflow. Epinephrine is available in three different forms: hydrochloride, borate, and bitartrate. Propine is converted by enzymes into epinephrine, which then lowers IOP. Because Propine is effective in lower concentrations than epinephrine, less of it is absorbed into the rest of the body.

In the eye, side effects seen with both of these drugs include irritated eyelids and conjunctiva in 10 to 15 percent of patients, and red eyes. This side effect is seen much less often with Propine because as a synthetic derivative of epinephrine, it is inactive when in contact with the external eye. It becomes active after passing into the eye, when it is then converted to epinephrine. Black deposits in the conjunctiva can also be observed in patients who have used epinephrine for a prolonged period of time. (These deposits are usually harmless; however, they can occasionally cause eye irritation and may need to be surgically removed.) Epinephrine and Propine can also cause cystoid macular edema, a fluid swelling of the macula, which can blur someone's central vision. (This has been noted in patients who've had cataract surgery or other procedures resulting in the loss of the eye's normal lens.) Fortunately, this side effect is usually reversible when the medication is stopped.

The pressure-lowering effect of epinephrine begins in one hour, peaks at about four hours, and lasts about twelve hours. Propine begins working within thirty minutes and has its maximum effect in one hour. Both are usually used twice daily. Because other antiglaucoma drops are known to be more effective, epinephrine and Propine are rarely first-line drugs for glaucoma. They are often used in combination with these other drugs, or alone in patients who can't tolerate other antiglaucoma drugs because of sensitivities or the risk of serious systemic side effects.

Note: Because both of these hormones have an effect on the cardiovascular system, epinephrine and Propine should be used with caution in patients with a history of rapid heartbeats or arrhythmia. They can induce tachycardia, extra heartbeats, elevated blood pressure, and chest pain due to angina. If you have a history of heart problems, it's essential that you discuss these risks with your eye doctor and your cardiologist.

Antiglaucoma medications related to epinephrine and Propine are isoproterenol, salbutamol, and norepinephrine.

Timoptic and Other Beta-Blockers

Timolol maleate (Timoptic) is known as a *beta adrenergic blocking agent*, or *beta-blocker*. Although its exact mechanism of action is not well understood, generally we know that Timoptic lowers intraocular pressure by blocking beta adrenergic receptors in the eye, which are important in the production of aqueous fluid.

Timoptic is a very effective antiglaucoma drug and today is one of the most popular drugs used in the United States to treat glaucoma—either alone or in combination with other medications. Like pilocarpine, Timoptic is more effective in lightly pigmented eyes. Studies have shown it to have a mean reduction in eye pressure of 30 to 33 percent. Several different medical centers looking at Timoptic use in patients with elevated eye pressures have also found that it reduced eye pressure below 22 millimeters of mercury more effectively than either pilocarpine or epinephrine used alone.

Timoptic has been available in solutions of 0.25 percent and 0.50 percent. Its pressure-lowering effect peaks after about two hours and lasts up to twenty-four hours. Typically it's given twice a day. Timoptic-XE 0.50 percent is a form now available as a suspension that has been shown to have a longer duration of action and is recommended as a once-a-day drop. As with other glaucoma drops, Timoptic seems to lose its effectiveness over time. Therefore, it is very important to have regular eye exams, so that your eye doctor can change your medication if this happens.

Timoptic's side effects in the eye are rare, but they include reduced tear production (which can cause dry eyes or make an existing dry-eye condition worse), red eyes due to hypersensitivity reactions, or corneal irritation.

Timoptic is related to propranolol (Inderal), metoprolol (Lopressor), and nadolol (Corgard), which are beta-blocker drugs often used to treat cardiovascular disease. Therefore, the systemic side effects of Timoptic are potentially life-threatening. *Again, it's a must for heart patients to discuss these implications thoroughly with their doctor.* Why? Because a drop placed in the eye can flow into the tear sac and then pass into the nose and eventually down to the back of the throat, where it's swallowed and absorbed into the body—possibly inducing or aggravating certain cardiovascular and pulmonary problems. In particular, Timoptic can lead to a slowing of the heart rate, congestive heart failure, decreased blood pressure, or lightheadedness and irregular heartbeat. Spasm of the lung's air passages is another important side effect. Fatigue, confusion, impotence, and depression have also been associated with Timoptic. Timoptic can also decrease the levels of "good" cholesterol (HDL) in the body. People with elevated "bad" cholesterol should discuss this with their doctor before using this drug for glaucoma.

Timoptic is also related to other beta-blocking ocular agents, including betaxolol (Betoptic), timolol hemihydrate (Betimol), carteolol (Ocupress), levobunolol (Betagan), and metipranolol (OptiPranolol). Each has advantages and disadvantages. Deciding which beta-blocker to use for a specific patient is not easy. Doctors need to take into consideration side effects, pressure-lowering effect, and price.

Betoptic is a beta-blocker that is more selective in its mode of action, causing fewer breathing problems. It is therefore often used in people with glaucoma who have a history of chronic obstructive pulmonary disease, or those who have developed breathing difficulties with Timoptic. Betoptic, because it is absorbed less by the body than other beta-blockers, appears to cause less fatigue, drowsiness, and depression. A drawback to its use, however, is that in new glaucoma patients and in those on chronic glaucoma therapy, Betoptic has been found to produce less intraocular pressure lowering when compared with other, less-selective, beta-blockers.

Betimol is a variation of Timoptic. Clinical studies have demonstrated that these two drugs have very similar potency and side effects. *Ocupress* has been found to have special receptor activity and, for reasons not clearly understood, may be a safer choice in people with coronary heart disease and with serum lipid imbalances. *Betagan* is a less selective beta-blocker with a long half-life (longer-lasting effect), in theory making it a better once-a-day product than Timoptic. It requires a larger drop size than Timoptic, and many doctors believe that it is therefore relatively expensive. *Opti-Pranolol* in many markets is the least expensive nonselective beta-blocker, with similar efficacy to Timoptic. Although ocular inflammation has been found to be a rare side effect of all topical beta-blockers, it appears to be most common with OptiPranolol.

Beta-blockers are very important drugs for the treatment of glaucoma. They are not all the same, and therefore careful consideration must be given when selecting them for patients.

Patients taking drops for glaucoma, especially Timoptic, should know about a technique called *punctal occlusion*, a way of administering eye drops that's been proven to minimize these potentially serious side effects by reducing the amount of medication that finds its way from the eye into the throat and circulation. Briefly, here's the technique: Place your forefinger at the nasal, or inside, corner of your eye, blocking the tear duct. With your other hand, put a drop of medication in the eye. Wipe away any excess drop with a tissue *before* releasing your forefinger's compression of the tear duct.

Iopidine and Alphagan

Apraclonidine (Iopidine) and brimonidine (Alphagan) represent a fairly new class of topical antiglaucoma drops called *alpha agonists*. They appear to lower intraocular pressure primarily by decreasing the production of aqueous humor, but they may also secondarily increase uveoscleral outflow (see the discussion of latanoprost below). Because Iopidine and Alphagan selectively stimulate *alpha-adrenergic receptors*—receptors that aren't found in large numbers in the heart and lungs—they have little effect on heart rate, blood pressure, and breathing. This means that they can be used —with caution—in people with cardiac and pulmonary problems, unlike beta-blockers such as Timoptic (see above), which can cause severe side effects in these individuals.

Both drugs begin lowering IOP within an hour, peak in about three hours, and are effective for eight to twelve hours. They are usually administered two or three times a day. Unfortunately, Iopidine's effectiveness significantly decreases with time—even after just a month. Because of this, it's mainly recommended for people already on maximal antiglaucoma medication (in combination with these or other medications), for a short period of time to control eye pressure in people awaiting a laser procedure or surgery. Iopidine has also been used to prevent postoperative pressure elevation after YAG laser procedures (see below). Alphagan was developed to be effective for a longer period than Iopidine and therefore is the better choice for long-term glaucoma management. It is also more selective for alpha receptor sites than Iopidine, further decreasing the chance for systemic cardiopulmonary side effects.

As mentioned above, although Iopidine and Alphagan have minimal effects on the heart and lungs, they should still be used with caution in people with hypertension, abnormal or slow heart rates, recent myocardial infarctions, history of strokes, or chronic renal failure. They may also cause an adverse reaction in people taking certain antidepressants. In the eye, the most common side effects of these drugs includes redness, itching, discomfort, and tearing.

Latanoprost

Latanoprost (Xalatan) is an exciting new antiglaucoma medication that recently became available. It is one of a new class of drugs, called *prostaglandin analogs,* now available to people in the United States. Latanoprost appears to act by increasing uveoscleral outflow or increasing aqueous humor absorption by the uveal tissues of the eye, particularly the ciliary body. Fluid in the eye is thus passed to the outside of the eye by way of the suprachoroidal space and sclera, and intraocular pressure is thereby lowered. This medication does not appear to have any effect on the production of aqueous fluid. Previous antiglaucoma medications have acted primarily by lowering intraocular pressure by decreasing the production of intraocular aqueous fluid or by increasing the outflow of aqueous drainage through the anterior chamber angle.

Latanoprost's unique primary mode of action makes this medication particularly useful as an adjunct with other glaucoma medications that work to lower eye pressure through different mechanisms. Furthermore, when latanoprost is used alone it has been shown to be potentially more effective than Timoptic, which is now commonly accepted by many as the initial treatment for glaucoma. This effect was also observed when latanoprost was used only once a day compared with Timoptic used twice a day. The ability to use latanoprost once a day, preferably at night—since intraocular pressure is usually at its highest during the early-morning hours—presents an added advantage, since people may well be more likely to use their glaucoma medication following this schedule. (Patient compliance—getting patients to use their medication—is a very common problem. Doctors and patients need to work together to address whatever it is that's interfering with compliance, whether it's schedule of drug applications, costs of medications, side effects of medications, or something else.)

You might wonder why all glaucoma patients aren't placed on latanoprost when they are first diagnosed. The reason, as you can probably guess, is side effects. Latanoprost does not often cause systemic or ocular side effects. Systemic effects—shortness of breath, a slowing of the heart rate, and so on—were observed less often with latanoprost than with Timoptic. On the other hand, latanoprost caused more eye redness than Timoptic. Of particular note, some people taking latanoprost who had mixed eye color—an iris that was blue-brown, gray-brown, green-brown, or yellow-brown—developed increased iris pigment, so that a green, blue, or light-colored eye turned brown. The long-term effects of this pigmentary change, if any, are still unknown. This has made many eye doctors hesitant to use latanoprost as a first-line drug in people with glaucoma.

Carbonic Anhydrase Inhibitors

Carbonic anhydrase inhibitors, or CAIs, block the production of aqueous fluid by inhibiting an enzyme called *carbonic anhydrase*, which acts on the eye's ciliary body. *Acetazolamide (Diamox)* and *methazolamide (Neptazane)* are well-known carbonic anhydrase inhibitors. They're prescription medications available in pill form as well as in intravenous and intramuscular preparations.

The pressure-lowering effect of Diamox usually begins in one to two hours, peaks at three to five hours, and lasts up to eight hours; Diamox also comes as a sustained-release capsule, which can last up to twenty-four hours. Neptazane is available in 25-milligram and 50-milligram pills. It begins working in about two hours, lasts about ten to eighteen hours, and is usually prescribed to be taken two or three times a day.

Recently, carbonic anhydrase inhibitors have become available as eye drops as well. *Dorzolamide hydrochloride (Trusopt)*, available in a 2 percent solution, is recommended for use three times a day. Its side effects in the eye include allergic reactions of the eyelids and conjunctiva. Also, because Trusopt is absorbed by the body, patients may note a bitter taste after administering a drop.

With pills, ocular side effects of carbonic anhydrase inhibitors are rare; however, increased nearsightedness has been reported. Systemic side effects are much more common and can include numbness and tingling in the extremities, weight loss, fatigue, kidney stones, and lowered blood levels of potassium, which can cause systemic problems and adverse drug effects. A rare form of anemia can also be caused by CAI use. You should review the full list of side effects with your doctor before beginning this drug. Also, carbonic anhydrase inhibitors are sulfonamides, which means they shouldn't be given to patients with known sulfa allergies. They're also not recommended for people with severe liver disease, those with advanced lung disease, and pregnant women. Finally, because carbonic anhydrase inhibitors may have an "additive effect"—which may magnify these side effects—it's not a good idea to combine the drops with pills.

Other Medications

Mannitol, glycerin, and *isosorbide* are three other medications. These are mainly used as short-term treatments in special, acute situations to lower eye pressures as quickly as possible. Generally they are administered either orally or intravenously for a rapid onset of action and work by drawing fluid from the eye into the bloodstream. At the time of this writing, there are several other topical medications on the horizon for the treatment of glaucoma.

Other Forms of Treatment

Lasers

An increasingly important tool for treating glaucoma, lasers have proven effective in both closed-angle and open-angle glaucoma.

Lasers in treating closed-angle glaucoma: Briefly, the trouble in closed-angle glaucoma is that the anterior chamber angle is narrowed or plugged by the root of the iris. As a result, aqueous fluid can't flow from its site of production, in the posterior chamber, out of the eye through the trabecular meshwork filter in the corner of the anterior chamber angle, and it "backs up," raising pressure within the eye.

Lasers provide a mechanical solution to the problem by making a hole, or *peripheral iridectomy* (PI), in the iris to improve the flow of aqueous from the posterior to the anterior chamber. It's like providing the aqueous with a short-cut to the trabecular meshwork. The PI relieves the pressure behind the iris, deepens the shallow anterior chamber and narrowed angle, and helps aqueous exit the trabecular meshwork and enter Schlemm's canal. Peripheral iridectomies are performed either with cutting lasers (called YAG lasers) or with burning lasers (argon lasers).

Candidates for PI include people with acute angle-closure glaucoma attacks (the sudden onset of painful glaucoma described above) and chronic closed-angle glaucoma. Occasionally PIs are also performed prophylactically (as preventive measures) on people with narrowed anterior chamber angles to preclude the sudden or gradual buildup of pressure.

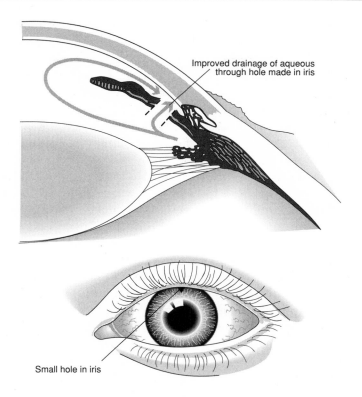

Improved drainage of aqueous through hole made in iris

Small hole in iris

Fig. 8.7. Peripheral iridectomy

A PI is painless, usually takes less than half an hour, and requires no preoperative testing or postoperative restrictions. Complications are minimal and may vary depending on the state of the eye at the time of the procedure. For example, bleeding from blood vessels in the iris is a common and usually limited occurrence after a laser PI. But in patients with an acute angle-closure attack, this complication can occur more often and may be more difficult to control. Other potential complications of peripheral iridectomies include a temporary elevation in eye pressure, inflammation of the eye (iritis), and temporary blurred vision. (As always, be sure to discuss all risks with your eye doctor before undergoing this or any form of treatment.)

Lasers in treating open-angle glaucoma: Argon lasers are also used in open-angle glaucoma. In several studies these "burning" lasers have been shown to lower intraocular pressures by as much as 10 millimeters of mercury for at least eighteen months in a statistically significant number of patients with elevated eye pressure. This effect varies greatly depending on the type of glaucoma being treated.

In this procedure, called *laser trabeculoplasty,* a specially designed mirrored contact lens is placed on an anesthetized cornea. The surgeon can then use a magnified slit lamp to get a good view of the trabecular meshwork. Carefully guiding the laser, the surgeon makes between fifty and a hundred "spots," or tiny burns, on the trabecular meshwork. Exactly how these burns lower eye pressures is not known, but current thinking is that they cause the minuscule fibers of connective tissue in the meshwork to contract, opening up sieve-like spaces through which the aqueous fluid can seep into Schlemm's canal. The treatment is painless and usually takes about half an hour.

Complications, as with laser PIs, are rare and mainly include a short-term rise in eye pressure and the development of scar tissue in the vicinity of the trabecular meshwork (which can make the drainage problem even worse). One drawback is that the results aren't immediate; it may take six to ten weeks before eye pressures get lower. Another is that, unfortunately, the effects don't seem permanent; studies have found that the results last for only about five years in about 46 percent of patients. In some cases people undergo repeat laser procedures, but results have not been shown to be consistently successful.

Therefore, laser trabeculoplasty is not a first-line choice in the treatment of glaucoma. It's usually done after medical therapies have failed to prevent advancing vision loss, or in an effort to delay the need for surgical intervention. Not infrequently patients still need some of their medications despite laser treatment. It is, however, an important treatment option in patients who aren't good candidates for surgery.

Glaucoma Surgery

There are several surgical approaches designed to lower eye pressure. Currently, these techniques are mainly used when medical and laser treatments fail—when, in other words, IOP can't be lowered sufficiently to halt the loss of vision.

Trabeculectomy, the most commonly performed surgical procedure for glaucoma, is basically the surgical creation of a new drain in the eye—a custom-built "trap door" in the sclera of the eyeball. The aqueous fluid collects under the conjunctiva, forming a "blister" of fluid, and is gradually

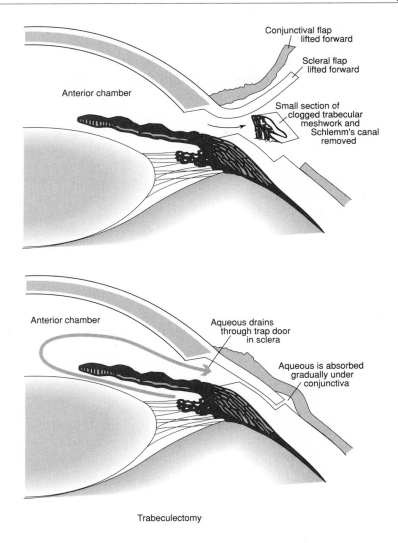

Trabeculectomy

Fig. 8.8. Trabeculectomy

absorbed into the circulation on the outside of the eyeball. Eventually a permanent fistula, or hole, develops at the trap door, maintaining a constant outflow of aqueous from the eye and lowering IOP with or without medication.

Note: This surgical technique is not without risks and should be performed only by those experienced in this surgery and the management of potential postoperative complications.

Surgically, a trabeculectomy tries to create a fine balance in the eye between *too much* and *too little* outflow of aqueous under a surgical tissue flap (the trap door). Thus, the days and weeks after this type of surgery can often be stormy. For example, *too much filtration* can initially lead to abnormally soft eyes and flat anterior chambers. If not corrected, this situation can lead to eye problems and result in permanent vision loss. The postoperative management of trabeculectomies—as the eye heals and establishes filtration through this new drain—often requires vigilance and patience by doctors as well as patients.

Another risk is that in some people scar tissue may form in this artificial drain, sealing the trap door. Doctors often use medications such as 5-FU and mitomycin during or after the procedure to help avert this problem in patients considered to be at higher risk. (Doctors can tell by examining them which patients are at higher risk.)

Other, rare, complications include infection, bleeding, and the development of a cataract in the operated eye. Before consenting to a trabeculectomy, it's important to weigh carefully the benefits of lowered IOP against the potential risks of the procedure.

These risks aside, the long-term results of trabeculectomies for maintaining eye pressure are good. No further progression of glaucoma can be expected in 80 percent of people after surgery, with 90 percent maintaining stable vision. As many as 40 percent of people may not ever need any medications for pressure control after the surgery, although many still require some eye drops.

What's Best for You?

Which brings us to this question: Could we do a better job of managing glaucoma?

Traditionally in the United States, glaucoma treatment has begun with a *single eye drop* to lower intraocular pressure. If this does not fix the problem—if it fails to lower pressure and halt vision loss—then another eye drop is usually added to the regimen. Each drop is evaluated alone or in combination with other eye drops, as doctors struggle to find the best regimen for each patient. And even when that perfect mix is found, patients must still be carefully monitored, because—in a phenomenon frustrating to both doctors and patients—these medications often lose their effectiveness over time or the glaucoma simply becomes harder to control.

Now, on to Plan B: if eye drops don't work to control intraocular pressure, or if the nerve fibers in the optic disc continue to deteriorate despite lowered eye pressure, then doctors usually consider topical or oral CAI medications. Plan C includes lasers and surgery, which are usually reserved for advanced glaucoma or for eyes that don't adequately respond to drops and pills. But studies done in other countries have suggested that this may not be the best way to go. Instead, these studies suggest, the most effective way to control glaucoma may be to perform a surgical trabeculectomy *before* attempting management with medical and laser treatments. *Trabeculectomy may ultimately produce better intraocular pressure control for a longer period of time, with less overall cost to the patient and with fewer side effects.*

The National Institutes of Health recently began the Collaborative Investigational Glaucoma Treatment Study, or CIGTS, designed to evaluate whether newly diagnosed glaucoma patients truly are best treated by the traditional medical approach (beginning with eye drops) or by surgical trabeculectomy. The study should give us an answer to this important question within the next several years.

Also, although it's generally accepted that IOP must be lowered in patients with glaucoma, *by exactly how much* is different for each patient. To make matters more complex, studies have shown that other factors, such as the level of IOP and the degree of optic disc cupping at the time of diagnosis, are also very important. It's probably due to some of these other factors that glaucoma continues to worsen in some patients despite vigorous lowering of IOP. People with normotensive glaucoma (see above), on the other hand, seem to be more susceptible to developing optic nerve damage at intraocular pressures considered to be normal for the majority of the population. Even more perplexing, some people, despite elevated intraocular pressures, never seem to develop vision loss or other signs of glaucoma.

The Ocular Hypertension Study, a national prospective clinical trial, is currently studying this latter group of patients. The results of this study may give us a better grasp of the relationship of eye pressure to the development and progression of glaucoma and help us understand some of these important contributing factors.

Some Questions You May Have about Glaucoma

Can glaucoma be caused by reading too much, wearing contact lenses, or even a poor diet?

Although no one really knows why some people develop glaucoma, it definitely does not appear to be related to any of these activities. Age, family history, and race are the most significant risk factors for developing glaucoma.

Will I go blind from glaucoma?

When glaucoma is discovered early, the vast majority of people with glaucoma will not go blind from it, because of the excellent array of treatment options available today. Early detection is the key to good glaucoma management, and regular eye exams by qualified professionals are very important.

Does glaucoma run in families?

Yes; at least, having a family history of glaucoma raises someone's risk of developing the condition. Other factors that may make someone more prone to developing glaucoma are having diabetes, being African American (African Americans have a particularly high prevalence of glaucoma), being over age fifty-five, or being very nearsighted.

I have hypertension. Does this mean my eye pressure is high as well?

Although elevated blood pressure can cause elevated eye pressure, for most people these are two separate issues; most of the people who have elevated eye pressure don't have it because they also have hypertension. Elevated eye pressure is also not related to any of the things we commonly think of as raising our blood pressure—increased stress, anxiety, or diet.

Can my eye pressure change from one day to the next?

Absolutely—and not only from one day to the next, but from one hour to the next! Eye pressures are usually highest in the morning. Because of this constant fluctuation, it's important to vary the times of your eye examinations, so that your doctor can get a better overall impression of your eye pressures right after taking medications as well as some time after taking medications.

If I forget to take my drops, will this really cause me to have more problems from glaucoma?

Missing an occasional eye drop will not greatly affect your glaucoma, since many of the medications have prolonged effects. Mild spikes in eye pressure due to a missed drop also do not appear to cause great damage to nerve fibers. But stopping your eye drops for long periods—like weeks or months—can lead to irreversible visual field loss.

I have a cataract and glaucoma. Can I have surgery for both at the same time?

Yes. Today's modern microsurgical techniques make it possible for surgeons to perform both of these delicate operations at the same time. However, this "combined" surgery is performed only after the eye doctor carefully considers the severity of the person's glaucoma and cataracts.

9

Age-Related Macular Degeneration

Macular degeneration may be the most baffling and frustrating eye disorder there is.

The official name of this condition is age-related macular degeneration (ARMD), but there's no official, universally accepted definition to go along with it. It's mainly found in adults over age fifty. Some people get it worse than others, but every older person has it to some degree. At its most devastating, ARMD advances unrelentingly, causing severe visual impairment and often overwhelming challenges to the quality of life. It is the cause of severe visual impairment in at least 2 percent of Americans over age sixty-five.

How does all this happen, who's at risk for developing ARMD, and can anything be done to stop its damage? The answers to these questions begin in the retina.

WHEN THE RETINA BEGINS TO FAIL

Basically, ARMD can be thought of as the aging of the outermost layer of the retina, the *retinal pigment epithelium*. Although we often say that the retina is like wallpaper lining the back of the eye, this doesn't tell the whole story. Unlike a single sheet of wallpaper, the retina has many integrated layers of tissue and cells, all intricately connected to each other, all working together, with the brain, to turn random images of light into coherent vision. (Remarkably, all of these layers of the retina are literally paper-thin, between 0.1 and 0.5 millimeter thick.)

The retina's foundation is the *sclera*, the "white" of the eyes. The retina and its supporting tissues line the entire surface of the inner white sclera inside the eyeball (see figure 1.1A). The next layer is the *choroid* (which isn't really part of the retina at all), rich in blood vessels. The choroid is like a blood-filled sponge—a network of vascular tissue that serves as a lifeline to the retinal layers that lie upon it, a crucial supplier of nutrients and oxygen. The choroid's constant and rapid blood flow helps maintain a fairly steady temperature and oxygen supply within the retina.

Next comes *Bruch's membrane*, a thin wafer that separates the choroid from the retinal layers above it. Right on top of Bruch's membrane, like a single layer of bricks on cement, are the retina's *pigment epithelial cells*. These important cells transport vital nutrients and other chemicals back and forth between the choroid below and the retinal tissues above. They also serve as trash collectors, removing by-products of the photoreceptors, which lie above and beside them.

The *photoreceptors* are the crucial cells in the retina that convert light energy into nerve impulses that travel to the brain and produce vision. These specialized cells come in two basic forms: rods and cones. The *rods* make it possible for us to see in dim light. The *cones*, which function in bright light, also provide visual acuity—so that we can read, for example— and color vision. These photoreceptors, plus the several (about seven or eight) layers of tissue and nerves that lie above them, plus all of their con- nections leading to the brain, make up the *sensory retina*. At the sensory retina's innermost core lies the *nerve fiber layer*, the final pathway of all nerve impulses that leave the eye. Here nerve fibers meet to form a "nerve trunk"—like electrical wires intertwined to form a thick cable—called the *optic nerve*, which connects directly to the brain.

As you can see in figure 1.1, panels A and B, the retina stretches to

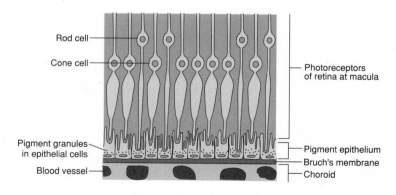

Rod cell

Cone cell

Photoreceptors of retina at macula

Pigment granules in epithelial cells

Blood vessel

Pigment epithelium

Bruch's membrane

Choroid

Fig. 9.1. Microscopic section of the macular region

cover about two-thirds of the inside of the back of the eyeball. Its most significant region by far is the *macula*, located just next to the optic nerve and between the arcades of the major superior and inferior temporal retinal blood vessels. The macula is responsible for central vision, including such functions as reading and fine visual acuity. Made up largely of cones, it's also important for color vision.

Many retinal problems can affect the macula, creating difficulties with central fine vision, reading, and color vision. The macula's *foveal region*, right in the middle, is primarily responsible for our sharpest vision. This region contains an especially dense concentration of cone cells; the cone cell population gradually decreases as we move toward the *peripheral retina*, which consists mainly of rods and is important in night vision. The peripheral retina, as its name suggests, is also very involved in side vision. (People with macular disease often have poor central vision but normal side vision, because their peripheral retina remains healthy.)

TYPES OF MACULAR DEGENERATION

As noted above, there is no universally accepted definition of age-related macular degeneration. But most eye specialists agree that ARMD includes certain changes in the retinal pigment epithelium and Bruch's membrane of the macula. All of these changes are seen in most older individuals, but they may be found in some people as early as their forties and fifties.

There are two basic kinds of ARMD: dry and wet.

The Dry Form

The dry, or *atrophic*, form of ARMD features slowly progressive, degenerative changes in the retinal pigment epithelial cells, Bruch's membrane, and the choroid. It's not generally agreed upon as to which of these layers begins to deteriorate first. One theory, held by many eye researchers, is that age-related macular degeneration is an exaggerated form of the normal aging process of the retinal pigment epithelial cells. Remember that we described these cells as a single layer of bricks built upon Bruch's membrane? Well, in normal aging—think of any time-worn brick house—these "bricks" gradually undergo degenerative changes. They weaken, change shape, lose their color, and, occasionally, disintegrate. As these retinal pig-

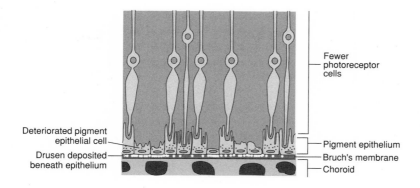

Fig. 9.2. Microscopic section of dry age-related macular degeneration

ment epithelial cells slowly change, so do the overlying photoreceptors. Over time they too lose their shape and configuration; they also begin to dwindle in number. Since photoreceptors are the main cells responsible for vision, it's not surprising that gradual visual impairment can result from all these changes. To make matters worse, a vicious cycle seems to develop: as the retinal pigment epithelial cells deteriorate, so do photoreceptors, and

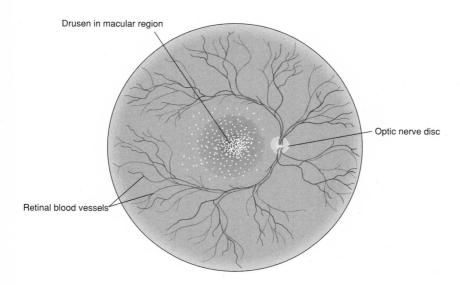

Fig. 9.3. Drusen of the retina

A.

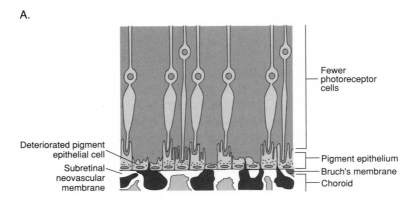

Fewer
photoreceptor
cells

Deteriorated pigment
epithelial cell

Subretinal
neovascular
membrane

Pigment epithelium

Bruch's membrane

Choroid

Fig. 9.4.   (A) Microscopic section of wet age-related macular degeneration, showing new blood vessels growing from choroid into retina; (B) visual effects from age-related macular degeneration and disciform scar

as photoreceptors degenerate, they release debris, which builds up beneath the retinal pigment epithelium, generally near Bruch's membrane, causing further cell malfunction and loss.

Accumulated deposits form *drusen*, which look like tiny yellowish dots in the retina (see figure 9.3). Drusen exist, studies have shown, in the eyes of most adults. But over time, in people with ARMD these deposits can become more pronounced and can crop up more frequently, prompting changes in the retinal pigment epithelial cells. And this, in turn, begets more retinal degeneration. (Drusen are often considered the hallmark of dry, or atrophic, ARMD. However, perplexingly, some people have changes in their retinal pigment epithelium without obvious drusen.) Eventually, as photoreceptors also become involved in this slow degenerative process, vision begins to deteriorate. *Note:* Although vision may be significantly impaired, people with this form of ARMD usually don't progress to the point of being legally blind.

The Wet Form

The wet, or *exudative*, form of ARMD is a faster, more aggressive process that can have a much greater impact on vision. It's not nearly as common, but its impact can be much more serious. (Although only about 10 percent of people with ARMD have this form, it accounts for 80 percent

B.

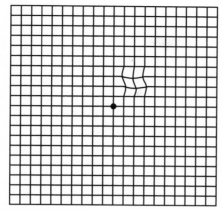

Distortion of Amsler grid from age-related macular degeneration

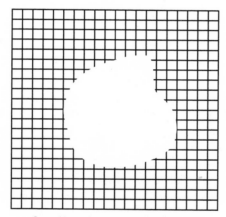

Central loss of vision from disciform scar

of the severe vision loss caused by the disorder.) Unfortunately, both the dry and wet forms of ARMD can occur in the same person—even in the same eye!

For reasons we don't yet understand, about 10 percent of people with "dry" changes can suddenly develop fresh threats to the macula: newly formed blood vessel membranes that begin in the choroid. Some scientists believe that these membranes may develop in response to inflammation in the choroid or Bruch's membrane, as a result of the degeneration described above. Others suggest that retinal pigment epithelial cells somehow inhibit the growth of new blood vessels in the choroid—and that as these cells degenerate, this inhibiting effect is lost, allowing unbridled growth.

Whatever the reason, these blood vessel membranes, called *subretinal neovascular membranes*, begin in the choroid under the retina. As they grow, like unchecked weeds in a garden, they tend to poke through Bruch's membrane and to invade the retinal pigment epithelium. Simply put, they can devastate the retina. They can cause fluid to seep through Bruch's membrane, forming little raised "blisters," called *retinal pigment epithelial detachments*. They can also cause fluid to collect in the sensory retina, disrupting the function of the rods and cones. These membranes, which often bleed and grow fibrous tissue, can cause severe scarring of the macula—and, thus, visual impairment. This central macular disfiguration is often referred to as a *disciform scar.*

WHO'S AT RISK?

ARMD affects an estimated 3.5 million older Americans. (One Massachusetts study, the Framingham Eye Study, conducted on a group of predominantly Caucasian individuals, estimated that age-related macular degeneration affected about 6 percent of adults between ages sixty-four and seventy-four, and nearly 20 percent of those over age seventy-four. Other studies have suggested that the incidence is 10 percent and 30 percent, respectively.) The National Eye Institute of the National Institutes of Health blames ARMD (mostly the wet form) for more than sixteen thousand new cases of legal blindness *each year.* ARMD is considered the major cause of severe vision loss in older adults in the United States and other countries including Canada, England, and Australia. Unlike cataracts, which cause a *reversible* form of vision loss, age-related macular degeneration's damage is irreversible. Even glaucoma and diabetic retinopathy, two other well-known causes of serious vision problems in people over age fifty, are much more treatable.

Who's at risk? Well, despite several studies attempting to identify predisposing factors, there's not much enlightenment in this area. The most obvious risk factor remains age. We do know a few generalities. The disease is more common in women than men. Heredity also seems to be a risk factor; if you have a family history of age-related macular degeneration, you should have a careful eye examination done by a specialist familiar with the diagnosis and treatment of this disorder. People with blue eyes, especially Caucasians, seem more susceptible.

Other risk factors linked to ARMD—but definitely not proven to cause it—include cigarette smoking, cardiovascular disease, and high blood pressure. Lifetime exposure to sunlight may also be a factor, some studies have suggested. People may become more susceptible directly, through the sun's damage to retinal cells, or indirectly, through an inability of the retinal cells to repair themselves after sunlight-caused damage. (Just as the sun damages unprotected skin, it can also damage unprotected eyes.) Although in theory sunglasses may modify sunlight's effect on the retina, no definitive, long-term studies have been conducted to prove this.

The role of vitamins and minerals has also been a subject of scientific controversy. Theoretically these may also protect the retina against sun damage. Studies in animals and humans have suggested that there may be an association between retinal phototoxicity (cell damage caused by light) and levels of such vitamins as A, E, and C.

Because the wet form of ARMD can result in such devastating vision loss, scientists have tried to identify specific risk factors associated with its development. One thing they've found is that the *type* and *extent* of drusen and retinal pigment epithelial changes can help predict the development of subretinal neovascular membranes. Large, soft drusen—especially when found in both eyes and accompanied by significant epithelial changes— raise someone's odds of developing these membranes. People who already have a subretinal neovascular membrane in one eye are also more likely to develop one in the other eye.

PREVENTION: CAN NUTRITION MAKE A DIFFERENCE?

As to prevention—again, much speculation, little concrete information. Most studies on the treatment of subretinal neovascular membranes have served mainly to emphasize our limitations and inability to control this devastating process. This has led many to search for new treatment pathways, and to seek preventive measures.

One of these new avenues of study is nutrition—a long-neglected area of research. Frankly, aside from what our mothers always told us about the benefits of eating carrots, we don't know much about the preventive effects of vitamin supplements on such problems as macular degeneration and cataracts. On the other hand, we do know a fair amount about the effects of vitamin *deficiencies* on vision and eye health. From animal studies we've learned that dietary deficiencies in vitamins A and E can cause the retina to degenerate. Other studies, in rats, have suggested that vitamin C may have a protective effect against sun damage to retinas. How does this information relate to the onset of age-related macular degeneration? We don't know. The Baltimore Longitudinal Study of Aging, the Eye Disease Case Control Study, the Beaver Dam Eye Study, and other human studies have suggested—but not proven—a link between age-related macular degeneration and such antioxidants as vitamin E, vitamin C, and beta-carotene.

Another clinical trial, investigating the effect of oral zinc supplements on the progression of ARMD, has suggested a beneficial effect. The Age-Related Eye Disease Study, conducted by the National Eye Institute, is a large, multicentered clinical trial designed to probe these suggested links between diet supplements and such eye diseases as cataracts and ARMD in forty-five hundred older Americans, who will receive either nutrient supplements or a placebo. (Neither the investigators heading the study nor the patients will know who's getting what.) The supplements contain concentrations of antioxidants and trace metals. Participants will be examined regularly, at least twice a year, for ten years. The results of this study should give us much better insight into the role of nutrition in eye disease.

SIGNS AND SYMPTOMS OF ARMD

Age-related macular degeneration, like many other eye disorders, is at first a dangerously silent, stealthy process. By themselves, drusen and retinal pigment epithelial changes usually don't affect vision. Even when drusen become large and pronounced, they rarely cause a noticeable problem; neither do pigment epithelial changes in the retina. However, central reading vision does become affected over time as these changes become more severe and involve the foveal region. For many people the first signs of trouble may be that when they're reading or looking at straight edges, such as table tops or patterns on clothing, the lines look crooked or wavy; this is usually more pronounced in one eye than the other. Later, reading becomes particularly difficult as letters and words become distorted. Other people notice that their eyes have trouble adjusting from bright sunshine to a dimly lit room; people with advanced age-related macular degeneration often need a few minutes to adapt to this change in lighting.

The Importance of Early Detection and Regular Monitoring

If you've been diagnosed with age-related macular degeneration, it's essential that your vision be monitored regularly. Your eye examinations should include a careful dilated retinal evaluation by an ophthalmologist who is very familiar with this disorder and its clinical stages. If you're considered to be at high risk for developing subretinal neovascular membranes, you may need eye examinations as often as every three to four months. If your retinal changes are less advanced, you may need to be examined only every four to six months.

Many eye doctors advocate home tests of visual acuity and function as a do-it-yourself means of monitoring macular degeneration's progression. The most popular means of doing this is called the *Amsler grid* (see figure 9.4B). As described in chapter 3, this is a black-and-white grid, observed at a distance of about fourteen inches with your normal reading glasses or bifocals (see figure 3.4). You should test each eye separately and as often as every day if you're a person at high risk for wet ARMD. Be sure to report anything unusual to your eye doctor immediately; this includes a loss of clarity, distortion, or waviness of the lines. Any changes may indicate a progression in macular degeneration—most important, the development of subretinal neovascular membranes; and these, if detected early enough, may be amenable to treatment.

Why is early detection important, if macular degeneration isn't usually treatable? A good question. Although there is no treatment for the dry form of ARMD, lasers can sometimes be used successfully to treat the new membranes that develop in the wet form. *And if this is the case for you, early detection and treatment may mean the difference between useful sight and legal blindness.*

For patients with age-related macular degeneration, a basic eye exam is often inadequate to establish whether these membranes are present underneath the retina. In patients in whom these membranes are suspected— from the patient's history, for instance, or because of retinal changes— imaging techniques including fundus photography and a fluorescein angiogram can help detect their often elusive presence. The fluorescein angiogram (see chapter 3), an essential tool in evaluation and treatment, helps us distinguish between normal and abnormal blood vessels in the retina. Since these new blood vessels develop *below* the retinal pigment epithelium—which means we can't see them with the naked eye—the fluorescein dye study helps reveal their location and extent, especially for laser treatment. It's also used after laser treatment, to make sure that the membrane has been successfully treated, and to monitor patients closely after treatment, to spot the earliest sign that the problem is recurring (see below).

Other monitoring techniques have been investigated over the years but have proven less successful than fluorescein angiography. One promising new technique, however, may be computer-enhanced indocyanine green angiography, which uses video imaging to study blood flow in the choroid and retina.

TREATING ARMD

This is a short section, because the vast majority of eyes with macular degeneration, dry or wet, can't be helped by any form of treatment. In fact, there are currently *no* treatments available for the dry form, the one that affects most people with macular degeneration.

Lasers

Although laser treatment has been shown to be successful for patients with the wet form of macular degeneration (the subretinal neovascular membranes), few people—an estimated one out of every ten—are diagnosed soon enough or considered good candidates for the procedure.

Much of our information on the natural history and treatment of subretinal neovascular membranes comes from the Macular Photocoagulation Study, a large clinical trial conducted by the National Eye Institute. In this study, argon lasers, in a procedure called *argon laser photocoagulation treatment*, were used on membranes of various sizes and locations in the macula. Investigators in the study found that 60 percent of the patients with well-defined subretinal neovascular membranes *close to but not involving the foveal region* of the macula developed severe visual impairment within three to five years. As might be expected, this percentage increased in patients with subretinal neovascular membranes directly underneath the fovea.

Laser treatment has been shown to be effective for some, but not all, patients with subretinal neovascular membranes. In the study, people with well-defined subretinal neovascular membranes *outside the foveal region* did better—in other words, they had less severe vision loss—with laser treatment than people who received no treatment. *Note:* Some people who received laser treatment still lost their vision, sometimes because of the laser treatment itself. Also, the laser treatment didn't always prevent vision from deteriorating further. Thus, in this study, laser treatment merely *reduced* someone's odds of severe vision loss. It didn't eliminate the risk entirely, but it did seem to help many of the people who received it.

Another fact of the laser treatment is that, even in the best cases, it destroys retinal tissue. For a surgeon to do a good job attacking the subretinal neovascular membrane, it's inevitable that some of the healthy retina will be lost as well. And often this results in a permanent visual blind spot. (The size and location of this blind spot depend on the position and extent of the subretinal neovascular membrane.) Another frustrating fact of laser treatment is that the membranes often grow back. The recurrence rate has been estimated to be as high as 42 percent within the first year, and as high as 53 percent within the second year. So if you're considering laser treatment, make sure you discuss the risks—and exactly what you stand to gain and lose—thoroughly with your surgeon. For some people this treatment can be more devastating than the disease.

Surgery

At this time surgical approaches to age-related macular degeneration are purely investigational—and controversial. Retinal specialists attempting to treat subretinal neovascular membranes surgically haven't met with much success. Retinal transplants have also been tried by many, but so far we've been stymied by two basic problems. One of them is rejection: the eye—which does very well with corneal transplants, because they don't involve many blood vessels—tends not to accept someone else's retina without a fight. The other problem is with retinal cell regeneration and differentiation: the cells don't work as they should after they are replaced in the eye. And finally, the ultimate functional practicality of retinal transplants remains questionable, since transplanted cells must also be able to reestablish and maintain the many complex nerve connections to the brain. Computer microchips implanted on the retinal surface are also being investigated as a way of restoring vision in people with severe forms of macular degeneration.

But many people have high hopes for the future of surgical treatment of macular degeneration. Many scientists remain optimistic about the potential of retinal transplants—one day—to *restore* vision in people with severe macular degeneration.

Other Treatments

Another exciting area of research in macular degeneration—at least in the wet form of it—centers around medical treatments. Can drugs help quell the recurrence of new vessel membranes after laser treatment? Or better yet, can they block their growth in the first place? Thalidomide may somehow inhibit the growth of subretinal neovascular membranes, and scientists are currently studying the use of this drug in treatment. Other treatments under investigation include dye-assisted photocoagulation and radiation therapy. These techniques may enhance doctors' ability to more accurately and precisely treat subretinal neovascular membranes.

THERE'S NO GOOD WAY to measure age-related macular degeneration's true impact—its threat to patients' independence and the burdens it often creates for family, friends, and society.

But even though there's no cure, yet, for age-related macular degeneration, there are many things patients can do to retain independence and quality of life. For one thing, there are visual aids: glasses, magnifiers, low-vision devices, and large-print materials (see chapter 19). There are agencies and services whose whole purpose is to help people with "low vision." You owe it to yourself and your family to see what they have to offer.

And finally, there's counseling, which really can help. The tremendous value of counselors and support groups is often underestimated because too often the enormous psychological impact of vision loss is overlooked by doctors as well as patients. For many patients and their families, simply knowing that they're not alone can mean a world of difference.

PART IV

Other
Eye Problems
Diagnosis and Treatment

10

The Eyelids

Their job seems simple enough: Open, shut. Blink—and in the process protect the eye from foreign particles, keep it from becoming too dry. What could possibly go wrong here? Well, there are several problems that can occur in the eyelids, ranging from benign dermatitis to malignant tumors. Here are some of the most common.

ALLERGIC DERMATITIS (RED, SCALY, ITCHY EYELIDS)

We all know what "allergy eyes" are: inflamed, itchy, and watery (see chapter 12). But an allergic reaction can also cause scaly, red, itchy skin outside the eye, and on the eyelids.

Allergic dermatitis is what happens when the skin of the eyelids becomes inflamed by an allergic reaction. It usually involves a miserable cycle of itching, rubbing, and dryness—followed by still more itching, rubbing, irritation, and even peeling and cracking of the skin. (*Note:* Another condition with a similar name, infectious dermatitis, is a different problem altogether. As its name suggests, the trouble here is an infection in the skin, and you can tell the difference between these two forms of dermatitis pretty easily: allergic dermatitis itches; infectious dermatitis hurts. The treatment differs as well: infectious dermatitis is treated by antibiotics and warm compresses.)

Treatment: To break the unpleasant cycle of itchiness and peeling, you'll probably be told to apply cold compresses (to decrease swelling of tissues) four times a day (or more often, if possible), and to use topical drops or ointments as well as oral drugs such as antihistamines. Your doctor might also prescribe a steroid-containing ointment for use in and around the eye. *Note:* Because ointments and creams used *near* the eye almost always work their way *into* the eye, make sure that whatever you're putting on your eyelids is *specifically for eye problems*. (If your allergic dermatitis is just on your face but not near your eyes, you can use mild over-the-counter steroid skin creams. But beware of long-term use of any steroid preparation—even one prescribed for short-term use by your eye doctor. Using a steroid cream regularly for months or years—even when it's just applied to your eyelid and not technically *in* your eye—can lead to elevated eye pressure and glaucoma.)

Hives: Eat the wrong food, and you may experience yet another allergic reaction on the eyelids: hives. Like hives elsewhere on the skin, these crazy dots or bumps seem to appear out of nowhere. They're red, extremely itchy mounds that can be as small as a kernel of corn or as large as a quarter (or even larger). Their only redeeming feature is that they usually don't last long and tend to go away on their own, or with the help of cold compresses and antihistamines.

BLEPHARITIS (INFLAMMATION OF THE EYELIDS)

Have you ever looked into the mirror and noticed that your eyelashes had crust or flakes in them—especially near the bottom, where they grow out of the eyelid? Or perhaps you've noticed a perennial dusting of flaky particles inside your eyeglasses. Maybe you're prone to recurrent sties, or the edges of your eyelids seem chronically red or pink. Do your eyes sometimes feel gritty and your eyelids heavy, especially when you read—even a spellbinding novel? All of these problems can be associated with *blepharitis,* or inflammation of the eyelids—a distinctly unglamorous condition that can be summed up as "eyelash dandruff."

Several things can make this happen. By far the most common is seborrhea, a disorder of the oil-making sebaceous glands—in this case, the ones at the base of the eyelids—that causes them to secrete more oil than usual. People who have seborrhea elsewhere—on the scalp, brow, or face—and/or oily skin may also be prone to this form of blepharitis, which is not infectious.

People with seborrheic blepharitis often have a secondary bacterial infection on their eyelids, however. Because more than one problem is at work here, this is called a *mixed blepharitis.* This infection, in turn, can cause trouble of its own—namely, chronic conjunctivitis (see chapter 12),

Lid Hygiene and Warm Compresses

How to give your eyelids a gentle bath:

- Place a drop of baby shampoo—it's gentle on the eyes—on a clean cloth, add water, and make a mild lather. (Eyelid scrubs, available at drugstores, can also be used.)
- Close your eyes (this is important!).
- Gently rub your lashes, going "with the grain": use a *downward* motion on your upper lashes and an *upward* motion on your lower lashes.
- Rinse thoroughly with warm water.
- Repeat at least twice a day, or as directed by your eye doctor.

How to apply a warm compress:

- Make a barber's towel: place a clean cloth in warm—but not too hot—water, and wring it out slightly.
- Place the cloth over your *closed eye.*
- When the cloth becomes cool, repeat the previous steps.
- Keep this up for at least ten to twenty minutes at a time.
- Do this at least twice a day.

with recurrent corneal infections. Its symptoms may include extra sensitivity to bright light, pain, tearing, redness, blurred vision, and mucous discharge from the eye. Worse, the bacteria can infect the glands of the eyelid margins and lead to recurrent sties and chalazia (see below). Misdirected, broken, and missing eyelashes are also common with this infection.

Treatment: Blepharitis is often a chronic condition, so our two goals are to *get* it under control and then to *keep* it that way. Lid hygiene and warm compresses (see box) are the mainstay of treatment for blepharitis, especially the seborrheic form. Cleaning the eyelash bases and applying warm compresses regularly will cut the buildup of secretions by the overactive sebaceous glands. Over-the-counter dandruff shampoos, which control seborrhea of the scalp, eyebrow, and face, also may help—although again, because these may inadvertently get into the eye, they should never be used directly on the eyelid.

If you're dealing with a bacterial infection on the eyelid margin (as in a mixed blepharitis, described above), you may also need antibiotic and/or steroid drops or ointments. Many people with blepharitis must use some combination of treatment for months or even years to keep this condition under control—especially those with chronically recurring chalazia (see below). Even so, eye makeup and contacts can still be worn.

ANGULAR EROSION (CHAPPING OF THE EYELIDS)

Eyelids can get chapped too—just like lips. This painful breakdown of the skin occurs at the outer angle of the eye, where the upper and lower lids meet. A form of blepharitis, often associated with a bacterial infection, *angular erosion* tends to persist if it's not treated.

Treatment: Fortunately, angular erosion can be cured with an antibiotic and/or a steroid ophthalmic ointment. Again, though, steroids should not be overused on the eyelids. *Note: Redness and pain are symptoms your doctor should assess; make an appointment, and go see him or her.*

BELL'S PALSY (WEAKNESS IN THE FACIAL MUSCLES)

A sudden weakness in all or part of the facial muscles is called *Bell's palsy.* Although its onset—which often has no apparent cause—is sudden and terrifying, Bell's palsy often goes away by itself within a few weeks. But sometimes during its stay Bell's palsy affects the orbicularis muscle, the muscle that closes the eyelids—hampering the eye's ability to close all the way. Then, because the eyes are constantly exposed to the air, they become dry and irritated.

Treatment: Lubricating eye ointments can help, although they do tend to cause smeary or blurred vision; some people must also tape their eyelids shut at night to relieve the dryness.

If Bell's palsy lasts longer than a few weeks, your eye doctor can perform a procedure called a *tarsorrhaphy,* which involves partially closing the lids with sutures. This can be a temporary or a permanent step toward alleviating the symptoms and potential complications associated with a dry eye. (For more on dry eyes, see chapter 13.)

BLEPHAROSPASM
(TIGHT SQUEEZING OF THE EYELIDS)

The key word here is *spasm*. Like a spasm of any other muscle—in the hand, for instance, or the heart—*blepharospasm* is an involuntary tight squeezing of the eyelids. This may be a symptom of Parkinsonism, or a result of eye irritation. Or there may be no apparent cause (this is called *essential blepharospasm*). In minor cases, it's mainly a nuisance; but in its more serious form, blepharospasm can be disabling.

Treatment: Of the many different treatments that have had some success, the most promising is an injection of botulinum toxin directly into the muscle, which usually gives good relief for several months and can be repeated after it wears off.

For more information on benign essential blepharospasm, contact the Benign Essential Blepharospasm Research Foundation, Inc., P.O. Box 12468, Beaumont, TX 77726-2468, (409) 832-0788.

DERMATOCHALASIS (DROOPING EYELID SKIN)

Over the years eyelid tissue loses its elasticity. *Dermatochalasis* (pronounced der-ma-to-KAL-a-sis) is an age-related drooping or sagging of the skin in the eyelid. (In the upper eyelid, this is commonly called *hooding*. In the lower eyelid, many people use the accurate but unflattering term *bags*.)

Dermatochalasis in the upper eyelid ranges from a mild loss of the normal eyelid fold—mainly a cosmetic issue—to extensive sagging, in which eyelid tissue completely covers the eyelashes and eyes and may even interfere with vision. (The severity of dermatochalasis often becomes an important concern with insurance companies, which tend not to pay for consultations and surgery related to cosmetic problems. Many insurance companies require a thorough eye examination with a summary letter from the eye doctor, photographs, and visual field testing to demonstrate the degree to which the droopy eyelids are impairing vision before they'll agree to pay for surgery to correct the problem.)

Treatment: Surgery to correct dermatochalasis (called *blepharoplasty*) of either the upper or lower eyelids is usually performed by an eye doctor or a plastic surgeon. It is generally a safe procedure with few complications. (*Note:* Before having *any* form of surgery, discuss all your concerns with your doctor, and make sure you understand the risks and potential side effects involved.) Both eyes are usually done at the same time, so that the eyes will look "even."

During surgery of the upper eyelid, the excessive skin is removed. A crescent of skin between the brow and lash edge is removed along with some underlying fat, and then the edges of the skin are sewn together. (The operation to remove bags under the eyes is more involved but equally successful.) The stitches are removed within the first week to ten days. Discomfort is minimal, although you'll probably have some black and blue marks around the eyes for a week or so; these fade, as bruises often do, to interesting shades of green and yellow before disappearing. Ice packs can help decrease the swelling. Within a couple of weeks all signs of the surgery will disappear, and vision and appearance will improve.

PTOSIS (DROOPING EYELID)

Much less common and more complicated than dermatochalasis is drooping of the entire eyelid, not just the skin. This condition, called *ptosis of the eyelid*, usually occurs when the nerve that works the levator muscle (which raises the eyelid) is damaged. The muscle can be weakened by a stroke or a condition such as myasthenia, and even by normal aging.

Treatment: Surgical repair may be recommended when ptosis interferes with vision, or when it dramatically affects someone's appearance. *Note:* Find a surgeon who specializes in this type of surgery! This operation, which may involve shortening the levator muscle and removing some of the overlying skin or some of the conjunctiva, is far more complicated than dermatochalasis surgery. Good surgical repair of ptosis alleviates the problem. Botched or overdone surgery may mean that your eyelids won't close all the way—so your eyes will get dry and irritated from being exposed to the air. Although lubricating eye drops or ointments can help, this situation can be worse than the original ptosis.

ENTROPION AND ECTROPION
(THE EDGE OF THE EYELID TURNING IN OR OUT)

Sometimes the lower eyelashes turn inward and brush against the eye; this is called *entropion*. Sometimes they turn outward, so that the eyelid doesn't close properly; this is called *ectropion*. Either way, the problem is irritating. Entropion causes the lashes to rub against the conjunctiva and the cornea, irritating the eye. Ectropion exposes the conjunctiva and cornea to the air, causing dryness.

Entropion sometimes begins when the eye is already irritated by something else. You blink hard, trying to get rid of whatever's irritating your eye, and it just gets worse. Fortunately, this is usually a temporary condition that goes away when the initial problem—say, itchy eyes from hay fever—resolves itself. *Chronic* entropion, on the other hand, often develops as tissue deep in the eyelid ages and loses its strength, causing the edge of the lid to flip inward.

Ectropion too is a result of aging tissues. Many people who have it are bothered as much by the way it affects their appearance as by the way it makes their eyes feel; when the lid turns out so much that the lid's reddish inner lining shows, it can be very noticeable.

Treatment: Treatment for entropion may be as simple and low-tech as a piece of adhesive tape: placed securely on the skin of the lower eyelid, the tape sometimes pulls the edge of the lid down and keeps it from turning in. Happily, this treatment sometimes reverses the condition, which settles down almost as if the lid had been "retrained" not to turn in. But this doesn't always work; also, the skin on the eyelid can be irritated by the tape. When the tape treatment doesn't work, then surgical repair usually solves the problem.

With ectropion, surgical repair as an outpatient is almost always necessary to relieve the chronic irritation caused by this condition.

Surgery can greatly improve either condition.

MYOKYMIA (TWITCHING EYELID)

Have you ever felt your eyelid jump, or seen it twitch in the mirror? This rapid twitching, called *myokymia*, though usually temporary, can become a nuisance if it persists. (You can stop it by pressing your finger over the twitching area, but it will probably start up again when you take your finger away.) Myokymia is most often caused by stress or fatigue and is not a sign of disease.

Treatment: The main treatment for myokymia is simply to wait it out and try not to let it drive you crazy. Eventually, when you get more sleep and feel more relaxed, it will probably go away; it usually resolves within three to four weeks. *Note:* If it doesn't go away after three or four weeks, or if it seems particularly severe, then consult your eye care specialist for a thorough eye examination. Persistent myokymia may be the result of other conditions. Regardless of what's causing it, if the myokymia is persistent and bothersome, administration of botulinum toxin to the muscles around the eyes might be considered as a treatment.

SHINGLES (NERVE PAIN AND BLISTERING, CRUSTY EYELIDS)

Remember when you had the chicken pox? Well, that virus is still around, somewhere, in your body. And it may have other cards to play: it's the same virus that causes herpes zoster, or *shingles*, in adults. Anyone who has ever had chicken pox may develop shingles years afterward.

Remember how bad those chicken pox were? Shingles is worse. It can cause pain, often severe pain, plus blistering and crusting of the skin. These blisters follow the route of a sensory nerve, so you develop pain and then blisters down a path on the skin. If the sensory nerve on your upper face is affected, the pain and blistering will blanket your forehead and even the eyelids. Mercifully, although the pain is miserable, the eyes themselves are usually spared. However, in a few people, especially if the nerve to the end of the nose is involved, this sometimes affects the eye—usually after the skin lesions begin to get better. *If you have shingles on your face, you need to see your eye doctor. Without treatment, if your eyes are affected, you're at risk for developing uveitis, glaucoma, and other conditions that could cause permanent harm.*

Treatment: Systemic antiviral medications don't seem to affect the incidence or severity of "post-herpetic neuralgia" (the nerve pain that persists after the skin lesions have healed), but they do make the cutaneous lesions clear up faster and reduce the incidence of herpetic keratopathy and uveitis.

HORDEOLA AND CHALAZIA (STIES OR LUMPS ON THE EYELID)

A sty, also called a *hordeolum*, is an infection on your eyelid: a red, swollen area that hurts when you touch it. Sties can crop up on the outside of the eyelid at the base of a hair follicle (an external hordeolum, due to an

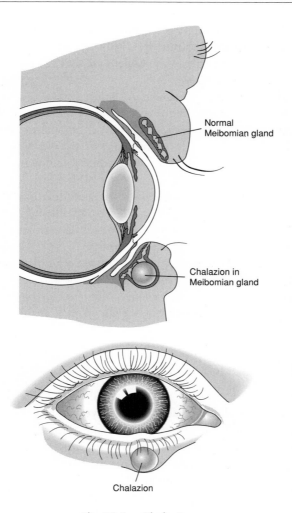

Fig. 10.1.   Chalazion

infected sebaceous gland) or on the eyelid's inner surface (an internal hordeolum, due to an infected Meibomian gland).

Sties can go away by themselves or with treatment. However, sometimes an internal sty evolves into a *chalazion* (pronounced sha-LAY-zeon), a usually painless lump that results from the body's inflammatory reaction to oily secretions in the clogged Meibomian gland. Chalazia typically don't affect vision, won't turn into cancer, and are essentially benign—more of a cosmetic nuisance than anything else. (However, if one of these lumps is located higher, in the middle of the upper eyelid, it can flatten the central cornea and distort vision.)

Treatment: The best treatment for sties is heat: a warm, wet cloth held over the sore spot for twenty minutes at a time, three to four times a day. Antibiotics are seldom needed. Steroid injections may be beneficial.

Most chalazia go away by themselves; we tell our patients that if it's small and not too bothersome, it's probably better left alone. However, if a chalazion gets big enough to be annoying, or if it affects your vision, you may need to have it removed surgically. The procedure is minor, involving local anesthesia, and simpler than having a cavity filled at the dentist's office. Within twenty-four hours your eyelid will be back to normal, except for some minor swelling and perhaps a black eye. *Note:* Although chalazia are usually minor, one-time occurrences, "repeat offenders" may indicate a more serious problem. Recurrent chalazia may actually be cancerous growths masquerading as benign eyelid lumps and may require a biopsy (a test in which a small sample of tissue is removed and analyzed).

EYELID TUMORS: DANGEROUS MASQUERADERS

Most of the eyelid's problems are annoying but benign. A few, however, are more serious. And unfortunately, some of these—particularly, malignant tumors of the eyelid—are sneaky, disguising themselves as blepharitis, chalazia, or sties. *Therefore, if you have any chronic eyelid problem that has not responded promptly to treatment, you should consult your eye doctor.*

Basal cell carcinoma, the most common eyelid malignancy, usually develops on the lower lid. It has many different patterns of growth: it can look like a bump, an ulcer, or a cyst, or it can even appear flat. As it grows, it may cause other eyelid problems, including entropion or ectropion, chalazion, or chronic blepharitis.

Squamous cell carcinoma is another common skin cancer of the eyelid. Squamous cell carcinoma too can mimic several benign eyelid problems.

Also like basal cell carcinoma, squamous cell carcinoma is thought to be caused by too much sunlight exposure; it often appears on sun-damaged skin, usually on the upper eyelid. *For this reason it is imperative that people who have had a basal or squamous cell carcinoma wear a wide-brimmed hat, sun-*

glasses, and sunscreen when outdoors. (Really, this is good advice for everyone, infants through adults.)

Sebaceous cell carcinoma is not as common but is even more serious—in fact, if not detected in time, it can be fatal. It too often resembles such common eyelid conditions as chalazion and blepharitis. So again, if you have recurrent or chronic chalazia or other eyelid problems, see your eye doctor, who may decide to order a biopsy.

11

The Cornea

The cornea is truly the eye's window. As described in chapter 1, it's the transparent, domed "watch glass" that sits over the sclera (the "white" of the eye). Through this clear porthole the iris and pupil are easily visible; looking further still beyond them, we can see all the way to the back of the eye—the vitreous, retina, and optic nerve (see figure 1.1, panels A and B).

Before we discuss some things that can go wrong with the cornea, let's take a moment to review its anatomy. The wafer-thin cornea—amazingly, only about 1 millimeter thick—is like a cake with five layers, each with its own special function. On top are *epithelial (outer lining) cells* (the "icing" on this cake, or the skin); this vital layer (also called the *epithelium*) protects the rest of the cornea and provides a smooth surface for tears. Next comes the cellophane-thin *Bowman's membrane;* then the tough, transparent *stroma,* the bulk of the cornea (the cake itself); then another layer of cellophane, called *Descemet's membrane.* These middle three layers act as scaffolding, providing structural support to the cornea as it arches over the front of the eye. Last is the single layer of *endothelial (inner lining) cells* (also called the *endothelium*). Because this important layer touches the aqueous of the eye's anterior chamber, it serves as a sort of "bilge pump," keeping the cornea free of excess moisture. When this pump malfunctions, the cornea can swell, and this can distort or even damage vision.

The cornea normally does not contain any blood vessels. However, it is rich in sensory nerve fibers: under the epithelial layer alone are about seventy of them, which helps explain why the cornea is so sensitive to pain. The epithelial cells act as a protective blanket, like enamel on a tooth, insulating the nerve fibers from the world. When that blanket is frayed—or, continuing the tooth analogy, when the enamel is cracked or has a cavity—those ultrasensitive nerves react. Painfully. Even a small loss of epithelial cells can be excruciating, if it exposes these nerve endings.

Now let's look at some common problems affecting the cornea.

CORNEAL ABRASION

Because of the abundance of nerves throughout its layers, even a slight injury or irritation to the cornea can result in a lot of discomfort or pain. An *abrasion*—a scrape of the epithelium, or outer surface—is the most common injury to the cornea. It can happen so easily—when the eye gets too close to a baby's fingernail, for instance, or the corner of an envelope, or a tree branch. All of a sudden it feels as if there's a hot poker in your eye. Other symptoms include redness, a feeling like there's a piece of grit in your eye, and extra sensitivity to bright lights. Because it's often difficult to see the actual injury with the naked eye, eye doctors rely on special fluorescent dyes, which target and highlight areas of damage, to help us determine the extent of the wound.

Fortunately, despite the severe discomfort and blurred vision that often accompany corneal abrasions, these injuries usually heal fairly quickly —sometimes in a matter of hours, sometimes within a few days—and don't leave any lasting damage.

Treatment: Basically, the cornea must heal itself, and all we can do is provide the best conditions possible. (Think of skin injured by a scrape or burn; it hurts until your skin lays down new layers of cells, which insulate the nerves beneath.) Thus, the main treatment for a corneal abrasion is simply to patch the eye. It's not quite as easy as it sounds—in other words, you shouldn't try to do it yourself with an eye patch from the drugstore— because to be effective, the eye patch must immobilize the eyelid and prevent it from rubbing over the injured area. The epithelial cells need time to multiply and coat the injury, which means that the patch needs to be tight enough to keep the eyelid still.

It takes several eye patches—generally three—to create enough bulk to secure the lid. (Eye doctors either stack three patches over the eyelid or use two, with the one directly on the eyelid folded in half.) The eye pads are fixed over the eyelid with at least four pieces of surgical tape, extending from the forehead to the cheek.

Sometimes, when eye patches can't be tolerated or when the abrasion doesn't appear to be healing, eye doctors apply a special "bandage" contact lens over the abrasion. (*Note:* Because there is a risk of infection with these lenses, this should be done only by an eye care specialist very familiar with this technique.) Bandage contact lenses allow the patient to avoid having to cope with the nuisance of wearing a large and bulky eye patch and enables the abraded eye to see while it heals.

There are different philosophies on fitting bandage contact lenses, but most often a large, medium- to high-water, thin, disposable soft contact lens (see chapter 5) is used. The lens is usually fit slightly loose to avoid adhesion to the cornea, and the large size allows for maximum coverage of the eye.

Contact lenses made of collagen are also available for patching an eye. These lenses are fit similarly to the soft contact lenses, but the collagen material dissolves on the eye within twelve to thirty-six hours, depending on the lens thickness. One of the advantages of a collagen lens is the lubricating effect that the dissolving collagen provides. However, these lenses do have a tendency to fall out as they dissolve.

Any contact lens has the additional benefit of acting as a drug delivery system for the eye. Eye drops prescribed for a corneal abrasion are absorbed by the contact lens and then slowly leach out from the lens onto the eye. This keeps the medication on the eye for a longer time and enhances the therapeutic benefit of the drops.

RECURRENT CORNEAL EROSION

As we said before, most corneal abrasions heal fairly quickly, without causing permanent injury to the cornea, the eye, or sight. However, an ornery few don't *stay* healed, apparently because the new blanket of epithelial cells doesn't stick to the injured area. This problem is called *recurrent corneal erosion.*

When an abrasion is particularly deep or damaging and healing is inadequate, the epithelial cells simply slide off—even months or years after the initial injury. And unfortunately, losing the protective insulation of the epithelial cells, again exposing the nerves underneath them, hurts about as much the second time as it did the first.

But we do have some clues as to who might be prone to recurrent corneal erosion—and therefore we can try to prevent it from happening. People who have had corneal abrasions due to fingernails, paper, or plant matter seem to be predisposed to developing recurrent erosion. We also know that the epithelial cells, if they're going to erode at all—and remember, in most people they don't—tend to come loose early in the morning, usually when people wake up. Why? Because your eyes dry out as you sleep. When the epithelial cells aren't secured to the cornea, they can be rubbed off by the simple act of opening your eyes in the morning. So if you have a history of eye discomfort when you get up—if you have pain and redness anyway, first thing in the morning—alert your eye doctor.

Treatment: Because dryness seems to exacerbate the problem, recurrent corneal erosion is usually treated successfully with additional lubrication—either artificial tear ointment or a specially prepared hypertonic ointment—in the eye at bedtime. (Some people need to use eye-drop forms of these ointments regularly during the daytime as well, to keep the cornea moist and foster healing.)

Interestingly, hypertonic drops and ointments work because of their high concentrations of salt. The salt draws excess water from the healing epithelial cells and enhances their ability to stick to the cornea. (Since too much dryness also makes cells fall off, this might be confusing, but bear in mind that there are different types of dryness. Dry eyes are the result of surface dryness, whereas cellular "dryness" or dehydration is the result of drawing excess water out of the corneal cells.)

Sometimes further treatments are necessary. One such treatment is the use of special "bandage" contact lenses similar to those used for abrasions (see above). And in particularly stubborn cases—if the recurrences are frequent, terribly painful, and debilitating—special surgical and laser procedures may be needed to help repair the damaged cornea.

CORNEAL ULCER

An *ulcer* is a focused, inflamed, painful response to infection. In the cornea, having an ulcer can feel a lot like having an abrasion—except that the redness, the sensation of having a piece of grit in your eye, and the difficulty tolerating bright light are usually worse.

Although countless bacteria exist in and around the healthy eye, normally they're effectively prevented from invading the cornea by the epithelium, which acts as a shield, and by the powerful bacteria-fighting agents in normal tears. But these natural barriers aren't impenetrable. They can be eroded by such things as eye trauma, dry eyes (particularly the severe form found in Sjögren's syndrome; see chapter 13), refractive surgery, improper eyelid function (a problem with Bell's palsy; see chapter 10), contact lenses, and even viruses including herpes zoster (found in chicken pox and "shingles") and herpes simplex keratitis (the same virus found in "fever blisters" on the lips). (Just as fever blisters often come about in response to physical or emotional stress, herpes keratitis can also reappear after months or even years.) *Note:* Viral infections of the cornea are very serious and can ultimately lead to scarring and permanent vision loss. In fact, herpes keratitis is the most common cause of corneal blindness in developed countries.

The slightest chink in the armor of the epithelial cells opens the door to the host of infectious agents crowding just outside—an unsavory cast of characters that also may include fungi and such bacteria as staphylococcus, streptococcus, and pseudomonas (often linked to corneal ulcers in contact lens wearers). Some bacterial strains are so nasty and virulent that once present in the eye, they can even grow *directly through an intact corneal epithelium*. Contact lenses greatly increase the risk of corneal ulcers when there is an infection present or there has been an insult to the eye, and in such cases should be removed immediately. Contact lens wearers should see an eye doctor at the first sign of a red eye or persistent eye discomfort.

Treatment: Because corneal ulcers are so serious, and potentially sight-threatening, your job is to get treatment as promptly as possible. Your eye doctor's task is to figure out what's causing the infection, and how best to treat it—with antibiotics, antiviral, or antifungal agents. Be sure to take the entire dose of antibiotic, if that's the treatment, since if you take less than the full dose, resistant microorganisms might grow and the infection could become much more difficult to get rid of.

CORNEAL DYSTROPHY

A *dystrophy* is an abnormal, possibly progressive, condition, often hereditary, usually present at birth. Many forms of dystrophy can affect the cornea, but the two most common are corneal epithelial basement membrane dystrophy and corneal endothelial cell dystrophy.

Corneal Epithelial Basement Membrane Dystrophy

Think of the basement membrane of the corneal epithelium as a slab of cement. On this cement, in nice, neat rows, are stacks of bricks—in this case, epithelial cells. The smoother the cement, the neater the stacks of bricks, and the better they serve as a wall against infection and as a smooth surface that, like a clean windshield, allows clear vision.

Basically, epithelial basement membrane dystrophy is a problem with the cement. It usually occurs in adults between the ages of forty and seventy, is slightly more common in women than men, and seems to be hereditary. The problem here is that the basement membrane becomes abnormally thick and irregular, forming a telltale pattern (as seen under the high magnification of the slit lamp) of ridges, cysts, and whirls—thus the descriptive name for this condition, "map-dot-fingerprint dystrophy." This causes the epithelial cells to buckle, break down, become "unstuck," and slough off.

Symptoms range from mild irritation to severe pain and redness in the eye. Because the underlying problem doesn't go away, and because symptoms are identical to those of recurrent corneal erosion, epithelial corneal dystrophy can even be thought of as a cause of recurrent corneal erosion.

Here too, as in recurrent corneal erosion, symptoms are usually worst in the early morning. Remember, while we sleep, when our eyelids aren't constantly blinking and applying new coats of lubricating tears, our eyes naturally become a little dry. But without that extra lubrication—if epithelial cells are poorly stuck to the cornea *already*—opening the eye is somewhat akin to scraping sandpaper across a layer of varnish; the eyelid rubs these cells right off. Ouch!

Treatment: Because this problem is so similar to recurrent erosion—and, in difficult cases, often just as frustrating—the treatment is much the same: keeping the eye properly hydrated so that the epithelial cells stay put.

The first line of attack is usually ointments—artificial tears and hypertonic saline preparations—at bedtime and drops during the day. An eye patch or "bandage" contact lens (described above, under "Corneal Abrasion") may also be necessary.

Because your eye, like your skin, responds to your immediate environment, it may also help to make your home and office more humid—with cool misters or vaporizers, or even a fish tank.

If the extra humidity and lubrication fail to stop these cells from falling off, the next step may be surgery—lasers or other techniques. For example, some people have been helped by surgery that gently clears away some persistently "unsticky" cells to make room for new, more adherent cells.

Corneal Endothelial Cell Dystrophy

Corneal endothelial cell dystrophy (Fuch's dystrophy) is a bilateral condition (one that affects both eyes); it usually manifests itself in people in their forties and fifties, is slightly more common in women than men, and is often hereditary.

Remember how the cornea's endothelium acts as a pump? Well, in this disorder the pump slowly fails. And as it does, the excess moisture that used to be siphoned away starts to build up. The cornea swells and becomes less transparent, and ultimately, vision can deteriorate.

The first symptom of this corneal swelling is usually blurry vision that's particularly noticeable when you first wake up. Here as well, too much moisture is a bad thing. During the day, when your eyelids are mostly open, water evaporates from the cornea; it's also removed by the pumping action of the endothelial cells, which siphon off excess water. All of this moisture removal helps keep the cornea clear. But when you're asleep, only one of these water-removing processes continues. There's no evaporation, because the eyelids are closed, so the endothelial cells have to work extra hard to keep the cornea dehydrated. In endothelial cell dystrophy, however, because the pump isn't operating at top form, excess water accumulates. Many people with this problem wake up with markedly swollen corneas and blurred vision—both of which improve gradually during the day, as the evaporation process commences again.

Note: Eye surgery, particularly cataract surgery, can hasten the deterioration of the endothelial cells in people who have this dystrophy. (Eye surgery is stressful anyway, but particularly when these cells are already vulnerable.) Surgery can cause severe corneal edema, which may even result in the need for a corneal transplant to restore someone's vision. So if you have a problem with blurred vision in the morning, make sure your doctor knows this before you have any kind of eye surgery.

Treatment: The best way to treat endothelial cell dystrophy is to identify, as soon as possible, the people at risk for developing it. If you have a family history of this disorder, tell your eye doctor. Regular examinations will be very important as a means of detecting early changes in your corneal endothelium. As soon as these changes progress and cause your cornea to swell and retain fluid, you can begin helping your eye's "pumps" by using hypertonic saline drops and ointments to draw out excess water.

Unfortunately, for many people dystrophy ultimately progresses to the point where ointments no longer work and vision is impaired. The next step, then, is a corneal transplant. Like a replacement window for your home, this is a fresh start, and it can improve your vision dramatically. (The transplant tissue, or "graft," comes from an organ donor, after death.) Corneal grafting was the first widely successful human transplant operation. The key to its success—particularly when compared with other tissue transplant operations—is the fact that corneas have very few blood vessels; thus, because there's little interaction with the rest of the body, the graft is less likely to be rejected as "foreign." Today the odds of success have been boosted even higher by improved tissue-matching techniques and the wider network of eye banks (foundations devoted to matching donor eye tissue with that of recipients in need).

CORNEAL ULTRAVIOLET LIGHT BURNS

Your eye can get sunburned, too. And like sunburn on the skin, injury to the cornea from ultraviolet light is acutely uncomfortable—but mercifully short-lived.

As their name suggests, these injuries to the cornea are caused by overexposure to ultraviolet light—from a sun lamp, from sunlight reflected off snow or water, or even from brief exposure to the intense flash of electric arc welding. (*Note:* Sunglasses are adequate protection against an ultraviolet corneal burn from snow or water, but not from strong sunlamps or "welder's flashes." A safe encounter with one of these powerful sources of ultraviolet light means wearing extremely dense, ultraviolet-blocking lenses.)

As with sunburn, it takes a while for the rays of ultraviolet light to start hurting your eye—usually about six to twelve hours—so you might wake up in the middle of the night with your eyes feeling like they're on fire and watering like crazy. The good news, again, is that—although intensely painful—most ultraviolet light burns of the cornea heal quickly. Immobilizing the eyelid with a patch (described above, under "Corneal Abrasion") helps the eye heal quickly.

12

The Conjunctiva

The conjunctiva is the thin, slippery membrane that covers the outside of the "white" of the eye and the inside of the eyelids. What can go wrong here? Two things, mainly. The most common problem is *conjunctivitis*, an inflammation of the conjunctiva caused by a virus, bacteria, allergies, or exposure to chemicals. Another common problem is *subconjunctival hemorrhage*, a dramatic red blotch on the "white." Reassuringly, these problems often look worse—sometimes a whole lot worse—than they really are.

CONJUNCTIVITIS

Viral Conjunctivitis: The Dreaded Pink Eye

Pink eye. Yuck! The name itself conjures up distasteful images of pinkish, swollen, watery eyes. Worse, it's highly contagious (ask anyone with small children), often sweeping through a school several times, for instance, before finally moving on to torment some other group of people.

Unpleasant as it is, however, you might say that pink eye has received a "bad rap." Not that pink eye isn't awful, but it's not the cause of every single case of eyes with inflamed, red, or pink conjunctiva. Actually, pink eye itself is a very specific problem, a viral conjunctivitis. (In fact, many people who believe they've endured pink eye probably had something else— symptoms caused by bacteria or by an allergic or chemical reaction.)

Pink eye, in the true ophthalmic sense, is caused by an adenovirus, one of the viruses responsible for the common cold. As noted above, it's extremely contagious, with a leisurely incubation period: symptoms usually manifest themselves seven to ten days after you come in contact with someone who's infected with it. It's a miserable condition. Besides being predominantly pink—as opposed to the bright red, mucus-oozing eye seen in bacterial conjunctivitis, for instance—the affected eye is also itchy and watery. These symptoms may spread to the other eye within a day or two; sufferers may also experience swollen lymph nodes in front of the ear or below the rim of the jaw.

Treatment: Like the common cold, pink eye usually has a long course: it can last weeks. Blurred vision, sensitivity to light, and watery, runny, itchy, swollen eyes are very common with pink eye. Antibiotics aren't much help, just as they're often ineffective at speeding recovery from a sore throat, runny nose, and other symptoms of the common cold. Thus, the treatment for pink eye conjunctivitis sounds a lot like that recommended for the common cold: lots of rest, plenty of fluids, aspirin or Tylenol for the discomfort, and antihistamines. Eye doctors often prescribe antihistamine eye drops and recommend cold compresses to ease eye puffiness and swelling. (Some doctors also prescribe steroid eye drops, but there's some question as to when this is appropriate.) Because true pink eye is so *very contagious*, you also need to take extra precautions in preventing its spread: don't share face towels, pillowcases, or washcloths, and don't leave tissues or other potentially infected items in places where they're likely to be touched by others.

Bacterial Conjunctivitis

If viral conjunctivitis is "pink eye," bacterial conjunctivitis might be considered "technicolor eye"—markedly inflamed, bright red eyes with a thick yellow mucous discharge. Its onset is quicker—within days of coming in contact with someone who has it—than that of pink eye. (Another difference is that swollen lymph nodes are rare with this form of conjunctivitis.)

How'd you get this? The possibilities are limitless. It is ridiculously easy to introduce infectious bacteria into your eye, because they're everywhere. Rub your eye after coming into contact with one of these organisms, and boom! Whatever you just touched may have been transferred right into your conjunctiva: potentially infectious bacteria from, perhaps, your mouth, nose, or scalp, from your grandchild's sticky fingers, from the stranger's hand you just shook, or even from the dog's head you just scratched. *Note:* The conjunctiva of the eye, like the mouth, *normally* contains bacteria. The bacteria that cause bacterial conjunctivitis are not the bacteria that are usually present in the eye, however; they are introduced from somewhere else.

Now, the eye has some pretty good defenses—namely, its protective eyelids, plus bacteria-fighting ingredients in tears and epithelial cells—that help keep normal bacterial flora in check. (Otherwise, conjunctivitis would be the norm, not the exception.) Trouble happens when the eye somehow becomes compromised: if the eyelids don't close the way they should, for instance, or if you have dry eyes, or a scratch, or chemical exposure, or some other injury—all of these things (and even viral conjunctivitis) can weaken the eye's resistance to infection.

Treatment: Antibiotics do a great job of treating bacterial conjunctivitis; the trick is figuring out *which* antibiotic you need. (It's not uncommon for an eye doctor to start a patient on one form of antibiotic eye drops and then change medications midstream if the infection doesn't respond within a few days.) Sometimes the eye doctor will take a culture of a severe or persistent infection, to identify the bacterium and determine its sensitivity to various antibiotics. (In rare cases, patients need to take antibiotics orally or even by intravenous injection.)

Note: As with any form of infection, good hygiene is crucial here. This means you'll need to scrub away any accumulated crust and debris along the eyelids and apply warm compresses regularly (see chapter 10).

Allergic Conjunctivitis

Your body's being invaded. At least it thinks it is, and it's reacting to the enemy—cat hair, pollen, mold, dust, even food—by making antibodies, sending specialist "warrior" cells into battle. Soon the skirmish gets ugly. Chemical weapons released by these warrior cells are called into play, causing the battleground—in this case, your eyes—to become even more inflamed. This inflammation, your basic allergic reaction, can range from mild to severe.

In the eye, allergic reactions are usually characterized by mild redness, itchiness, and swelling of the conjunctiva, and excess tearing. (This often happens in both eyes at once.) Most people who get this form of conjunctivitis are no strangers to allergies; they've probably had some allergy-related conditions—asthma, hay fever, or hives—all their lives.

For some people, allergic conjunctivitis is a predictable, seasonal event, rearing its ugly head without fail whenever the air is rich in oak pollen, for example. Other people never figure out what's driving their eyes crazy. And for some people, allergic conjunctivitis hits with the subtlety of a freight train, producing dramatic, instantaneous swelling of the conjunctiva that makes the eye seem to bulge from its socket. (This effect, called *chemosis*, is the eye's version of a sudden hive on the skin; with treatment it tends to go away as quickly as it came.)

Some eye care products can also cause allergic conjunctivitis. Eyeglass-cleaning soaps or detergents, for example, can irritate the eye if you don't rinse away every last trace of residue. Preservatives in eye drops—drops for treating dry eyes or glaucoma, for example—produce allergic reactions in many people. Also, some contact lens wearers develop a form of allergic conjunctivitis called *giant papillary conjunctivitis* (see chapter 5).

Treatment: Treatment is just what you might expect for an allergic reaction: antihistamines, decongestants, cold compresses, and occasionally such medications as aspirin, Tylenol, and Advil for discomfort. *Note:* Steroid eye drops should be used with caution! Regular, prolonged use of these drops can cause glaucoma. Also, take care not to *overuse* Visine or similar over-the-counter drops that "get the red out." Although these medications alleviate redness and itching at first, if used too frequently (four times a day for three or four days, for instance) they can produce "rebound redness" (similar to the rebound effect caused by overuse of nasal decongestants) when they wear off. This leads to *more* red in the eye instead of less.

Recently, several new kinds of eye drops have become available for treating allergic conjunctivitis (see Appendix); you might want to ask your eye doctor whether one of these is right for you. Some of these new drops can even be used prophylactically, as preventive measures for allergy sufferers during hay fever season and other high-risk times.

Conjunctivitis Caused by Chemicals and Irritants

Really, very few things in this world were meant to be placed in or near the eye. Thus, *any* exposure to chemicals or irritants—either directly spilled into the eye or carried in by smoke, fumes, or dust—can cause conjunctivitis. Reaction may be severe (such as that caused by exposure to strong household cleaners; see chapter 17), or it may be fairly mild (getting suntan lotion in your eye stings, for instance, but the discomfort usually doesn't last long).

Treatment: Even if you don't know what got into your eye, *wash it out!* It's best to use a chemically balanced irrigating solution if you have one on hand—drug stores sell several different brands, and you may want to buy one for emergencies—but the old standby, tap water, is also fine. If you can, remove any solid material from the eye by gently dabbing it with a cotton-tipped applicator. There's no such thing as using too much water. *Irrigation should be copious*, and if your injury was caused by an acid or alkali, such as lye and certain cleaning ingredients, you should bathe your eye *continuously for half an hour to an hour*. (For more on eye injuries, see chapter 17.) Afterward, try holding a cold cloth or ice bag to your eye for the pain; aspirin, Tylenol, Advil, or similar medications may also ease the discomfort. Then, call your eye doctor—*especially if the pain and irritation persist*. You may need additional treatment, including prescription eye drops (which help relieve pain but can also prevent a secondary bacterial infection; see "Bacterial Conjunctivitis," above).

LUMPS AND BUMPS OF THE CONJUNCTIVA: PINGUECULAE AND PTERYGIA

What the heck is this? Thousands of people visit their eye doctor each year because they've spotted something that wasn't there before: a raised cream-colored, white, or chalky growth on their conjunctiva. These tissue growths commonly appear on the surface of the conjunctiva nearest the nose (this is called the *nasal*, or medial, side), but they can also occur on the opposite side (called the *temporal*, or lateral, side) of the eye. They're particularly noticeable when the eye becomes inflamed (such as in bacterial or allergic conjunctivitis, described above). These areas are called *pingueculae* (pronounced ping-GWEK-ū-lee). When their growth extends onto the cornea, we call them *pterygia* (te-RIJ-ē-a).

But don't worry. As scary-looking as either of these conditions may be, and as alarming as their names sound, they are benign. Think of them as harmless "age spots" in the eye: they're an age-related degeneration of the conjunctival tissue, the result of decades of sunlight and general environmental exposure. *However, unlike sun-caused changes to the skin, these aren't dangerous.* Pingueculae are especially common in people living near the equator, whose lifetime exposure to sunlight is much greater than the exposure of, say, people in Scandinavian countries. (Interestingly, some scientists believe that the reason these growths are most often seen on the nasal side of the eye is that the nose's angle may actually concentrate ultraviolet rays on this area.) Wearing eyeglasses and sunglasses, which help protect the eyes from ultraviolet exposure, probably lowers your risk of developing pingueculae.

Pingueculae seldom grow, and they almost never cause discomfort.

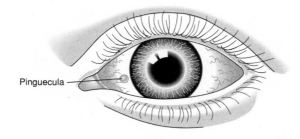

Fig. 12.1. Pinguecula

They're just a cosmetic nuisance. Again, unlike skin changes from the sun, pingueculae and pterygia *have no tendency to become malignant.*

On the rare occasion when a pinguecula does grow and slowly creeps onto the cornea (becoming a pterygium), it hardly ever affects vision. If it does, or if it irritates the eye, you may need to have it removed surgically; this can be done under local anesthesia. The problem here is that, despite meticulous surgical technique, these annoying things often grow back. The rate of recurrence after excision is as high as 40 percent. (In fact, when pterygia recur they tend to come back faster, and bigger.) In an attempt to lessen this high rate of recurrence, eye doctors are trying new techniques, including radiation, autologous conjunctival grafts (replacing the "bad" conjunctiva with tissue from another area of your own eye), and additional treatment with medications that inhibit cell growth.

But for now the bottom line with these nuisances is to leave pingueculae and pterygia alone, unless there's a clear need to remove them.

SUBCONJUNCTIVAL HEMORRHAGE

Speaking of scary-looking changes to the eye, hardly anything is more terrifying than looking in the mirror and seeing a huge red blotch in your eye. And yet amazingly, the most dramatic thing about a *subconjunctival hemorrhage* (one under the conjunctiva) is its appearance.

Here's the story: All over our body, all the time, tiny blood vessels break and are repaired. A blood vessel in the conjunctiva may break spontaneously for no apparent reason, or when someone coughs especially hard or vomits forcefully. An injury to the eye may also cause a subconjunctival hemorrhage (and in this case it's important to make sure that the injury didn't do any damage to the rest of your eye). Sometimes this causes a little discomfort, but most people feel nothing unusual at all.

Note: Many people think a broken blood vessel in the eye is a warning sign of dangerously high blood pressure, and that it means you're about to have a stroke. Not true. A subconjunctival hemorrhage looks terrible, but it doesn't mean that you have high blood pressure. (On the other hand, if you have two or three of these in a month, you probably need to see your internist or family physician; recurring subconjunctival hemorrhage can signal a health problem, such as high blood pressure or a blood-clotting disorder.)

13

The Complicated World of Tears

Tears aren't simple. They're complex creations of water, mucins, oils, and electrolytes; they also possess some protective bacteria-fighting substances that help reduce our risk of getting eye infections. Their functions are many and essential. For the cornea, they provide a smoother optical surface, so that our vision remains clear; they also help keep the cornea properly moisturized and rich in oxygen. For the eye in general, tears also act as "wiper fluid," allowing the eyelids to wash the eye free of debris with every blink.

Tears, believe it or not, are layered. The innermost layer contains *mucins*, which allow tears to adhere to your eye and coat it evenly. These mucins are produced by many tiny "factories" named *goblet cells* in the conjunctiva (the clear covering over the "white" of your eye) and inside your eyelids. (They are called goblet cells because they are shaped like goblets; goblet cells are present in all mucous membranes in the body.) The middle layer, which contains about 90 percent of the tear, is mainly water, with just a pinch of salt. Most of this watery layer is produced by the *lacrimal glands*, located just above and outside each eye. As a backup system, our eyes are also equipped with accessory glands, which provide extra water. The outermost layer contains fatty oils, called *lipids*, which slow the evaporation of the watery layer and thus keep tears in our eyes longer, just as a coating of lotion helps skin retain moisture. These oils are produced by the *meibomian glands* on the edges of the eyelid, just behind the lashes. (Here too there's an additional backup system of accessory oil glands.) A reduction in any of these layers can lead to dryness.

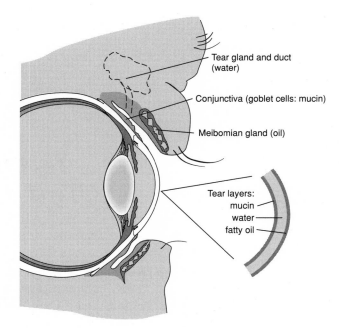

Fig. 13.1.   Side view of tear layers, showing goblet cells and meibomian gland

When you blink, your upper eyelid sweeps tears across the surface of the cornea, down toward the inner corner of each eye. The tears drain through a small opening in the eyelid called the *puncta*. Each eye has two of these small openings, one on each eyelid. The tears flow through the puncta into the *nasolacrimal duct*, a canal that drains excess tears into the nasal passages (which is why, when you cry, you also need to blow your nose). (This process of draining tears is different from the process of draining aqueous fluid from the anterior chamber of the eye, described in chapters 1 and 8.)

There are two different types of tearing: the first, *basic tearing*, is normal tearing, which helps maintain the eye. The second, *reflex tearing*, is a reaction to a stimulus, such as a foreign body in the eye or a strong emotion, happy, sad, or surprised.

When your eye is irritated, the reflex tearing mechanism causes the lacrimal glands to produce water—the goal being simply to wash away the irritation. Reflex tears, designed to solve a specific, temporary problem, contain much more water than basic tears; they're low in mucins and oils,

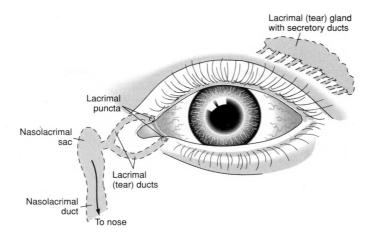

Lacrimal (tear) gland
with secretory ducts

Lacrimal
puncta

Nasolacrimal
sac

Lacrimal
(tear) ducts

Nasolacrimal
duct

To nose

Fig. 13.2.   Front view of tear gland and tear ducts

so the *quality* of these tears doesn't do much to lubricate the eye.

If your eye becomes significantly irritated—from dryness, say, or allergies—then reflex tearing will start. Your eyes will get very watery, but because the quality of these tears is so poor, the excess water won't really help with the dryness. But simply adding a drop of an artificial tear substitute to your eyes when they are watering excessively can change everything! The extra lubrication from the drops helps alleviate the dryness, and this in turn relieves the excess watering.

As people age, they sometimes have tear problems that cause discomfort: some people have dry eyes, and some have excessively wet eyes, from tearing.

DRY EYES

The diagnosis: you have dry eyes. And it's no fun having eyes that often burn, feel tired, gritty, irritated, itchy, or sticky.

For people who suffer from it, having dry eyes can be a constant source of discomfort that makes it difficult to get through the day. Having dry eyes means you're infinitely more sensitive to everything around you. Symptoms get worse, for instance, whenever it's windy, when the air quality is poor, when the humidity is low. Indoors, heating and air conditioning can wreak havoc on both your comfort *and* your vision.

Having dry eyes is a chronic problem, and currently there's no cure. But there are good treatments—drops, ointments, punctal plugs, and even "bandage" contact lenses—that can make you feel almost as good as new by helping control the dryness and the miserable symptoms it can produce. Before we cover how these work, let's take a moment to consider the problem.

Why Are My Eyes Dry?

There are two basic problems: either you're not making *enough* tears, or the tears you're making aren't as *good* as they used to be. Occasionally dry eyes may be caused by a third problem: the eye itself can't get the tears where they need to go.

Not Making Enough Tears

Perhaps your eyes don't make enough tears. This condition, called *KCS* (for *keratoconjunctivitis sicca*), usually occurs in both eyes but can be worse in one eye than the other.

One of the most common causes of tearing deficiency is simply age. Like skin and hair, our tears tend to "dry up" slightly as we get older; we just make fewer tears. For most of us this decrease isn't terribly noticeable, but for some people tear production can drop off significantly—enough to produce the classic dry-eye symptoms of irritation, redness, grittiness, burning, or eye fatigue. (KCS is also more common in older women than in other groups, probably because of the hormonal changes that occur with age.)

Other health problems can hamper tear production. One of these is *injury to the lacrimal glands*, from infection or trauma; the effect of the injury may be temporary or permanent. Another is *Bell's palsy*, a condition that affects the facial nerves; its effects too may be either temporary or permanent. People with this ailment are often unable to close one eye or blink on one side of the face, and that eye also produces fewer tears. As you may imagine, the combination of not being able to blink and making fewer tears causes major problems with dryness.

Autoimmune disorders can impede tear production. *Sjögren's syndrome* is the miserable trio of symptoms—dry eyes, dry mouth, and joint pain—that may be associated with other autoimmune disorders, such as rheumatoid arthritis, systemic lupus erythematosus, and scleroderma. (The term *secondary Sjögren's syndrome* is used to describe dry eyes associated with any other disease.) Other systemic ("whole body") diseases, such as sarcoidosis, leukemia, lymphoma, and chronic thyroid problems, often diminish tear production, as well.

Occasionally *medications* decrease the tear-making ability in some people. For instance, as you may already know too well, antihistamines and decongestants for allergies and colds dry out everything—eyes in addition to sinuses. Diuretics, taken to lower blood pressure and ease water retention, may decrease tear production. Hormone replacement therapy and even birth control pills also can lead to dry eyes. Other potentially eye-drying medications include certain eye dilators (atropine and scopolamine), motion sickness inhibitors (scopolamine), tricyclic antidepressants (amitriptyline, desipramine, imipramine, nortriptyline), oral acne medications (Accutane, tetracycline), and opiate-based pain medications (morphine). *Note:* Of course, even though these and other drugs may produce dry eyes, this isn't reason enough to stop taking them! If the eye-drying side effect really bothers you, talk to your doctor. It may be possible for you to switch to an alternative medication.

The Old Tears Ain't What They Used to Be

Even if your tear *production* is just fine, your eyes can still be dry if the *quality* of tears is poor. Remember the ingredients in each tear; they're all important, and when the balance of them is off, your tears (and your eyes) may suffer as a result.

Diseases in the eye or body can cause a drop in either the mucin or the lipid portion of tears. Vitamin A deficiency, trachoma (an infection that's very common in the Middle East), Stevens-Johnson syndrome (an inflammation of skin and mucous membranes causing scarring and dysfunction of those membranes), and chemical burns of the eye all cause a breakdown and scarring of the conjunctiva and sclera. This in turn destroys goblet cells and causes the production of mucins to dwindle. Without mucins, tears don't hold up as well; they break apart much more quickly on the surface of the cornea. (Imagine the difference in texture between watercolor and oil-based paint.) As a result, the cornea tends to dry more quickly.

One of the most common eye diseases to obstruct lipid production by the Meibomian glands is *blepharitis,* an infection of the eyelid (see chapter 10). When the eyelid becomes infected, bacteria (and the immune reaction they trigger) cause the Meibomian glands to clog and shut down. Again, the result is a more watery (and less oily) product: tears that evaporate much more quickly from the eye. Even worse, as these lipid-lacking tears evaporate, they leave behind a greater-than-normal concentration of salt, and salt burns the eyes.

Another common cause of dry eye from lack of lipids is sleeping with your eyes open *(nocturnal lagophthalmos)*. Sleep is the body's great restorer, a chance for everything, including eye moisture, to be replenished. If you don't close your eyes fully when you sleep, exposed parts of your eye tend to dry out. Symptoms are usually at their worst when you wake up, and get better during the day as normal blinking returns moisture to the eye. This is a fairly easy-to-treat problem; often, simply applying an artificial tear ointment before bedtime is enough to keep the eye moist overnight. (Nocturnal lagophthalmos is also a common problem for people with Bell's palsy; the lid of the disabled eye doesn't close at night, and this makes the already dry eye feel even worse. But taping the eye closed at night, along with the use of artificial tear ointments, can help replenish eye moisture.)

Distribution Problems

With tears as with any complicated manufacturing system, the breakdown may come not in quality control or production but in shipping or distribution. Sometimes the tears themselves are just fine, and they're made in adequate amounts, but the eye itself can't get them where they need to go.

Irregularities on the surface of eyelids or corneas, for instance, can cause dryness even if tear production is adequate. If the eyelids are scarred significantly—a problem in chronic blepharitis—the lid can't distribute tears evenly across the surface of the cornea; think of faulty wiper blades trying to sweep a car's windshield. Similarly, if the cornea is scarred, the lid can't do a good job of spreading tears. In either case, the tear-deprived surface of the cornea becomes parched.

Growing older can also cause *changes in the musculature and shape of our eyelids,* occasionally causing them to sag or turn outward (ectropion) or inward (entropion; see chapter 10). These problems too disrupt how tears are spread across the eye, and how they flow out of the eye. Often, when this happens, people experience symptoms of dryness. A person may also have tears that stream down his or her face. (This may sound like a flat-out contradiction of a diagnosis of dry eyes: after all, how can your eyes be dry when they're literally overflowing with tears?)

Finally, some people just don't do a good job of blinking; consequently, tears don't get spread across the eye as they should. With each complete blink, the upper lid should meet the lower lid. *Partial blinking* leaves the lower portion of the cornea constantly exposed and increases dryness over the course of the day.

Diagnosing Dry Eyes

The first step in diagnosing dry eyes is to measure both the quantity and the quality of your tears. Your eye doctor will probably begin a careful examination of your eyes with a *slit lamp biomicroscope*, a microscope that gives a three-dimensional magnified view of the front surface of your eye. The doctor will look for any irregularity on the surface of your cornea, any abnormality in the position and function of your eyelids, and any dysfunction of your Meibomian glands. The doctor may also use special stains—two types of dyes are used, fluorescein and rose bengal—to highlight damaged cells and dry spots on the surface of the cornea. (The principle here is similar to that behind those awful red dyes dentists sometimes use to illustrate where you're not adequately brushing your teeth. In this case, areas of damage and dryness absorb the stains and pinpoint the trouble spots on your cornea.)

Next, your tears will be scrutinized for volume and quality. Are they relatively clean, or do they contain "ocular debris" (skin cells, airborne particles, and mucin strands)?

Are you blinking well? Your doctor will also check to make sure that your eyelids are adequately spreading tears across the surface of the eye.

Tear *volume* can be measured with something called a *Schirmer test*. The description is worse than the actual test. "Schirmer strips" (sterile pieces of paper) are folded and hung over your lower eyelids. For five minutes they'll soak up your tears; then your doctor will measure the saturated area of each strip to determine whether you're making enough tears. Some doctors are convinced that the Schirmer test is very useful, while others question its value. We think that it actually does tell something useful about tear production.

Fluorescein dye, which sticks to the mucin layer of tears, may also be used to determine your "tear breakup time" (how well your tears maintain their integrity)—in other words, to find out whether your problem is an issue of tear *quality*. After putting a few drops of fluorescein in your eyes, your doctor will ask you to blink several times, to get an even distribution of your tears across the cornea. Next you'll be asked *not* to blink, while your doctor observes and measures how long it takes before the tears evaporate and dry areas are observed on the cornea. The *rose bengal test* (described in chapter 3) is another test in which a dye placed in the eye can help doctors diagnose a dry eye.

For more specific tests, your doctor may need to send samples of tears or tissue (this is painless) from your eye to a laboratory. Tears can be tested for quantities of salt, electrolytes, and proteins to help pinpoint the cause of dryness, and conjunctival tissue can be biopsied to look for changes within the cell structure that may indicate the source of the problem.

Treating Dry Eyes

Simply put, the basic goal in treating dry eyes is to keep the eye moist—in other words, to treat the symptoms, and not the cause. There are several ways to do this.

Tear Substitutes

Tear substitutes are used to rewet the ocular surface. Fortunately there are many good over-the-counter teardrops to choose from. Depending on why your eyes are dry, you'll probably find that some tear supplements work better than others. Some people need a drop that "mimics" tears to add more *quantity*. Others need drops containing extra lubricants to enhance the mucin layer and improve tear *quality*.

If burning is a problem, you can find drops that are hypotonic (containing less salt than natural tears). If your problem is more severe and you need drops particularly often (several times an hour), you may prefer preservative-free tear supplements, which are often easier on the eye. Tear ointments are especially useful for people who wake up at night or in the morning with dry, gritty, irritated eyes. They are inserted in the eyes at bedtime.

Note: Be careful using drops designed to "get the red out" and improve the cosmetic appearance of your eyes. *These treat a different problem.* Often these drops contain ocular decongestants and vasoconstrictors that shrink the dilated blood vessels that show up when your eyes are dry. These additional ingredients can affect mucin production, so although your eyes may look better, they'll still feel dry. Also, as many of us have learned the hard way with similarly acting nasal sprays, constant use of vasoconstrictors can lead to a temporary "rebound" reaction, in which these blood vessels actually dilate *more* and your eye looks even redder than it did before you used the eye drop. If your eyes are red because they're dry, appropriately rewetting them with an artificial tear supplement usually takes care of the redness as well.

Procedures to Fix Your Tear-Drainage System

If tear supplements don't ease all your symptoms, your doctor may suggest methods of making more use of the tears you have, by keeping them in your eye longer.

One approach is to close the puncta (the eye's "tear drain") to slow or lessen drainage of tears into the nose. Remember, you've got two of these in each eye, one on the lower eyelid, one on the upper. Your doctor may want to close only the one on the lower lid to reduce the outflow of most of your tears, but leave the upper lid's puncta open. One bonus here is that this procedure doesn't have to be permanent; your puncta can be closed temporarily, as a test to see whether such treatment will help or not. Your doctor can close the puncta with collagen plugs, which will slowly dissolve over the next few days. (If the plugs work and the dryness improves, then you can talk about more permanent treatment.) If the collagen plugs don't last long enough for you to measure the effectiveness of this approach to treatment, your doctor can use silicone plugs (which will close the puncta until they're removed). Then, if you and your doctor decide it will indeed help, the silicone plugs can be left in or the puncta can be permanently closed with thermal cautery. In thermal cautery the doctor applies a very hot wire to the puncta after first numbing the area with anesthetic. This shrinks the tissues in the area and causes scarring and permanent closure of the puncta.

"Bandage" Contacts

For some people, contact lenses can be helpful as a "bandage" that holds more water on the eye and smoothes the surface of the cornea (see chapter 11). However, the risks may outweigh the benefits of this type of therapy: the bandage contact lens is more likely to allow bacteria (as well as moisture) to accumulate in your eye, and this can cause even worse problems than dryness—problems like infections and corneal ulcers. If your doctor decides that this form of therapy is appropriate, you'll need to have your eyes checked frequently, so that any potential problems can be treated as soon as possible.

New Medications

Currently under investigation are tear-stimulating medications, either as eye drops or in pill form, which may be available soon.

TEARING

Tearing—by the way, the word we're using rhymes with *hearing*, not *herring*—isn't just crying, although that's certainly one reason for tearing. When eye doctors use the term, we simply mean "making too many tears"—in other words, having watery eyes.

Ideally the eye maintains a delicate balance between tear production and drainage. To review briefly: Most tears are secreted by glands in the upper eyelid onto the cornea, where they act as the eye's "window-washer" fluid, constantly bathing the cornea (see figure 13.2). They either evaporate or collect in the "gutter" created by the lower eyelid, called the *inferior cul-de-sac*. Blinking pumps the tears in this gutter ever downward toward the nose; first they drain through the puncta in each eyelid, into a common aqueduct to the nasolacrimal sac. From here tears flow into the nose and then to the back of the mouth, where they mix with saliva and are swallowed.

Many things can cause excess tearing. Most common are foreign particles (specks of dust, for instance) that get blown into the eye; the eye jump-starts its tear production in an attempt to wash out these invaders and cleanse itself. Eye infection, emotional stimuli (such as, literally, the "tear-jerker" movie), wind, smoke, and fumes—all of these can cause more tears to be made. Ironically, as mentioned above, even dryness in the eye can cause increased tearing.

But tearing can also result from *poor drainage* of tears from the eye—think of rain that pools in a blocked gutter. Sometimes irregularities in the shape of the eyelid can hamper tear drainage or hinder blinking (a critical means of keeping tears moving through the drainage system). A deformed punctal opening or blocked tear duct—this sometimes happens with aging—may also cause a buildup of tears. In this case, as a simple outpatient procedure, your doctor can dilate, probe, and irrigate or flush the nasolacrimal drainage system and reopen this passage. If this does not work, then thin silicone tubing can be used to dilate and reestablish the flow of tears through this system.

One important but often overlooked cause of tear-draining problems is an infection in the nasolacrimal sac called *dacryocystitis*. Remember, tears drain into this sac before they pass downward into the nose and throat. Sometimes bacteria find their way here as well, and the resulting infection can be difficult to treat because the sac is located so deep within the tissues around the eye. The nasolacrimal sac is hard to reach with topical drops, and oral antibiotics are often needed to knock out the infection.

The biggest problem here, however, is that because of the often-elusive nature of such infections, they can go undiagnosed for months—leading to scarring of the nasolacrimal sac and chronic tearing problems. When this occurs it may be necessary to open the scarred sac surgically. (This procedure is known as a *dacryocystorhinostomy*, or *DCR*.) Patients with tearing difficulty due to dacryocystitis must weigh their degree of discomfort against the anxiety, inconvenience, and cost of undergoing surgery. You may decide that having too many tears isn't so bad after all. As one patient points out, "It's better than having a dry eye."

Some Questions You May Have about Dry Eyes

Sometimes my vision gets blurry, but I can clear it with a few blinks. What's the problem?

If your eye is dry, the surface of your cornea can lose some of its smoothness. Dry patches form on the cornea, and this tends to blur vision in between blinks. But by blinking several times in a row—think of applying a roller of paint to a rough wall—you fill in those dry patches with tears and clear your vision. This problem is much improved too by artificial tear supplements, which help heal the dry patches and maintain more consistent vision.

Why do my eyes burn when I work at my computer?

You know that daze you feel sometimes when you stare at the computer for hours on end? You're not imagining it; many of us really do go into a kind of trance after prolonged computer use. We blink less, for one thing. Then, with a lower tear supply, the moisture in our eyes starts evaporating. When this happens, the normal amount of salt in our tears builds up, becomes more concentrated, and starts burning. Using an artificial tear supplement that is hypotonic (containing less salt than natural tears) helps ease this symptom. (It may also help if you make an effort to blink more often while you're working on the computer.)

Why don't my eyes feel dry all the time?

Look around you. For the comfort of your eyes, environment is everything. Temperature and humidity, for instance, both influence tears; sudden changes in either of these can cause dryness.

Indoor heating during the winter, especially the forced-air kind, can significantly dry your eyes, just as it dries your skin. A humidifier, even placing a fish tank in a dry room, can help immensely. (It really is true what they say: "It's not the heat, it's the humidity.") In the summer, air conditioning—which makes the rest of your body so much more comfortable—is designed not only to cool the air but to take excess water out of it as well. And either of these—the loss in humidity or the cool air—can dry your eyes.

Also, the big difference in temperature and humidity that hits us when we go from a heated or air-conditioned house into the seasonal weather takes its toll on the eyes. Until they catch up and adapt to the climate change, our eyes often feel dry as a result.

Spring and fall, the time for relief? No, the time for pollen! If you're one of the millions of Americans who suffer from pollen allergies, you're probably way too familiar already with the dry, itching, burning eyes that go along with the sneezing and scratchy throat. A big drawback to oral allergy medications is that they usually make this dryness worse. You may need allergy medications especially intended for eyes; these reduce the swelling and itching from allergies but also contain an artificial tear supplement to ease the dryness.

Sometimes I wake up at night with a pain in my eye. What could be causing this?

Two of the most likely suspects are dry eyes and recurrent corneal erosions (see chapter 11). However, another possibility is that you have a recurrent sinus infection. The sinuses surround the eyeball, which means that if they're inflamed, there can be real discomfort around the eye. See your physician to check for this.

14

The Uvea
Iris, Ciliary Body, and Choroid

Uvea is the Latin word for "grape," so it's a good name for this purple, blood-rich layer of tissue located just inside the eye. In fact, the uvea is sometimes called the eye's "grape" layer. Lying below the sclera (the "white" of the eye), the uvea is made up of three regions—the iris, ciliary body, and choroid—whose main function is to nourish and maintain the integrity of the eye and its tissues. (For more on the parts of the eye, see chapter 1.) The choroid supplies important nutrients to the retina, while the ciliary body produces aqueous fluid, which is essential to the health of the anterior segment and shape of the eyeball. The iris and ciliary body are also vital in helping the eye see properly.

The two most common problems in the uvea are uveitis and iris nevi.

UVEITIS (ARTHRITIS OF THE EYE)

Arthritis is an inflammation of the tissues in the joints, right? So how can it be a problem in the eye? Well, in some ways eyes have a lot in common with knees or elbows: both are relatively self-contained, with definite boundaries or walls that create fluid-filled cavities, or spaces, of connective tissue. (In our joints the job of the fluid is to help unyielding surfaces, such as bones and ligaments, move smoothly over each other.)

The eye's version of arthritis is called *uveitis*. This is the general term for inflammation of the uveal tissue structures in the eye—the iris, ciliary body, and choroid. Arthritis in the iris specifically is called *iritis;* in the ciliary body, *cyclitis;* in the choroid, *choroiditis*. Uveitis may strike one eye or both. When it does, it can cause redness, throbbing pain, and difficulty with bright light; it may even affect the vision. It can also be "silent" (if it affects only a small area in the back of the eye).

Just as in many cases of arthritis, determining exactly what causes uveitis can be baffling and frustrating. Some cases of uveitis, frankly, stump us; they seem to arise out of thin air. In other people uveitis may be linked to a host of medical problems including headaches, infections, allergies, deafness, numbness or weakness, vitiligo, skin rashes, oral or genital ulcers, bowel problems, joint aches or pains, or difficulty breathing. There's some speculation that smoking cigarettes and having a poor diet may contribute to the condition.

With uveitis, the first step for the medical professional is to take a very careful medical history. Be sure to tell your eye doctor about any other eye problems or general health problems you're having now or have had in the past (including surgery or trauma). Your doctor may recommend further testing, which may include a chest X-ray and TB test (if a lung problem is suspected), blood tests, stool evaluation, skin tests, or even a spinal tap. You may also need a biopsy (a test in which a small sample of skin or tissue is removed and analyzed).

Even after all these tests, uveitis can be a real challenge to treat; recurrences are common and are frustrating for both the doctor and the patient. Also, just as chronic arthritis can lead to joint-crippling deformities, uveitis can lead to other problems, including glaucoma, cataracts, and swelling in the retina, called *macular edema*, similar to the macular edema of diabetic retinopathy (see chapter 18).

Fortunately, steroid and nonsteroidal anti-inflammatory eye drops—often the first line of treatment—are very effective at treating most forms of uveitis. If the inflammation persists or comes back, your doctor may also inject steroids around your eye or prescribe additional medications including oral steroids, antibiotics, antifungals, antivirals, or even a drug that arrests cell growth (called an *antimetabolite*).

NEVI

Iris Nevi

Think of them as freckles in your eye. Like freckles, pigmented nevi on the iris come in all shapes and sizes; even the degree of pigmentation can vary greatly among nevi in the same eye. And, like freckles, they're almost always benign.

Nevi that are small and unchanging should be routinely checked whenever you get your regular eye examination—every year or two. But if nevi are large, or if there's a suspicion that they're growing, then they should be checked at least every few months, because nevi that are on the move—ones that are either growing or changing in shape and color—can cause problems like cataracts and glaucoma.

However, if you have iris nevi, don't worry. It's highly unlikely that they'll ever cause you any trouble. In fact, clinical studies suggest that only 5 percent of even the most suspicious-looking ones ever change—become malignant—within five years. Of course, you don't want even to take a chance with malignancy, so check the nevi from time to time in your bathroom mirror. Look for any changes in size and color and any changes in the shape of the pupil. You probably won't find any. But if you do, contact your eye doctor and have it checked out.

Also, your eye doctor may want to make a record of photographs of suspicious iris nevi, to monitor any changes over time.

Choroidal Nevi and Melanomas (Pigmented Growths under the Retina)

Nevi can also be seen *below* the retina, in an area of tissue called the *vascular choroid*. These choroidal nevi are fairly common and can be seen during a routine eye examination. They almost never cause any problems with vision, and they rarely become malignant. It's estimated that fewer than 15 percent of them ever grow at all over five years. (Here too, as with iris nevi, a photographic record is often an invaluable means of detecting changes and growth.)

Melanomas, malignant pigmented cancers, can also occur in the choroid or ciliary body. They usually develop spontaneously and almost never arise from preexisting choroidal nevi. Like all pigment lesions in the eye, they are slightly more common in people with skin melanoma. However, they are still very rare.

Choroidal and ciliary body melanomas don't usually produce any early warning symptoms; it's only as they enlarge that people may experience visual changes or even develop eye inflammation. Because these cancer cells begin to grow under the retina, at first they can be hard to distinguish from benign choroidal nevi or other common retinal changes and growths. When a diagnosis of a choroidal or ciliary body melanoma is made, there are various treatment options to consider. Depending on the size, location, and extent of the tumor, the appropriate treatment may be observation, radiation, or enucleation (removal of the eye).

As with any medical problem, it's essential to seek the advice of expert health care professionals with experience in diagnosing and treating your problem.

15

The Retina and Vitreous

In chapter 8 we described how the aqueous and vitreous cavities help maintain the eye's shape. *Vitreous*, you may remember, is the jellylike substance—a gooey mass of connective tissue—that fills the eye's posterior cavity (see figure 1.1A). The walls of this cavity are lined by the *retina*, the crucial layer of the eye that converts light energy into nerve transmissions and sends them to the brain, where they're converted into images that make sense. When things go wrong with the vitreous cavity or with the retina (or with the part of the retina called the *macula;* see figure 1.1B), your attention is required; although the consequences are not always serious, they can be, and you need to know what's what.

FLOATERS AND FLASHES

The retina and the vitreous cavity, always immediate neighbors, are particularly closely linked at several key sites, including certain blood vessels, the optic nerve, the far edges of the retina, and the macula. But sometimes—as a result of eye or head trauma, or simply of aging—the vitreous jelly can shift and separate from the retina, a condition known as a *posterior vitreous detachment*, or PVD. (Think of an old house that develops cracks as it settles.)

The repercussions of such shifts vary. Among the most common consequences are what eye doctors think of as "condensations" or "opacifications" in the vitreous, and what patients often describe as "hairs," "gnats," or "spiders" in their vision: *floaters*. Light entering the eye passes around these opacifications in the vitreous and casts a shadow on the retinal photoreceptors; therefore, we see a spot floating. Almost everybody experiences floaters at some point in life. If the shift in the vitreous jelly is associated with traction or rubbing on the retina, patients can also experience quick sparkles of light or lightning: *flashes.*

Both of these, by themselves, are harmless. A shift in the vitreous alone is no cause for concern. Floaters can go away fairly quickly, or they can last for months to years. Usually, with time, they become less annoying and more tolerable. Flashes due to the rubbing or pulling of the vitreous on the retina are also usually short-lived.

So why worry about the sudden onset of floaters or flashes? If the traction against the retina is significant, the shift of the vitreous can cause the retina to rip slightly. *Such a tear can lead to a retinal detachment.* And retinal detachments can lead to permanent loss of vision. Therefore, suddenly experiencing flashes or floaters means you need to be evaluated by an eye care specialist, so that any holes or tears in the retina can be repaired before they cause permanent damage. *Note:* Flashes and floaters associated with retinal detachment usually happen only in *one eye* at a time, not both! (For more on this serious problem, read on.) Bilateral flashes (in both eyes) are an unusual phenomenon and are usually associated with visual forms of migraine, with or without an accompanying headache (see chapter 18).

A DETACHED RETINA

We often describe the retina as the wallpaper lining the back of the eye, even though, as we've discussed earlier in this book, it's infinitely more complicated than a single wafer of paper. For one thing, the retina isn't one sheet, it's an elegant, intricate network of layers. Its job is to take the light rays that enter the eye, convert them into nerve impulses, and then telegraph them, via the optic nerve, to the brain, where they're decoded into images that make sense.

Simply put, we see because of the retina. An eye without a working retina is blind. Therefore, when the retina becomes detached, or unhinged from the back of the eye, it must be treated immediately, because the repercussions are so great.

Fortunately, there are some warning signs of a detached retina. At first, you may experience the sudden onset of flashes—bursts of light, like fireworks or sparklers, that last only seconds at a time. Remember, the flashes we're talking about happen *only in one eye, not both eyes at the same*

Warning Symptoms of a Retinal Tear or Detachment

- A gradual or sudden increase in floaters in one eye. Like pieces of lint on a movie screen, these intrude on vision and may resemble cobwebs, spiders, or even circles.
- A gradual or sudden increase in flashes in one eye. Fleeting bursts of light, like fireworks or lightning, these may be especially noticeable in the dark.
- The gradual or sudden appearance of a dark cloud or "curtain" over your field of vision, from any direction.

If you experience any of these symptoms, call your eye doctor *immediately!* These may be signs of a retinal detachment.

---

time. Another cause for concern is the sudden development of annoying spots or specks in the eyes—floaters—which may resemble gnats, flies, spider webs, or even a recognizable shape like a ring or heart. (Typically, these are seen best against a solid background, such as the sky or a white wall.)

Floaters and flashes are most often due to a shift in the vitreous, the gooey jelly that fills the eye. Sometimes this vitreous shift leads to a break in the retina, in the form of a tear or hole. Then, gradually, the retina begins to detach, or peel off, from the back of the eye as the vitreous starts to seep through this opening. When this happens, patients can notice a slow loss of sight in that eye, as if a curtain were being drawn up or down across their vision. (This generally begins on one edge and may move centrally; moreover, if the detachment moves to affect the macular region at the back of the eye, central vision may also become affected.)

Ways the Retina May Become Detached

There are three basic things that can go wrong here.

Rhegmatogenous (or mechanical) retinal detachment: In this most common type of detachment, a hole or tear develops in the sensory retina, allowing liquid vitreous (most of the vitreous is a gel; however, as we get older, some of it becomes more liquid) to seep through the sensory retina and sever it from the retinal pigment epithelium. Those at risk for this type of detachment include people with specific forms of peripheral retinal thinning such as lattice degeneration, or people with severe nearsightedness or aphakia (the lack of a lens in the eye). People with a history of blunt trauma—

from boxing, for instance—or penetrating eye injury are also at risk.

Tractional retinal detachment: In this less common condition, fibrous scar tissue on the sensory retina's inner surface contracts—just as scar tissue does elsewhere in the body—pulling the sensory retina away from the retinal pigment epithelium. This problem is seen in people with diabetic retinopathy after a vitreous hemorrhage that produces scar tissue. It also may occur after eye trauma, or even as a complication following surgical repair of a rhegmatogenous retinal detachment.

Exudative retinal detachment: In this form, there's neither a hole for vitreous to pass through nor shrinking scar tissue to tug on the retina. Instead, fluid oozes from the choroid, through Bruch's membrane, and accumulates under an *intact* retina, like a blister. This may happen as a response to inflammation or in such conditions as uveitis (see chapter 14) or age-related macular degeneration (see chapter 9).

Fixing a Detached Retina

How hard is the task of repairing a detached retina? Imagine trying to unfold a crumpled piece of Kleenex in a glass of water without tearing it. This delicate, precise surgery requires steady hands, high-powered magnification, and special instruments.

The good news is that remarkable advances have been made over the last several decades in our ability to treat each form of retinal detachment. We would like to illustrate this with a brief discussion of the surgical treatment of rhegmatogenous detachment.

Rhegmatogenous detachment: The goal here, clearly, is to reattach the sensory retina to the retinal pigment epithelium, and retinal surgeons do this by compressing the sclera, the "white" of the eye—either with a buckle or with tiny sponges—to force these two layers back together. (A buckle is often required to indent the scleral wall from the outside of the eye enough to put these two retinal layers on the inside of the eye back in touch with each other, so that they can reattach to each other.) Surgeons also may inject gas bubbles into the vitreous cavity to help push the sensory retina up against the retinal pigment epithelium. (*Note:* Because the eye may have to be specially positioned to make these bubbles "float" into the best position, some people need to spend hours in one position—on their side or even upside down—as the retina heals after surgery.) It's almost always necessary to close the hole or tear in the sensory retina, and surgeons use lasers or cryotherapy (localized freezing techniques) to "spot-weld" around any retinal breaks. Sometimes this same treatment is used prophylactically on eyes prone to retinal detachment, to avoid a detachment before it occurs. Some people also may need to have excess retinal fluid drained from beneath the detachment so that the sensory and retinal pigment epithelial layers can reattach to each other. Modern microsurgical techniques using sophisticated small instruments for work inside the eye may also be used in reattaching the retina.

When the Eye's Blood Supply Is Blocked

It's simple: every single ounce of tissue, every tiny cell we have, needs oxygen to live.

Oxygen comes through the blood, and blood is piped throughout the body via our arteries and veins. Arteries deliver oxygen-rich blood throughout the body; like rivers, they branch into ever-smaller streams to reach every part of us. Veins make the return trip back to the heart and lungs, where more oxygen is pumped into the bloodstream; then the arteries deliver it all over again.

Blood reaches the eye through the big aorta and carotid arteries, which basically transport blood up through the neck; then, a smaller vessel, called the *ophthalmic artery*, carries it up into the eye. This important artery branches into smaller arteries as it nears the eye. Some supply blood to the choroid layer underneath the retina's pigment epithelium; others penetrate the optic nerve outside the eyeball and travel inside it to reach the eye's innermost workings. Most crucial of these branches are the *central retinal artery*, which supplies oxygen-rich blood to the retina's inner layers (these are known as the sensory retina), and the *central retinal vein*, which takes the oxygen-depleted blood out of the eye back toward the heart.

Blockage of the Retinal Blood Supply

These major retinal blood vessels, then, are pipelines—or, more precisely, lifelines—entering and leaving the eye. As you may imagine, a clog in one of these pipes can be devastating. Say the blockage is of an incoming, oxygen-bearing artery: deprived of oxygen, the retina immediately begins to react—to degenerate and swell. If the clog is in an outgoing retinal vein, the reaction is equally abrupt, like a sudden traffic jam on a major interstate—an almost-instantaneous backup of blood and fluid into the retina.

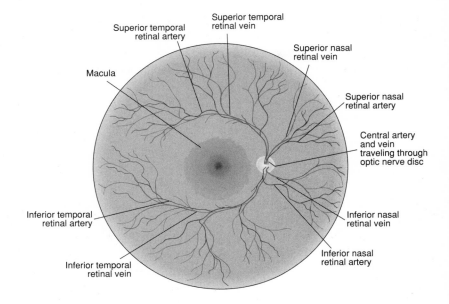

Fig. 15.1. Arteries and veins in the retina

Retinal vessel blockage—either arterial (with incoming blood) or venous (involving outgoing blood)—is a significant cause of visual problems in all ages, but especially in people over sixty-five. Just how common are these blockages? Nobody knows for sure; one difficulty in making estimates is the fact that many people don't notice a problem if it occurs in the nondominant eye or on the far edge of vision. Although their specifics differ, depending on whether an artery or a vein is involved, these blockages share one important common denominator for the retina: they mean big trouble.

Retinal Artery Blockages

Before we discuss retinal artery blockages, picture a river with four branches, or a road with four forks. The main line, or river, is the central "trunk" of the retinal artery; each of the four arteries, which branch at the head of the optic nerve, supplies one quarter of the retina. These are the *superior temporal, inferior temporal, superior nasal,* and *inferior nasal* arteries (see figure 15.1). There are many variations, but this is the basic pattern.

As you may imagine, the degree of injury—and its effect on vision—

depends on the location of the blockage, or "occlusion." A clog at the central retinal artery, the main line, can cause an eye to lose all vision instantly. If the problem is in a branch artery, vision loss is confined to the particular quadrant of the visual field served by that branch. (*Note:* Remember from chapter 1 that the retina's image is *inverted and reversed* by the brain. This means that a blockage of, say, the superior temporal retinal artery will cause a corresponding loss of vision in the inferior nasal visual field.)

In either case—whether it's a central or a branch artery involved—the resulting loss of vision is usually sudden, painless, and complete. There's an *infarction*, just as in a heart attack or stroke. Blood supply is cut off, and oxygen-starved tissue begins to swell, deteriorate, and then die. Almost always, this tissue loss is permanent.

As if this weren't devastating enough, there are other implications here. Is this clogged artery a symptom of a really big problem in the rest of your body? In other words, is there an even worse infarction—a heart attack or stroke—waiting to happen? Also, could the same thing happen in the other eye, causing total blindness?

The most common cause of central and branch retinal artery blockages in older people are cholesterol plaques lining the carotid arteries, a result of atherosclerosis ("hardening of the arteries"). Atherosclerosis is also an important factor in heart attacks and strokes. In the most likely scenario, a piece of the cholesterol plaque breaks off, floats downstream through the ophthalmic artery, and makes its way into the eye through the central retinal artery. At each fork in the road, the passage becomes tighter. Because they're so narrow, the central retinal artery and its branches in the retina are particularly prone to obstruction by these runaway cholesterol plaques.

Other causes of central and branch clogs in the retinal arteries include calcium deposits from damaged heart valves, leftover bits of a blood clot after a heart attack, and even foreign particles injected during IV drug abuse. Also, blood disorders such as sickle cell disease, other health problems such as migraines, collagen vascular diseases such as systemic lupus erythematosus, giant cell arteritis (see chapter 17), and even too-low blood pressure, by allowing these vessels temporarily to collapse, may cause these blockages. (In giant cell arteritis, the other eye is at especially high risk for a similar blockage.)

Fortunately, the chances of recovering vision are much better in branch blockages (80 percent of the time, vision returns to at least 20/40). However, even though they may recover much of their lost vision, many people with branch blockages do have some permanent vision damage.

Artery blockages in the retina are almost impossible to treat, because medical care must be almost immediate. *Within the first hour after the artery becomes clogged*, either the blockage must be removed or blood flow to the retina must be improved through the use of medications to dilate the arteries. After that, the lack of oxygen to the retina causes permanent and irreversible damage—and treatment days or even hours after the fact won't help. *Note:* Some patients do recover a little of their lost vision weeks afterward; when this happens, most doctors believe, it's because of relief from the swollen retinal tissue, not from a return of blood flow to already dead tissue.

Because, as mentioned above, this blockage might indicate other serious health problems that need prompt medical attention, patients with retinal artery blockages need a careful physical exam—perhaps including an evaluation of the carotid arteries and heart— beginning with a thorough and complete medical history. So, although this problem may begin in the eye, your family physician, internist, or cardiologist definitely needs to see you as soon as possible.

Retinal Vein Blockages

As you can see from figure 15.1, the retinal veins form almost a mirror image of the retinal arteries, only the flow is reversed. Instead of bearing oxygen-*rich* blood into the eye, the veins take oxygen-*poor* blood out of it. So instead of depriving retinal tissue of blood, a blockage in the veins causes blood to back up and pool there, like a clogged drain in a sink with the water still running. This can happen either *acutely* (a total block, causing sudden symptoms of vision loss) or *gradually* (a partial block, progressively slowing the outflow over months to years).

Again, there are two types of blockages: central and branch.

Central Retinal Vein Blockages

The main vessel, or "trunk," of the retinal vein lies at the optic nerve head. As with the central artery line, an obstruction here can cause major trouble: a huge backup of blood into the retina, usually resulting in a sudden loss of vision (see figure 15.2). When the blockage is more gradual, symptoms are less severe but may still end in vision loss.

The two big complications associated with central retinal vein blockages are *damage to the macular region* in the retina, causing swelling and per-

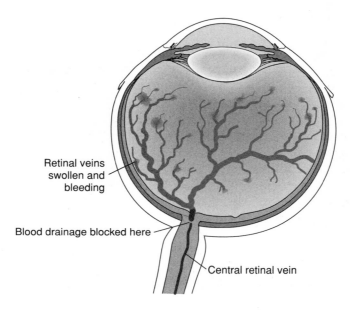

Retinal veins
swollen and
bleeding

Blood drainage blocked here

Central retinal vein

Fig. 15.2.   Central retinal vein blockage

manent vision loss, and *neovascular glaucoma,* a rare but devastating form of glaucoma that can happen days to months after the fact (especially within the first ninety days). Fortunately, most people with a central retinal vein occlusion do not develop neovascular glaucoma. This extremely serious condition can be excruciating. Even worse, it can cause patients to develop uncontrollable elevated eye pressure and chronic discomfort. Neovascular glaucoma may require laser, cryotherapy, or surgical treatment to alleviate pain and preserve the eye, even when there is no hope of recovering vision. Because of this, although there's practically no way to treat a central retinal vein blockage—laser treatment for the macular damage has not been proven effective—patients need careful monitoring afterward, in case neovascular glaucoma develops.

Again, as with artery blockages in the retina, problems in the veins may indicate larger health problems, particularly hypertension, cardiovascular disease, and diabetes. Thus, patients also need a general medical workup to avert any further trouble, either in the other eye or elsewhere in the body.

Branch Retinal Vein Blockages

The central retinal vein splits into two main branches, which serve the *superior* and *inferior* halves of the retina. Blockage in either of these veins causes trouble in the corresponding half of the retina. These major branches are fed by the *temporal* and *nasal* retinal venules (smaller veins), and by their own tributaries. A blockage in any of these branches causes swelling and a backup of blood and fluid—but smaller, more focused areas of damage.

As in central retinal vein blockages, macular swelling, or edema, is a common complication that may lead to vision loss. (The threat of neovascular glaucoma is much less common in these smaller blockages.) *Note:* Branch blockages here usually don't mean both eyes are at risk; in fact, if you've had one in one eye, your risk of having a similar blockage in the other eye is only about 10 percent. Branch retinal vein blockages tend to occur mostly in people with hypertension or cardiovascular disease.

Within the first six months after the branch retinal vein blockage, there is often so much pooled blood that it's difficult to determine the extent of injury to the retina. As this hemorrhage gradually clears, your eye doctor will probably want to use fluorescein angiography to assess the damage, and to see whether macular edema is present.

As the excess blood and swelling recede, some people spontaneously regain their vision; others may need laser treatment to treat the macular edema. Because some people do get better on their own, most doctors hesitate to attempt laser treatment for the first six months or so, to give the retina a chance to heal itself.

MACULAR CYSTS AND HOLES

It's rare, but sometimes—for reasons that aren't clear, despite much speculation—people develop a small cyst or hole in the center of the macula. (The macula, remember, is the most important part of the retina, the part that's responsible for our central vision.) Some people experience absolutely no change in vision; others may suffer a total loss of central vision.

What's happening here? Could the vitreous gel be pulling at this area, causing these changes? Are they early forms of degeneration of the retinal pigment epithelium, part of the more severe changes seen in age-related macular degeneration? Again, nobody knows.

Often people first notice the problem—manifested as a subtle distortion—when they're reading. The lines of the crossword puzzle, for instance, start to bend. Letters of words in a book may seem distorted or appear to be missing. If you're experiencing any changes like these, see your eye doctor for a complete eye examination, including a dilated retinal evaluation.

To date, the treatment for macular holes and cysts has met with limited success. Both laser and surgical treatments have been attempted. Some doctors have even tried to seal these holes by injecting growth factors that promote healing into the back of the eye—with debatable results. These treatments, because of potential complications, are usually reserved for people with poor visual acuity due to the hole or cyst. For many people the only help we can offer is to monitor the condition and provide education, support, and counseling for low-vision problems, if this becomes necessary.

Fortunately, macular cysts progress slowly, if at all, and macular holes essentially never lead to a retinal detachment.

MACULAR WRINKLING

There are many names for this phenomenon, including macular pucker, epiretinal membrane formation, surface wrinkling retinopathy, and cellophane maculopathy. The basic problem is the growth, over the surface of the macula, of a membrane—think of a cellophane wrap over a plate of cookies—that causes it to contract and wrinkle. Usually these membranes are harmless. But occasionally they can progress, leading to marked distortion of the retina, and sometimes impeding vision.

Abnormal membranes can be found after vitreous hemorrhages or eye trauma, or after eye surgery (to repair a retinal detachment, or remove a cataract, for instance); they may also be associated with certain retinal diseases, especially those that cause inflammation. They can show up, *for no apparent reason*, in healthy eyes—one or both—as well.

For most people these membranes remain stable for years, causing no deterioration in vision (85 percent of people retain a visual acuity of 20/70 or better, and 67 percent have 20/30 or better; fewer than 5 percent ever progress to 20/200 or worse). However, if epiretinal membranes do grow to a point where they begin to distort the retina and cause vision problems, symptoms usually begin with mild distortion or blurred vision.

There is a treatment—surgical stripping of epiretinal membranes from the retina—for certain patients. However, most retinal surgeons will attempt this procedure only if it's clear that the vision problems are definitely being caused by the membrane, and, depending on the membrane's location and growth, that removing it will actually improve someone's vision. Microsurgical vitrectomy techniques have come a long way in recent years and have also proved very effective in removing advanced epiretinal membranes. However, as with all procedures, there are risks involved—including infection—and you and your doctor will need to discuss them thoroughly before deciding whether this procedure is for you.

16

The
Optic Nerve

Here we are, in the eye's nerve center—a massive cable that links the eye to the brain, allowing us to make sense out of what we see. Like a mighty river fed by countless streams, the optic nerve cable, made up of more than a million tiny fibers, starts small—in the ganglion cells of the sensory retina. These fibers connect to the retina's interior, where they form the nerve fiber layer, and then amass in a giant bundle at the back of the eye to form the optic nerve. The next stop, via the sclera at the eye's "back door," is the brain.

As you can see from figure 1.1A, the optic nerve is the only game in town: every single visual impulse that travels from point A, the eye, to point B, the brain, must take this route. Thus, even the slightest disruption—from inflammation, poor blood flow, infection, trauma, or a tumor—can have devastating consequences for someone's vision. Two important optic nerve problems that warrant special mention here are *optic neuritis* (inflammation of the optic nerve) and *ischemic optic neuropathy* (a tiny stroke in the optic nerve).

OPTIC NEURITIS

Optic neuritis is an inflammation of the optic nerve. It can be caused by infection and immune-related illnesses, or its cause can be *idiopathic* (a medical term that means, essentially, "We don't know why this has happened").

When the optic nerve becomes inflamed, the impact on vision is prompt: a marked decrease in central or fine visual acuity, or loss of visual field. Usually only one eye is affected at a time. Other symptoms almost always include pain or tenderness of the eyeball, with discomfort as the eye muscles pull or rub on the optic nerve sheath surrounding the optic nerve. In optic neuritis, it may be difficult to see straight ahead, colors may appear washed out, and lights may seem dim; trouble with depth perception is also common. Exercise, a hot shower, or any other activity that raises body temperature may make the vision problems worse.

In a typical episode of optic neuritis, the decline in vision tends to level off within a few days; eyesight improves gradually over the next four to six weeks. At least 85 percent of people with an episode of optic neuritis regain useful vision, and any loss of central, peripheral, or color vision is often mild, detectable only on testing. Also, the majority of patients with optic neuritis never suffer another episode. Only in very rare cases, when involvement has been particularly severe, does it happen that vision fails to recover from the initial decline.

Although, as mentioned above, most cases of optic neuritis are idiopathic, many ailments can also take their toll on the optic nerve, including viral illnesses (such as mumps, rubella, and cytomegalovirus), bacterial infections (such as cat-scratch fever and TB), sinus infections, and inflammations elsewhere in the body or eye. Also, because the optic nerve is, in effect, an extension of the brain, it seems to be susceptible to some of the brain's own disorders, particularly multiple sclerosis.

Multiple sclerosis is what's called a *demyelinating* condition: it erodes myelin, the protective sheath of insulation around the nerve fibers, leaving the bare "wire" exposed. No one understands why it happens, but for some reason spots of myelin just melt away, disrupting the conduction of electrical impulses, causing delayed transmission, and leading to such classic symptoms as numbness and tingling in the arms and legs, difficulty walking, and double vision (due to an effect on the nerves that control the eye muscles). *Note:* One episode of optic neuritis certainly doesn't mean that you have, or that you are going to develop, multiple sclerosis. However, up to 95 percent of people who do develop multiple sclerosis will have an episode of optic neuritis at least once in their lives. (It's also worth noting that multiple sclerosis has many degrees of severity. Many people live completely normal lives with very mild forms of the disease. In fact, scientists believe, some cases of multiple sclerosis are never even diagnosed because the symptoms are so minor!)

Treatment: Treatment begins with an exhaustive medical history and a physical examination—and that's the easy part, because there is no one widely accepted treatment for optic neuritis. Sometimes you can see the inflamed optic nerve in an eye exam. Rarely does treating an *underlying* disease or condition alter the course of optic neuritis; only time can tell whether vision will return after the inflamed optic nerve gets better on its own.

For years controversy surrounded the use of *steroids* (medications known to decrease swelling in the body) in various dosages and regimens against optic neuritis. In a search for better, more definitive answers, the National Eye Institute sponsored the national Optic Neuritis Treatment Trial (ONTT), a large, multicentered clinical trial designed to study the effects of steroids on optic neuritis. The study's striking results have completely changed the way we treat people with optic neuritis. Scientists found, to their surprise, that steroids did not significantly improve vision after the episode, nor did they lower the odds of recurrence. But in people with optic neuritis *and* brain scan evidence suggesting multiple sclerosis, they found that steroids *helped slow the course of multiple sclerosis.*

Today, as a result of these findings, all patients newly diagnosed with optic neuritis are advised to have an MRI (magnetic resonance imaging) of the brain (a painless, noninvasive test) as soon as possible. If the scan suggests the possibility of multiple sclerosis, then high-dose intravenous steroid therapy should begin soon—within eight days of the onset of optic neuritis symptoms. Even though this probably won't help the optic neuritis, it appears to help protect brain cells against further demyelination. The results of the ONTT are still being evaluated, and data from four-year and five-year follow-ups suggest that the protective effect of steroids, unfortunately, may begin to wane after three years: the people taking steroids begin to catch up with those not taking steroids in the incidence of clinically definitive multiple sclerosis. This is an evolving field, though, where much research is being done all the time. The ONTT at least established that the use of high-dose IV steroids seems to delay the onset of MS in the short term.

ISCHEMIC OPTIC NEUROPATHY (POOR BLOOD FLOW TO THE OPTIC NERVE)

When the supply of blood—and the vital oxygen it carries—is shut off, the result is called *ischemia*. This can happen, in mild or severe form, anywhere in the body. In the heart, major ischemia can cause a heart attack; fleeting ischemia can cause the intense chest pain of angina. In the brain, severe ischemia causes a stroke; temporary ischemia can lead to TIAs (transient ischemic attacks), or "mini-strokes." In the eye, episodes of *temporary* ischemia—usually from atherosclerotic narrowing of the carotid artery, hindering blood flow to the retina—can cause "gray-outs" (also called *amaurosis fugax;* see chapter 18). And *severe* ischemia—a shutoff of blood flow thought to result from artery disease within the optic nerve—can lead to the eye's version of a stroke: nerve cell damage and a sudden, dramatic, and usually permanent loss of vision in one eye. This is called *ischemic optic neuropathy.*

There are two distinct varieties of ischemic optic neuropathy. The first is *nonarteritic ischemic optic neuropathy* (nonarteritic ION). It's a long name, but the word *idiopathic* (meaning "we don't know") ought to be in there somewhere, because although we know what happens to the optic nerve, we don't know why, or what causes it. Equally serious but with systemic implications is *arteritic ischemic optic neuropathy* (arteritic ION). We do know what's causing this: an inflammatory condition of the blood vessels supplying the optic nerve and of other blood vessels throughout the body.

Nonarteritic Ischemic Optic Neuropathy

People with nonarteritic ION experience a scary, painless sudden loss of vision, sometimes the upper or lower half of their visual field. There are no early warning signs. The problem seems to be age-related: it tends to strike people in their sixties. Many of these people also have hypertension or diabetes. It is assumed that these diseases play a role in causing nonarteritic ION, although we don't know exactly how. (Some experts speculate that the problem is caused by atherosclerosis, or "hardening" of the eye's blood vessels.) Unfortunately, most of the vision loss is immediate and permanent; recovery of the lost vision is rare. Plus, in about 10 percent of people, nonarteritic ION strikes the second eye as well—and sadly, we have no means of preventing this loss.

Arteritic Ischemic Optic Neuropathy

Arteritic ION happens when the blood vessels that feed the optic nerve become inflamed. The inflammation chokes, or sometimes blocks completely, blood flow to the optic nerve. It is not an isolated problem: this same inflammation also occurs in blood vessels elsewhere in the body, causing symptoms that may include headache, scalp tenderness, jaw discomfort when chewing or talking, fever, malaise, weight loss, and muscle weakness in the arms and legs. This generalized inflammation of the blood vessels—also known as *temporal arteritis* or *giant cell arteritis*—is usually confirmed by a blood test called a *sedimentation rate*.

Temporal, or giant cell, arteritis is characterized by a classic headache along the artery at the temples; when samples of the affected artery are examined under the microscope, we can see telltale enlarged (or giant) cells in the blood vessel walls. A biopsy of the temporal artery is usually needed to confirm this diagnosis. Your doctor may need samples of *both* temporal arteries (called a *bilateral biopsy*) to be certain. Fortunately, unilateral and bilateral biopsies don't interfere with blood flow to the head or face. Giant cell arteritis is thought in some patients to be related to a larger disorder known as *polymyalgia rheumatica*, characterized by pain and discomfort in the large muscles of the shoulders, neck, and thighs. Both conditions tend to occur in older people, often in their seventies, most commonly in women.

In arteritic ION the vision loss is usually more severe than in the nonarteritic form. Some people experience transient visual disturbances, or fluctuations in vision, before the acute loss of vision with ION—probably caused by intermittent blockages of blood flow.

Treatment: There is no proven treatment for arteritic ION, although many patients experience a modest improvement in vision over time. The big thing to worry about here, as in nonarteritic ION, is the second eye. In 70 percent of people with arteritic ION, the second eye becomes involved within days to weeks after the first eye. *Therefore, when arteritic ION is suspected, high-dose oral steroid therapy should begin immediately in order to protect the other eye.* This *prophylactic*, or preventive, steroid therapy is often needed for months or years to keep the giant cell arteritis under control. Unfortunately, however, prolonged use of steroids can cause problems of its own. Be sure to discuss these with your doctor, who will almost certainly want to monitor you closely, to check for the development of any steroid-related side effects.

PART V

*Other Things
You Need to Know*

17

Eye Trauma and Emergencies

It stings, it hurts, it's red, it's watery—but is it an emergency? You need to know, because if it *is* an emergency, it is essential that you get prompt care, either from your eye doctor or at the emergency room of a hospital. Doing so or not doing so can make a big difference.

So, let's start this chapter off with a list of *emergency situations*. All of these require immediate attention:

- Any *severe* eye pain or discomfort
- Chemicals in the eye
- Eye trauma (like getting punched in the eye)
- A feeling like there's a foreign body in the eye
- Sudden loss of vision
- Any postoperative eye discomfort or change in vision
- Sudden onset of double vision

Now, here are the symptoms of an *urgent situation*. If you have any of these symptoms, you need to see a doctor within twenty-four to forty-eight hours:

- Gradual loss of vision over days or weeks
- Recent onset of light flashes and floaters
- Red eye without loss of vision or severe pain
- Recent onset of sensitivity to light

In this chapter we'll take a close look at some of these emergency and urgent situations. Other situations (like flashes and floaters) are covered in other chapters (check them out in the Index).

CHEMICAL BURNS

It hurts like crazy; it may also cause permanent damage. When chemicals get splashed or sprayed in the eye, you need emergency attention—fast. How bad is the injury? Can the eye recover? This depends not only on which chemical has injured your eye and on how severe the injury is, but also on how quickly you get medical help.

There are two main categories of chemical burns in the eye: those caused by alkalis, such as lime, lye, and ammonia, and those caused by acids, such as battery acid.

Alkali burns generally do the most damage. These chemicals react rapidly with fats in the cell membranes, the protective barrier covering the eye's outer surface. Weakening this natural shield allows the chemical to penetrate even deeper, into the cornea—often causing serious corneal swelling, inflammation, and even cataracts. Sometimes the cornea becomes so severely scarred that it can't even be fixed by a corneal transplant; the result is permanent vision loss.

Acid burns, surprisingly enough—even those caused by such harsh chemicals as battery acid—are usually tolerated better than alkali burns by the cornea. Because they tend not to damage the cell membranes, they usually don't penetrate deep into the cornea. Therefore, the risk of major corneal scarring, as described above, is much lower.

Detergents are other chemicals that often find their way into the eyes. More often than you might think, people inadvertently mistake liquid dishwashing soap for a contact lens cleaning solution, causing painful inflammation. Despite the irritation and swelling they may produce, detergents in the eye, as chemicals go, are usually pretty harmless. Even when, as sometimes happens, they injure the cornea's epithelium (its outermost layer of cells), the eye almost always recovers completely.

Treatment: No matter what caused the injury, your immediate response should be copious irrigation. In other words:

Step 1: Wash it out! The long-term health of your eye depends on how quickly you can begin rinsing it. You can use tap water, contact lens wetting solution, or saline. Tap water is usually the fluid most readily available in large quantities; it's best to splash water into the eye with your hand, rather than stare up into the gushing faucet.

Step 2: Don't stop. Keep irrigating vigorously for about thirty minutes.

Step 3: Go to the eye doctor or emergency room. An eye exam at this point will reveal the extent of the damage and the need for further treatment.

(This may include further irrigation, debridement—removal of foreign particles or injured tissue—medication, or an eye patch.)

"BLACK EYE" AND OTHER TRAUMA

No matter how you got it—by falling, being punched, or getting elbowed while shooting hoops—the same injury that causes the classic "shiner" can cause severe internal eye damage, which may include bleeding within the eye, iritis (arthritis-like inflammation in the eye), glaucoma, double vision (due to difficulty moving the eye), a detached retina, and even temporary or permanent loss of vision. If the floor of the orbit is fractured, this could cause muscle damage, which may limit eye movement and create the appearance of a sunken eyeball—either of which may require surgery. So don't be your own expert and simply apply the beefsteak. First, let your eye doctor or local emergency room physicians check it out.

CORNEAL ABRASIONS AND FOREIGN BODIES

Even though these can be some of the most uncomfortable eye problems, they're also among the most easily treated.

Why does it hurt so much? It's because a host of sensory nerves make their home in the cornea and conjunctiva. Their job is to sound the alarm, alerting the eye's defense mechanisms to dryness, foreign bodies, injury, even temperature change. The eye then responds—by blinking or producing tears, for example.

When a foreign body, such as a tiny fleck of metal or rock, invades the cornea and becomes embedded in it, these same sensory nerves can make a splinter feel like a log. *Note:* They can also cause misleading sensations, making you think that something actually lodged in the center of the cornea is under the upper eyelid, when in fact it's the movement of the eyelid over the foreign object in the cornea that's so painful.

Treatment: Most foreign bodies stay on the surface of the cornea. They're fairly easily removed, under high magnification at the slit lamp, using a cotton-tipped applicator, needle, or other instrument. Your eye doctor will want to make sure that the foreign body is a lone invader (or, if it's not, to remove any other specks or splinters), that it hasn't perforated the eyeball, and that there's no associated infection, trauma, or injury. (This may require a dilated eye examination.)

Preventing Eye Injuries: Caution and Common Sense

There are some easy, commonsense steps you can take to prevent one of the most common causes of eye problems in this country: eye injuries, which result from an unbelievable variety of activities. Obviously, it's not possible to prevent a car crash or freak accident. But it doesn't take long, when you take care of patients in a busy hospital emergency department, to grasp a few lucid points. One of them is that using a grinding wheel or chain saw without goggles can and does result in eye injuries. Letting your kids run around holding scissors with the points exposed is *not* a good idea. Nor is putting in contact lenses at a bathroom counter cluttered with household chemicals. Being a little neurotic about protecting your eyes from injury just makes good sense.

To prevent the risk of infection after the fact, your doctor may also give you an antibiotic eye ointment under a pressure patch worn for twelve to twenty-four hours. Fortunately, because the corneal epithelium grows so fast, the cornea usually repairs itself, quickly covering any dents or scratches left when a foreign body is removed. Usually the cornea heals in twenty-four hours, with no permanent visual defect. (If, however, the foreign body manages to penetrate the center of the cornea, it may cause a corneal scar, and this may affect vision permanently.)

Recurrent corneal erosion (see chapter 11): Materials with rough surfaces—paper, wood, even fingernails—can cause a corneal abrasion. Either by becoming lodged within the eye or simply by rubbing or poking the cornea, they can significantly alter the corneal epithelium's basement membrane. Picture a slab of cement, with a single layer of epithelial cells as bricks upon it: damage to this cement affects the way these cells stick to the basement membrane and eye. They may become loose and "slough off," especially at nighttime. (When this happens, the eye feels like it's being injured all over again, hence the term *recurrent corneal erosion.*)

Recurrent corneal erosions are common and can be very annoying. Fortunately, they usually don't last too long, and plenty of help for the discomfort—including drops, ointments, patches, surgical debridement or scraping, and even lasers—is available. Your eye doctor may want to see you at least one more time to rule out any infection or other complications.

VISION DISTURBANCES

We've already talked about flashes and floaters (see chapter 15). But other, equally distressing, transient disruptions in the visual field are strange patterns—wavy lines, broken glass, or jagged edges—that often show up first at the edge of vision and then march toward the center and back again. These are often found to be a form of migraines, *with or without the headache* (see chapter 18). Many things can combine to cause this, including stress, caffeine, certain medications, hormonal surges (including those in pregnancy and menopause), and diet. The good news is that when the migraine goes away, so do these weird patterns.

SUDDEN LOSS OF VISION OR VISUAL FIELD

Don't wait for this to get better on its own: *seek help immediately!* In the world of eye problems, it doesn't get much more serious than this. *Note:* By "loss of vision" we mean here *partial or total loss of sight in one or both eyes*—not just something funny going on with your vision, such as floaters, migraine patterns, second images of cataracts, or blurry vision caused by dry eyes or infection (although these too are important and also require medical attention).

One Eye, or Both?

If you are suffering vision loss, your eye doctor's first step will be to figure out what's causing the problem. In addition to receiving a thorough eye exam, you'll be asked a lot of detailed questions. The first will probably be, Is this happening in one or both eyes?

This is terribly important, because *if you're having simultaneous loss of vision in both eyes, chances are that the trouble isn't originating in your eyes.* One cause of a sudden vision loss in both eyes (called a *bilateral* loss) is a breakdown in the pathways that connect the eyes to the brain. The occipital lobe is the brain's vision center; a stroke or infarct (caused by a blocked blood vessel) here can cause a sudden, and often permanent, bilateral loss of vision. Migraines too can cause temporary bilateral visual loss (see chapter 18).

If the vision loss is in one eye (called *unilateral* loss), the important question is, Is the problem temporary? The most common cause of transient unilateral loss of vision is "fleeting blindness," or amaurosis fugax. In this case, the loss often progresses from the edge to the center of vision, like a dark curtain closing. Then, seconds to minutes later, the curtain opens again, with vision returning gradually but completely within about twenty minutes. This odd and often frightening problem is believed to be caused by platelets or other tiny impediments that briefly interrupt blood flow in the retina. Many people who suffer from fleeting blindness have carotid artery disease—atherosclerosis in the carotid artery, another problem not to be taken lightly. They should undergo a careful physical examination; if significant blockage or buildup is discovered, these patients may need a surgical procedure called an *endarterectomy*, the surgical cleaning out of cholesterol plaque from the carotid artery. Other causes of transient unilateral vision loss include atypical migraines, hypotension, anemia, arteritis (see below), and elevated intracranial pressure from a variety of causes, including tumors and bleeding in the brain.

If the vision loss in one eye is permanent, the next big question is, Where's the loss—in your *central* or your *peripheral* vision? Because the optic nerve or retina can be involved in both cases, a thorough eye examination, including a dilated optic nerve and retinal evaluation, is crucial for pinpointing the problem.

Several things can cause sudden loss of central vision in one eye, including inflammation of the optic nerve, blockage of a main or branch retinal artery (see chapter 15), blockage or inflammation of other nerves in the eye, a detached retina, or a subretinal neovascular membrane (see chapter 9)—a problem often associated with macular degeneration. *Note:* It is rarely caused by cataracts, glaucoma, or diabetic retinopathy, and it's *never* caused by inadequate eyeglasses.

Giant Cell Arteritis

Giant cell arteritis, also called *temporal arteritis*, is a fairly common condition in people over age sixty-five that can lead to sudden permanent vision loss in one or both eyes. A disorder of the body's autoimmune system, giant cell arteritis is an inflammation that affects blood vessels—particularly those near the eye. Symptoms of giant cell arteritis, or inflammation of the blood vessels supplying the optic nerve, may begin with transient visual disturbances—brief episodes of losing central or peripheral vision, like temporary blackouts in an overheated city. Eventually these blackouts may become permanent, resulting in the total loss of central vision, or loss of the top or bottom half of the visual field.

What's happening here? The inflammation shuts off blood flow to the nerve, a condition called *ischemic optic neuropathy* (see chapter 16). Although there's no blood clot involved, the nerve damage is like that brought on by a stroke or heart attack: without oxygen, the optic nerve quickly begins to deteriorate, causing permanent damage—and, perhaps, irreversible loss of vision. Giant cell arteritis often causes other problems, including headaches, tenderness in the temples or scalp, trouble hearing, jaw pain, and trouble chewing. Clearly, if you're having any of these symptoms— particularly the vision disturbances described above—call your doctor immediately. Another worry is that giant cell arteritis often affects both eyes; therefore, early diagnosis and treatment are crucial.

Diagnosis and treatment: Your eye doctor will begin with a careful medical history. If giant cell arteritis is indeed suspected, you'll need a blood test called a *sedimentation rate* (also known as a "sed" rate). This test isn't definitive, but it can show whether the body's immune system is working overtime, as it does in arteritis. However, a similar immune response happens in other diseases, including arthritis and cancer; therefore, if the sedimentation rate confirms that giant cell arteritis is a possibility, your doctor will perform another, more specific test: a temporal artery biopsy. There are two temporal arteries, one located near each temple; the biopsy —which causes no lasting effects, poses minimal risks, and is performed under local anesthesia—will probably be done on both sides.

The treatment in giant cell arteritis, to protect the other eye from ischemic optic neuropathy, or to preserve vision in the first one, is high-dose steroids; your doctor may even prescribe them before performing the biopsy. Because steroids can cause many problems of their own (see chapter 20 and Appendix), they're never prescribed lightly; because treatment for this disorder is often long-term, lasting months or even years, your eye doctor or internist will want to monitor you carefully for any sign of side effects.

Nonarteritic Ischemic Optic Neuropathy

There is another form of ischemic optic neuropathy that also affects people in their fifties and sixties; because it is not related to arteritis, its name, by default, is *nonarteritic ischemic optic neuropathy* (see chapter 16). It differs from the arteritic form in that it often affects only one eye, it's associated with only mildly elevated sedimentation rates, steroid therapy doesn't help, and—perhaps most important—vision loss is usually not as severe or as permanent. Its cause is not known, though it seems to be found more often in people with hypertension. Unfortunately, there is no widely accepted treatment for this condition.

18

General Health Problems That Can Affect the Eyes

Sometimes the problem doesn't begin in the eye at all. The disease is *systemic*—that is, it affects the whole body. But as far as the eye is concerned, the consequences of some of these general health problems are as serious as any specific eye disease could ever be. Some of these disorders are discussed in this chapter, beginning with the big threat to eyesight posed by diabetes.

DIABETES

Diabetes cuts a wide, devastating swath through the body. No cell or organ, it seems, is immune to its ravages, and the eyes seem particularly vulnerable. In fact, among Americans of working age, diabetes is the leading cause of new cases of blindness.

Diabetes can cause trouble in the lens, eye muscles, iris, and other eye structures. People with diabetes are more prone to developing cataracts and glaucoma. But within the eye, diabetes has its worst effect on the retina.

What diabetes does to the retina—and this encompasses a broad spectrum of mutations, ranging from pinpoint blood clots to retinal detachments, which may result in blindness—is known as *diabetic retinopathy*. Fortunately, most people with diabetes do not wind up blind from diabetic retinopathy; only about 3 percent of all people with diabetes eventually develop severe vision loss. But most people with diabetes do, at some point, experience some eye complications.

Before we discuss these, let's take a minute to review diabetes itself, which is in fact two diseases: *Type I*, or *insulin-dependent diabetes*, and *Type II*, or *non-insulin-dependent diabetes*. Only about 10 percent of all people with diabetes have Type I, which is usually diagnosed in childhood or adolescence. Because these people have the disease throughout their lives—as opposed to those with Type II, who tend to develop it later on—the disease has plenty of time to cause trouble. Diabetic retinopathy is especially prevalent in this group. (In one study of people with Type I diabetes, 25 percent had some retinal changes after three or four years; but after fifteen years of having diabetes, a staggering 80 percent showed signs of diabetic retinopathy.)

The vast majority of people with diabetes have the Type II variety. Because the classic symptoms of this disease—increased thirst, frequent urination, weight loss, and lack of energy—are often ignored, not recognized as warning signs, or confused with other ailments, it may be years before the condition is discovered. And because of this delay, in many people retinopathy is found soon after the diabetes is diagnosed. (Fortunately, it doesn't seem to be as severe as the retinopathy found in Type I disease.)

What Diabetes Can Do to the Retina

Diabetes attacks the small blood vessels of the body—the essential pathways that help supply blood and nutrients to the brain, peripheral nerves, kidneys, and eyes.

Briefly, diabetes targets the small blood vessels' *basement membrane*—which, as its name suggests, is their foundation, or cement. On top of this basement membrane, lining the inside of the blood vessels, are *endothelial cells*. Other tiny yet important cells are *pericytes*, whose job seems to be to help the basement membrane support the retinal blood vessels. In the eye, diabetes causes the basement membrane to thicken and the number of pericytes to dwindle, particularly in the retina. This in turn makes the blood vessel cells more porous and less able to carry oxygen and nutrients to the retinal tissues—which over time become malnourished and sickly. And this, basically, is diabetic retinopathy.

The damages here can be classified into two general types: *nonproliferative diabetic retinopathy* (tiny blood bulges, or microaneurysms, pinpoint hemorrhages, cotton-wool spots, changes to the wall of blood vessels, macular edema, and shunts), and *proliferative diabetic retinopathy* (an unwanted surge in the growth of blood vessels, or *retinal neovascularization*).

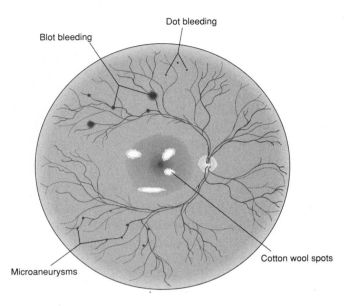

Fig. 18.1. View of the retina with nonproliferative diabetic retinopathy

Nonproliferative Diabetic Retinopathy

The retinal changes of nonproliferative diabetic retinopathy, described below, can be ranked according to their severity. They may be mild to moderate, moderate to severe, or very severe. These ratings are particularly important when determining when someone should undergo laser treatment.

Microaneurysms, tiny blood vessel outpouchings that look like small red dots in the retina (particularly in the macula), can go away all by themselves. But they also have a tendency to leak fluid into the retina, contributing to a far more serious condition called *macular edema* (see below).

Dot hemorrhages are pinpoint areas of bleeding in the retina. *Blot hemorrhages* are larger, irregular, and roundish. Both of these types of bleeding also may be absorbed by the retina without causing any long-term damage.

Cotton-wool spots, or *soft exudates*, are localized areas of retinal *infarction* (loss of blood flow to an area of tissue). These happen when tiny capillaries clamp themselves shut, halting the blood supply to nerves in the retina. The nerve tissue then swells (under the microscope, this looks like wisps of cotton on the retina).

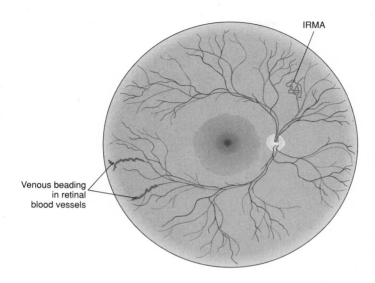

Fig. 18.2.   View of the retina with intraretinal microvascular abnormalities (IRMA) and venous beading

Venous beading can cause the normally smooth walls of retinal blood vessels to look bumpy. Other results of retinal blood vessel changes are *abnormal blood flow patterns* and *shunts* (small, tubular areas of mutated capillaries that look like spaghetti). These are called *IRMA*, or *intraretinal microvascular abnormalities*. (Both of these are common in advanced forms of nonproliferative diabetic retinopathy.)

Macular edema is the most common cause of visual impairment in people with diabetic retinopathy. Nearly all of the retina's surface area is devoted to peripheral, or side, vision. A surprisingly small area—about 10 percent—is responsible for our fine central, or reading, vision. This is the macula (see figure 1.1B). And the heart of this minute but critical region, the *fovea*, is a tiny area (less than 2 millimeters wide) of nerve cells—yet this is the epicenter of vision, the site of our most important sensory vision cells.

Macular edema doesn't just erupt overnight. As diabetic retinopathy takes its slow toll on the retinal blood vessels, they get progressively weaker and form tiny microaneurysms—particularly in the macula. These microaneurysms—which actually are abnormal areas of the blood vessel walls—leak; they ooze a nasty, fatty fluid into the retina. The swelling this causes is called *macular edema*. Imagine trying to watch a TV screen behind a fish

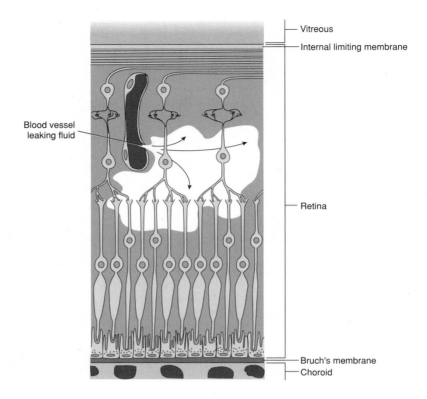

Vitreous

Internal limiting membrane

Blood vessel leaking fluid

Retina

Bruch's membrane
Choroid

Fig. 18.3. Microscopic section showing macular edema

tank: the water would blur the picture. Well, the same thing happens in macular edema: The fluid obscures central vision. Reading is blurry. Looking straight ahead is blurry. And frustratingly, eyeglasses can't do anything to help. No matter how sharply light rays are focused onto this swollen retina, the retina's machinery simply can't function any better because the leaking fluid is in the way.

Although sometimes this fluid buildup gets reabsorbed on its own, mostly it doesn't. And over time this edema can cause irreversible damage to the retinal sensory cells, resulting in permanent vision problems. Fortunately, with early and appropriate treatment (see below) to slow the leakage and reduce the fluid, macular edema rarely causes blindness anymore. Remember, all of these changes to the retina may be either mild or very severe, or something in between.

Proliferative Diabetic Retinopathy

Sometimes the problem isn't bleeding from existing blood vessels, it's bleeding from a "baby boom" of new blood vessels that have formed in the retina. These proliferative changes, primarily *retinal neovascularization*, also cause vision problems. To complicate matters, a person can have diabetic macular edema, proliferative or nonproliferative diabetic retinopathy, or any combination of these.

Nobody knows exactly why these new blood vessels spontaneously begin to grow in the retina. We do know that the new vessels usually stem from old ones, and that this happens after someone has had diabetes for many years. One theory is that as the retinopathy progresses—to the point of extensive capillary closure, poor blood flow, and severe nonproliferative complications including venous beading and IRMA—new blood vessels begin to sprout up, as if to reroute blood flow and offer the retina a fresh source of oxygen and nutrients. These offshoots grow either in the peripheral retina or on the optic disc. They develop particularly quickly in patients who have other health problems—breathing problems such as emphysema, for example, or the extra burden of pregnancy. (Pregnancy may also spark new blood vessel growth because of surges in hormones, changes in the body's blood flow, or changes in the blood's oxygen levels.) Interestingly, some eye conditions, such as advanced glaucoma, actually seem to protect the retina from these problems. Carotid disease, which can affect the blood flow to the eye, may also increase or decrease someone's risk of proliferative retinopathy.

In general, this neovascularization is believed to occur in response to blood vessel changes caused by a lack of oxygen. Many investigators believe that the oxygen-starved retina releases a chemical cry for help—a substance that's been termed the *angiogenic* or *vasoproliferative factor*—to the ailing retinal blood vessels. In response, they grow, spewing tiny new blood vessels into the retina.

If you think about it, this process is pretty similar to what the body does elsewhere to repair injuries: we cut ourselves, and then the body efficiently heals the cut, laying a foundation of new blood vessels, connective tissue, and skin cells over the wound. The big problem in the eye is that *these newly formed blood vessels are not normal.* They're tiny, spindly, flimsy blood vessels—not at all like the mature vessels found in a healthy retina. Also, they grow in a haphazard pattern, with an unfortunate tendency to poke through the retina into the vitreous gel. In short, they're puny imita-

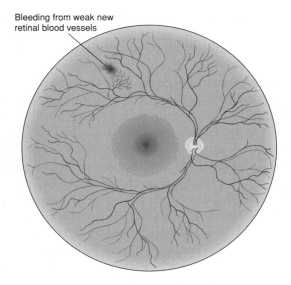

Bleeding from weak new
retinal blood vessels

Fig. 18.4. View of the retina with proliferative diabetic retinopathy

tions of the original blood vessels, with a bad habit of breaking and bleeding into the retina and vitreous.

It is this awful bleeding of the new crop of blood vessels that leads to proliferative diabetic retinopathy's most devastating complications. These new vessels appear to rupture at the drop of a hat—in response to sudden jerks of the head, for instance, or even to eye movements like those in normal REM (rapid eye movement), or "dream," sleep. Coughing, throwing up, sneezing, not to mention anything really traumatic, such as having a baby—you name it, and it will cause these blood vessels to break. Then they bleed, either directly into the retina or between the retina and vitreous jelly, resulting in *intraretinal* or *preretinal hemorrhages.* Blood can also gush out into the vitreous, producing a hemorrhage there—*vitreous hemorrhage.*

Whatever the cause for this bleeding, or wherever the hemorrhage, the change in vision is usually immediate. Patients may have a localized loss—a "hole" in part of their visual field—or they may see "spots" and "cobwebs," which gradually worsen to a dense haze or, in the case of a vitreous hemorrhage, a total loss of vision.

Given enough time, the body can usually remove this blood from the retina or vitreous. However it may not necessarily accomplish this quickly enough—or, even worse, the body's "cure" may be as bad as or worse than the initial problem. As cells inside the eye begin the cleanup process, they may also produce scar tissue in the retina and vitreous. (Scar tissue is the body's basic way of protecting itself against almost any injury.) Sometimes this scar tissue gets carried away, attaching itself to various areas of the retina, optic disc, and vitreous gel.

As scar tissue heals, it tends to contract. In the eye this contraction can tug on the retina, leading to a retinal detachment (see chapter 15). This kind of *tractional retinal detachment* is particularly devastating when it occurs in the macula. At its worst, it may result in permanent and severe vision loss.

Who's at Risk?

Although most people with diabetes eventually develop some degree of diabetic retinopathy, some have relatively minor trouble while others may wind up with severe impairment (but again, most never go blind from it).

By far the most significant risk factor is *how long someone has had diabetes:* the longer the diabetes has a chance to cause trouble—and here, people with Type I are at a major disadvantage—the greater the odds of developing some form of retinopathy.

Can severe damage be prevented? Actually, there is much you can do to lower your risk of eye complications from diabetes. One huge favor you can do for yourself is to *control your blood sugar.* The Diabetes Control and Complications Trial, a national clinical study of the effect of glucose control on diabetic complications, showed that in people with Type I diabetes, intensive insulin therapy delayed the onset and slowed the progression of diabetic retinopathy. (Similar studies on Type II diabetes are under way.) Keeping a tight watch on your blood sugar, with medication or insulin injections and a careful diet, appears to make a major difference in preventing vision problems.

High blood pressure, obesity, infections, and pregnancy are also known to raise someone's odds of having serious complications from diabetic retinopathy (or from diabetes in general, for that matter). Most of these are within your control: watching your weight and blood pressure, and promptly attending to any infections. Though not always easy, such control is certainly possible to achieve—particularly when the consequences of *not* doing so can threaten your eyesight.

In addition to taking care of your body, take special care of your eyes. Get a routine eye examination at least once a year (and more often if you're having vision problems). The American Academy of Ophthalmology has made the following recommendations:

Age of Onset of Diabetes	Recommended First Exam	Routine Follow-up
0–30	Five years after onset	Annually
31 and older	At time of diagnosis	Annually
Before pregnancy	Before conception or early first trimester	Three months

Find an eye doctor who's very familiar with diabetic eye disease and its many complications. If you have any doubts, *seek a second opinion.* The stakes—your eyes—are too high for anything less than expert medical care.

Diagnosing Diabetic Retinopathy

As always, an eye examination should begin with a careful history. This should include a discussion of any eye trouble you may be noticing right now: fluctuations in blood sugar often cause intermittent bouts of blurred vision, difficulty with night vision, and trouble reading. (If your diabetes has only recently been diagnosed, you may also experience these problems as your blood sugar is being regulated. Therefore, it's probably best to wait a couple of months after your blood sugar is under control before you get a new prescription for glasses.)

Your doctor should also learn the specifics of your disease: how long you've been known to have diabetes, how well it's been managed over the years, any other medical problems—such as hypertension or kidney disease—you've experienced, and anything else that may be important, including any medications you're currently taking and any allergies you may have. (Also, if the disease runs in your family, be sure to tell your eye doctor if any other relatives have had diabetic retinopathy.)

In the eye examination, your doctor will probably want to check, among other things, your visual acuity with and without your glasses or contacts; to check your distance and reading vision; and to inspect your eyes carefully for signs of glaucoma (which is more common in people with diabetes). Then, using a slit lamp (see chapter 3) to illuminate your eye, your doctor will look for any evidence of external eye infections or cataracts. After this, your doctor will probably dilate your eyes to get a complete view of the retina. Your doctor may also use a *direct ophthalmoscope* (a hand-held tool that looks like a flashlight) to examine your optic disc, macula, and retinal blood vessels, and an *indirect ophthalmoscope* (the "coal miner's lamp" that shines a high-powered light through a special lens) to see the retina's far edges. (For more on what to expect from a detailed eye exam, see chapter 3.)

Sometimes other techniques are needed to measure someone's degree of retinopathy—particularly when macular edema is suspected but not obvious, or if the edema is so extensive that it's tough to distinguish the exact areas of leakage. If this is the case, you may also need a test called a *fluorescein dye study*, which involves intravenous injection of a dye into the blood vessels. Your doctor will take a timed series of photographs of your retina, tracing the dye's progress as it enters the blood vessels, passes through them, and exits the eye. If you have macular edema, this study will show your doctor where the trouble spots are by highlighting the leaks. This study is painless, with few side effects—the most common one being that the orange dye temporarily gives the skin a mildly jaundiced tint and turns your urine a startling shade of yellow for about twelve hours. Some people also feel a brief twinge of nausea at the time of injection, as the dye rapidly circulates through the body.

Treating Diabetic Retinopathy

The good news is that, thanks in large part to extensive research efforts directed by the National Eye Institute, we've made great strides in treating this complicated problem over the last thirty years—so much progress, in fact, that today most people with diabetic retinopathy don't suffer severe visual impairment from it.

Treating Macular Edema

The breakthrough weapon against macular edema is the argon laser, and the treatment is called *photocoagulation*. Basically, the doctor uses a laser and, guided by the results of the fluorescein angiogram, "spot-welds" the seeping blood vessels in the macula. If the leaks are small, the laser is applied directly; if leakage is widespread, the laser is used in a grid pattern, like a patchwork quilt, over a broader area. An average treatment session will require between fifty and one hundred pinpoint-sized laser "spots."

Note: Your doctor will probably tell you this, but it's worth repeating just the same: all laser treatments for diabetic retinopathy, macular edema, or proliferative disease are done *to keep vision from getting worse, not to make it better.* So don't be disappointed if a laser treatment for diabetic retinopathy does not improve your vision.

Another important point: laser treatment doesn't absolutely guarantee that someone with macular edema won't suffer significant visual impairment, but it does lower the odds considerably. In a large clinical trial, called the Early Treatment Diabetic Retinopathy Study, sponsored by the National Eye Institute, patients who underwent laser treatment had significantly less visual impairment than those who received no treatment (14 percent versus 32 percent at three years).

The procedure is tricky. Because the area in question, the macula, is so small that any false step can have a devastating and permanent effect on someone's eyesight. Most of that burden rests on your doctor, who must know exactly where to place the laser. But part of the burden is yours. Your job, throughout the procedure, is to sit *completely still*—without moving your body or eye. (Special anesthesia can be given to help keep your eye from moving; see below.) The treatment session may take anywhere from fifteen to forty-five minutes. Then, when it's over, you can immediately return to your normal activities; usually there aren't any postoperative restrictions.

The laser treatment is performed as a same-day procedure, usually at your doctor's office or in an eye clinic; there are no preoperative testing requirements. Immediately before the procedure, you'll be given dilating eye drops to enlarge your pupil and give your surgeon a clear view of the retina. Since the procedure is performed using a special contact lens on the eye, you'll also be given anesthetic drops to numb your cornea. Some people also receive an injection of local anesthesia—like the novocaine you get in the dentist's office—near and behind the eyeball to prevent discomfort and minimize eye movement.

The actual laser treatment is delivered, with high-powered magnification, through a slit lamp biomicroscope (like the kind used in a routine eye examination). With each laser "spot," or burn, you'll probably notice a click and a bright flash. Although there's usually no pain, some patients do feel a little discomfort.

Afterward you may experience a mild headache and some temporary blurring of vision; both of these should clear up gradually over the next twenty-four hours. (If symptoms persist longer than a day, call your eye surgeon.) A lightweight patch, worn for the first day or so afterward, can help by decreasing light sensitivity and relieving the blurring. You may also be given some steroid eye drops to ease any postoperative swelling. *Note:* Although you can resume your normal activities—reading, exercising, working, and driving—right away, it's a good idea to have someone drive you home; you won't feel "100 percent" for about a day. (For more on side effects, see below.)

It generally takes about three months for the laser treatment to have an effect on macular edema. If by the end of that time your edema has not substantially subsided (and this is often the case after the first go-around), then you may need a "touch-up" session, or several (it's not uncommon for someone to need three or four separate treatments), until the fluid is judged to be minimal.

As we've discussed, macular edema can be especially difficult to treat in people with poorly controlled diabetes, people with hypertension or fluctuating blood sugars, and people who are pregnant or who have kidney problems or infections such as bacterial foot ulcers. Whatever you can do to improve the rest of your health will certainly boost your odds of having successful treatment.

Treating Proliferative Diabetic Retinopathy

Many years ago eye doctors noted that people with diabetes who had large areas of retinal scarring—from such problems as infection or trauma—seemed less likely to develop proliferative diabetic retinopathy. This led investigators to create *artificial* scars on the retina, to see if this had the same protective effect.

It did. In the late 1970s, after encouraging results from earlier studies, the National Eye Institute's national Diabetic Retinopathy Study confirmed the theory: somehow, scarring—done with argon lasers—indeed slows or stops out-of-control blood vessel growth in proliferative diabetic retinopathy. The study's results were striking. Four years after undergoing argon laser treatment, patients were *less than half as likely to develop severe vision loss* as those who hadn't received this treatment. *Note:* Again, as with macular edema, the laser is not a cure-all for proliferative diabetic retinopathy; it's not guaranteed to prevent severe vision loss, but it does significantly lower the odds.

Laser treatment for proliferative diabetic retinopathy is more extensive than the "spot-welding" used for macular edema (although many features of the procedure, including anesthesia, are the same; see above). The technique here is called *panretinal photocoagulation;* instead of fifty to one hundred laser "spots," or burns, it may involve eight hundred to two thousand pinpoint-sized burns and may take two or three sessions to finish.

The idea, basically, is to scar most of the retinal tissue. Nobody quite understands *why* this helps slow rampant growth of new blood vessels. It may be that the scarring decreases the amount of angiogenic factor (the retina's "chemical cry for help" mentioned earlier) released by the retina; or that it improves blood flow in the mature vessels; or that it lowers the retina's need for oxygen (and thereby reduces its need for new blood vessels). Whatever the reason for its effect, this treatment has been tremendously helpful for people faced with proliferative disease. (For more on the side effects of laser treatments, see below.)

Treating Vitreous Hemorrhage and Tractional Retinal Detachments

As discussed above, the fragile offshoot blood vessels of proliferative diabetic retinopathy bleed at the slightest provocation. When they spill blood in the retina and into the vitreous cavity—producing a *vitreous hemorrhage*—they can cause scarring on the surface of the retina and in the vitreous jelly. Unlike the deliberate scarring done with the laser to combat proliferative retinopathy, this scarring is dangerous for vision. Over time it gradually contracts, as all scar tissue does, and takes the retina along with it, causing it to separate from the back of the eye. This is a *tractional retinal detachment* (see chapter 15), a serious process that can severely impair vision and even lead to blindness.

However, we now have a successful way to treat vitreous hemorrhage: a procedure called *vitrectomy.* Using specially designed instruments—scissors, picks, and tiny lights for guidance—retinal surgeons can now remove the vitreous hemorrhage from the back of the eye, carefully stripping away scar tissue and relieving the pulling on the retina. The success of this surgery was investigated and confirmed more than a decade ago by the National Eye Institute's national Diabetic Retinopathy Vitrectomy Study. This large study particularly showed the benefit of early vitrectomy for a severe vitreous hemorrhage in a person with Type I diabetes, but not in a person with Type II. Laser photocoagulation or cryotherapy of the retina may also be used during vitrectomy surgery to treat any underlying proliferative retinopathy.

Coping with Diabetic Retinopathy

Diabetes takes its toll on the whole body—including your emotional well-being, which can have a great influence on the course of your disease. Depression and anxiety are very common in diabetes, and understandably so—particularly in people who are newly diagnosed or who have just been told they have diabetic retinopathy. Sometimes emotional problems and difficulty coping—which may be triggered by having *any* chronic disease—can sap patients' motivation and jeopardize their ability to control the diabetes. If there's a possibility that your emotional reactions may be interfering with the management of your illness, don't hesitate to seek professional help. Also, your doctor may be able to recommend local support groups. It can help tremendously simply to talk about what you're going through with people who are experiencing the same kinds of problems.

Some Questions You May Have about Laser Treatments for Diabetic Retinopathy

Does laser treatment have any side effects?

Usually only minor, temporary ones, such as mild swelling, blurred vision, and light sensitivity. However, laser treatments for macular edema, if placed close to the center of the macula or in a pattern to cause a dense scar, sometimes result in small areas of "blind spots," which are usually most noticeable when you're reading. Panretinal treatment for proliferative diabetic retinopathy, because it's performed mainly in the peripheral retina, can make it more difficult to see at night and may slightly reduce your peripheral and color vision. Clinical studies have demonstrated that laser treatments for diabetic retinopathy may also cause a slight loss of visual acuity.

Like any procedure, laser treatment isn't without its risks—which may include bleeding, increased macular edema, improperly placed laser burns that result in severe vision loss, and increased retinal scarring—and you shouldn't go into it without a thorough understanding of these. Also, as we've said before, because this is your eyesight at stake, you should have the utmost confidence in your surgeon. However, the risks and complications of laser treatment in diabetic retinopathy are rare. For most doctors and patients, they're far outweighed by the good that these treatments do in preventing retinopathy from getting any worse.

Will laser treatments improve my vision?

Probably not. The main goal of laser treatments for diabetic retinopathy is to slow or halt the progression of this eye disease—in other words, *to keep your vision from getting any worse.* So you shouldn't go into this surgery expecting to come out with perfect vision—and if your doctor leads you to believe that this is a possibility, you may want to re-think letting him or her anywhere near your eyes with a power tool. It's true that a tiny percentage of people do notice a visual improvement after laser treatment for macular edema, *but this is the exception, not the rule.*

Vitreous hemorrhages often cause annoying symptoms of "cobwebs," spots, or floaters in the eye, and laser treatments can't do anything to get rid of them; they're in the jellylike vitreous. As the blood is gradually absorbed, or as it settles, they may become less noticeable, but rarely do they resolve completely. A vitrectomy, if necessary, can remove this blood from the back of the eye and replace the vitreous with water. (This surgical procedure *can* diminish floaters or spots in the eye.) But again, as with any surgical procedure, a vitrectomy is not without its own set of risks and should not be performed until you have thoroughly weighed the benefits and risks.

How many laser treatments will I need?

It depends on your eyes. Some people may require only one, two, or three treatment sessions per eye to treat macular edema. Others may need ten or twelve treatments over the course of several years to control macular edema and proliferative retinopathy.

Perhaps more important than how many sessions you'll need—whatever that number may be—is that you and your doctor talk about it thoroughly first, and that you have a reasonable idea of what to expect. It's easy to get frustrated if you expected a couple of sessions to clear up a problem that turns out to need eight or even a dozen. You'll also need your fair share of patience, because healing doesn't happen overnight; your eye will need time to recover—about three months—after each session before your doctor can determine whether you need another one.

HYPERTENSION

An estimated fifty million Americans have hypertension, or high blood pressure. For most of them, controlling blood pressure is a daily struggle. Over time, hypertension takes its toll throughout the body, particularly in the brain, heart, kidneys, and eyes.

In the eye, hypertension hits the retina hardest, causing tiny arteries there to become even more narrow, impeding blood flow. Although we consider these to be "classic" changes of high blood pressure, they're often difficult to distinguish from similar "arteriosclerotic" changes that come with normal aging. (Arteriosclerosis, or generalized narrowing of the arteries, is certainly not limited to the eye; it happens in blood vessels throughout the body.) In fact, hypertensive and arteriosclerotic changes can even be seen *in the same eye*. And hypertension can make arteriosclerosis even worse.

Over a span of years, even relatively mild elevations of blood pressure take their toll on the body's vasculature, and we can see evidence of this in the eyes. The consequences of skyrocketing blood pressure, especially if it rages uncontrolled for months or even years, can be dramatic and severe: retinal hemorrhages, infarcts (total blockages that prevent blood from reaching tissue) in the nerve fiber layer, and even retinal exudates (fluid leakage into the retina from these blood vessels). One good note, from a diagnostic standpoint, is that these latter changes aren't subtle and rarely go undetected during an eye exam. They're almost impossible to miss—which means we can work with your internist or family physician to begin treatment for your blood pressure as soon as possible.

CAROTID ARTERY DISEASE

The carotid arteries are to the brain what the aorta is to the heart: a lifeline—actually, twin lifelines that carry oxygen-rich blood to the head. As they travel upward, these great rivers branch, forming the internal and external carotid arteries. The *internal carotid artery* is important here because one of its own branches, the *ophthalmic artery* (again, there are two—one for each eye), supplies blood to each eyeball. The ophthalmic artery, in turn, divides again, becoming the *central retinal artery*, whose job it is to nourish the inner retina, and the *posterior ciliary arteries*, which feed the choroid, among other structures. Without life-sustaining blood, these tissues become diseased or die—which is why any ailment affecting the carotid artery can have great ramifications for the eyes.

Atherosclerosis ("hardening of the arteries") is the most common malady of the carotid arteries. As in the atherosclerosis that leads to heart attacks, this most common cause of artery disease is a historical record of a lifetime's habits. Every fatty meal, every day or week or decade without exercise, every pack of cigarettes puffed—it's all here, in the greasy, brittle buildup of cholesterol and fibrous tissue lining the walls of these blood vessels. Over time, atherosclerosis leads to a narrowing of the artery's opening (called the *lumen*) and a drop in blood flow to the retina and brain. Imagine a garden hose that becomes clogged inside with dirt: the water has trouble getting through. When this happens to blood in the brain, the results can be serious and may include transient ischemic attacks (TIAs), or "mini-strokes"; temporary weakness or loss of sensation on one side of the body; aphasia (difficulty with speech or writing); a loss of vision in one eye (called *amaurosis fugax*); and severe eye pain (not unlike the intense pain of angina in the heart).

Amaurosis Fugax

Amaurosis fugax is a form of TIA, or "mini-stroke," that occurs in one eye. An artery is blocked, and tissue is damaged, but the blockage is only fleeting; it clears itself, and blood flow is restored. Amaurosis fugax is the most common symptom of carotid artery disease. You're driving a car or working in your yard, and all of a sudden your vision becomes dim or dark in one eye—like a "blackout," a "brownout," or a gray veil or curtain. Mercifully, this usually lasts only about five to ten minutes, and seldom more than thirty minutes. Vision returns to normal slowly, as if a veil or curtain were being gradually lifted from the eye. There may be another episode within a few days. *Note:* This event is not usually accompanied by other problems such as dizziness, lightheadedness, headache, trouble talking, or forgetfulness. If you have more prolonged or permanent dysfunction involving, for example, your speech or vision or the use of an arm or a leg, this may be due to a stroke.

This temporary vision loss is a warning sign—so don't ignore it! About one-third of people with untreated TIAs or amaurosis fugax eventually have a stroke. Amaurosis fugax is often caused by small particles—chunks of cholesterol or bits of platelet—that break off from a "hardened" artery and float up to the eye. Usually they become lodged in the small retinal vessels and block blood flow for a few scary minutes before becoming dislodged and moving on downstream. If this doesn't happen—if they don't move on—they can cause a branch or central retinal artery occlusion (see chapter 15), a far more severe blockage. (It happens in the eye just as in the brain: a TIA is a small stroke that usually does no lasting damage, but a major stroke can result if there is no return of blood flow—if, in other words, the blockage is not temporary and the damage is more extensive.)

So again, don't disregard a temporary loss of vision. You will need a thorough medical history and physical examination by your family doctor or internist. It may be that your problem is not caused by carotid artery disease. Several other disorders can also produce temporary vision loss, including giant cell arteritis (see chapter 17), migraine, elevated intraocular pressure, blood-clotting problems, and low blood pressure. In any case, this is nothing to leave "to take care of itself."

Ocular Ischemia

Atherosclerosis is a nasty, troublemaking condition in the eye. Amaurosis fugax is one of the problems it causes; ocular ischemia is another. Remember the clogged garden hose described above? In this case the poor hose's opening becomes increasingly narrowed for prolonged periods, and the garden it's supposed to water becomes increasingly parched. Here, the hose is the carotid artery, and the garden is the eye itself. ("Ischemic" tissue is parched, as well; it's starved for blood, oxygen, and nutrients.) Ocular ischemia can be devastating: it can lead not only to loss of vision but even to loss of an eye.

Many patients with ocular ischemia may never realize they've got a problem. Here's another reason for regular eye exams: *We can usually detect the problem early enough to treat it.* On a routine eye examination, we can see small, scattered hemorrhages (tiny red dots) and other changes in the retina that suggest poor blood circulation in the eye.

Other patients may have a symptom that's impossible to ignore: the eye's version of angina. Like angina associated with heart disease, *ocular angina* is an intense, intermittent pain caused by ischemia. (Think of this pain as the ischemic tissue's very loud cry for help.) Other people with poor ocular circulation may experience a few minutes of visual difficulty when they go from dark areas into bright light. (However, this may also be due to other ocular problems such as cataracts, age-related macular degeneration, or even the need for a new glasses prescription.) (See chapter 15.)

In advanced ocular ischemia, *neovascular glaucoma* may also develop. This can lead to uncontrollable high eye pressures, causing chronic severe eye pain and discomfort, and result in blindness. In order to preserve eyesight, some people need special treatment: laser photocoagulation or a retinal freezing technique called *cryoablation*, two techniques for creating retinal scars that can be effective in controlling neovascular glaucoma.

Diagnosis of Carotid Artery Disease

If your eye doctor or family physician suspects that you have carotid artery disease, you'll need a complete medical history and physical examination. Your carotid arteries will need to be examined specifically, and this may involve several tests. The most widely used of these tests is *Doppler ultrasound* (also called *sonography*). Ultrasound, a medical version of the sonar used on submarines (and a technique often used on pregnant women to monitor their unborn babies), can help your doctor check blood flow in the carotid artery.

Ophthalmodynamometry (pronounced op-thal-mō-dy-na-MOM-e-tree), a less commonly used test (it's being replaced by the more sensitive Doppler technique), can also measure carotid blood flow. It estimates the amount of pressure on the eyeball necessary to block circulation in the retinal arteries. (The less pressure needed to block retinal blood flow, the slower the circulation in the carotid artery.) You may require still other tests, such as *carotid arteriography* in which a doctor injects dye into the blood vessels and takes special pictures as the dye flows through the carotids. (You may have heard of an arteriogram, used to measure heart disease; this is the same technique.) Although more definitive than Doppler studies, "invasive dye studies" also carry more risks, including bleeding, infection, and potential formation of a blood clot. Thus, they're not the first line of diagnostic testing and are used only in special cases.

Treatment of Carotid Artery Disease

The first step in treating carotid artery disease is to minimize your chances of further damage from poor blood flow. So, how to improve blood flow to your eye? One approach your family physician or internist may recommend is *anticoagulation*: "thinning" the blood with medications, including aspirin, Coumadin, and ticlopidine or Ticlid. Another approach is mechanical: "cleaning out" the clogged artery, in a procedure such as *carotid endarterectomy*. It's the carotid version of a Roto-Rooter technique: a surgeon opens the blocked artery and removes the gunk accumulated on its wall.

Who should get a carotid endarterectomy? This controversial question has been much studied over the last decade, because of the potentially serious complications—such as cerebral and retinal stroke—associated with the procedure. A large, multicentered clinical trial compared the benefits of carotid endarterectomy with the use of antiplatelet medication to decrease clotting and improve blood flow. This study found that in patients with symptoms—such as TIAs, including amaurosis fugax—of carotid artery disease and a *greater than 70 percent stenosis, or blockage, of the carotid artery,* endarterectomy significantly lowered their risk of having a stroke. A more recent study found that endarterectomy was even beneficial in certain patients who hadn't yet developed these symptoms of carotid disease. Endarterectomy has also been successful in helping people with poor blood flow to the eye as seen in ocular ischemia (see above). In these people, the procedure helped maintain their vision, relieved angina-like eye pain, and even, in severe cases of ocular ischemia, preserved the eyeball. With endarterectomy, patients with ocular ischemia and significant carotid artery disease can regain useful vision if the conditions are caught early enough.

HEADACHES

Headaches, like fingerprints or snowflakes, are unique. Nobody's is exactly like anybody else's—in fact, even in the same person, rarely are two headaches exactly the same.

Headaches can be contained, or localized, to a particular area of the scalp or head; they can be dull or sharp, intermittent or prolonged. They may be accompanied by other symptoms such as nausea, vomiting, dizziness, or "visual phenomena"—seeing wavy lines, or having double vision. Because of the infinite variety here, your doctor isn't going to be able to help much unless you get specific. Your description of your pain and other symptoms, plus your doctor's thorough questions, will help establish the type of headache and its cause (see box).

Your doctor may ask you to keep a headache diary, recording such things as the time of day, any events that happened just before the headache, and the duration. Also, if you have chronic, recurrent, or severe headaches, you may need a thorough physical checkup, plus blood tests, sinus X-rays, and a magnetic resonance imaging (MRI) scan of the head.

Tension Headaches

Most headaches are caused by tension. Your basic tension headache begins as the muscles tense up in the back of your head or neck. This pulling then radiates to both sides of your head and around front, to your

Establishing the Type and Cause of a Headache

Here are a few questions you can expect your doctor to ask you about your headache:

- Where was the pain? In the temples? The top of the head?
- When did it start? How bad was it? (In other words, were you still able to function, or did you need to lie down?)
- How long did it last?
- How often do you get such headaches? Twice a month? Once a week?
- Do you have any other symptoms when you get a bad headache?
- Has any medication—aspirin, Advil, Tylenol, an antihistamine—helped or not helped?
- Does anything seem to trigger it—stress, reading, medications, certain seasonings or foods (such as any food or drink containing caffeine)?
- Do the headaches seem to occur at a certain time of day?
- Does the headache wake you up from sleep?
- Do you awaken in the morning with the headache?
- Does it vary with changes in position? (A yes to these last three questions may suggest headaches due to elevated intracranial pressure.)
- Does anyone else in your family suffer from bad headaches? (A family history of headaches can help your doctor diagnose a migraine.)

forehead. This has been called a "bandlike" tightness, because it feels as if someone's clamping a vise around your head. It can also occur in migraine sufferers, sometimes making it difficult to distinguish between the two types of headache. However, although the symptoms may be similar, *tension headaches are always related to stressful moments.* They don't get worse or better if you turn your head or body a certain way, as migraines can. They usually aren't affected by light or accompanied by *photophobia* (abnormal sensitivity to light) or other associated neurologic symptoms such as nausea, dizziness, loss of vision, numbness, or muscle weakness.

If it's any comfort, you're not alone. Almost everybody gets a tension headache at least once in a while. Also, this form of headache can almost always be relieved by over-the-counter painkillers—aspirin, Tylenol, Advil, and the like. (However, if your tension headaches are persistent and if they're affecting the quality of your life, you may need additional medication or therapy.)

Sinus Headaches

Another common cause of eye pain and headache is acute or chronic sinusitis. The sinuses are empty cavities in the skull. (These empty air-filled cavities evolved, scientists believe, to help lighten the load, since a skull of solid bone would be a bit heavy to balance on our relatively frail necks.) Among other things, the sinuses warm the air we breathe and play a role in speech. There are several sinuses in the skull, most of them located over, under, and next to the eye; some sinuses even share an adjoining wall with the orbit. Therefore, because they're such close neighbors of the eye, any infection or inflammation in the sinuses can also irritate the eye or eye muscles next door. If you have a history of sinusitis, and if you're experiencing occasional eye pain or pressure, the two might be related. You should see your eye doctor or family doctor. Such inflammation or infection is typically treated with decongestants and/or antibiotics, but if chronic or recurrent, the condition may require surgery.

Refractive Error Headaches

What's a refractive error? It's a problem with the way your eyes focus light—in other words, why most of us need eyeglasses or contacts to help us see. This is not a major cause of headaches, and finding the right prescription for nearsightedness, farsightedness, or astigmatism rarely puts an end to persistent headaches. Therefore, before simply writing you a new prescription, your doctor needs to make sure something else isn't going on here, either another medical problem or another eye problem. You'll need a complete eye evaluation, including a dilated retinal examination, to rule out other eye ailments, including conjunctivitis, corneal abrasions and ulcers, iritis, cyclitis, posterior scleritis, acute closed-angle glaucoma, optic neuritis, eye tumors, and other eye inflammatory diseases. All of these can cause headaches or eye pain. (See the Index for specific page references to these problems.)

How do you know if it's a refractive headache? Does it happen when your eyes are hard at work—for example, reading, doing needlework, or working on an intricate ship model? Since these headaches are usually due to someone's need for glasses—in most cases reading glasses—or the need for a different prescription, you may experience "tired eyes," or discomfort around or behind the eyes after prolonged reading or computer work.

You don't get refractive headaches first thing in the morning, when your eyes are relatively refreshed. You don't get them when your eyes are relaxed—on weekends, for example, when you're leisurely gardening in your backyard. Headaches related to the eyes are dull and aren't associated with the nausea, vomiting, or "visual phenomena" found in migraines. However, they can lead to a tension headache from the anxiety they cause.

Migraines

Believe it or not, although the name is synonymous with headaches, you don't have to have a headache to have a migraine. You could just see things—geometric shapes, flashbulbs, jagged lines, heat waves, sparkling, watery images, "Swiss cheese" patterns, and other phenomena.

Nobody really knows what causes migraines. However, scientists think they're caused by changes in the blood vessels of the brain. They can be triggered by a dazzling variety of stimuli, including stress, caffeine (coffee, tea, cola, chocolate), cheese, nuts, red wine, MSG (monosodium glutamate, common in Chinese food), or birth control pills; all of these are known to cause the brain's cerebral blood vessels to constrict, or clench. This constriction can decrease blood flow to certain parts of the brain, causing a relative ischemia, or lack of oxygen. Then, in response, the cerebral blood vessels compensate by dilating: they stretch the surrounding brain tissue. All of this, in people who are prone to migraines, can cause chaos: the visual problems mentioned above, or feelings of nausea and dizziness, or a terrible, disabling headache, or combinations of these symptoms. Symptoms may even change from episode to episode, and many people who experience visual or other migraine symptoms never even get a headache. There seem to be infinite variables at play here.

Migraines can strike at any age. Generally, they're classified into four types: common, classic, cluster, and complicated.

Common Migraines

Common migraines are severe headaches that usually begin on one side of the head as pounding, stretching, or throbbing. They can spread to involve half or all of the head. The intense headache pain can even occur behind the eyeball, mimicking sinus or other eye problems. Many sufferers of common migraine have a premonition that one's about to hit; this is called an *aura*, and it can come in the form of visual events, a mood change, a series of yawns, trouble with speech, or other neurologic symptoms.

Common migraines can be extremely incapacitating headaches, lasting hours or even days, often causing people to seek refuge in a quiet, dark room until the pain goes away. They may be associated with nausea, conjunctival redness, watery eyes, a "foreign-body" sensation in the eyes, or ultrasensitivity to light.

Classic Migraines

Classic migraines have better-defined warning symptoms than common migraines. These migraines also tend to include visual or "sensory-motor" disturbances, such as numbness or weakness of an arm or leg, before or during the headache. Sufferers describe a visual aura such as shining lights, flashbulbs, sparkles, geometric patterns, zigzag lines, heat waves, or "Swiss cheese" areas of vision loss. These visual phenomena can last minutes, hours, or even days. People may even experience a buildup, crescendo, or march of these phenomena—in other words, the little wavy lines may begin as a small area off to one side of your vision and gradually increase until they involve half or all of your visual field. Sometimes the aura before the headache isn't visual; instead, people may experience numbness around the mouth, an unusual sensation over half of the body, dizziness, or even temporary disorientation. Classic migraine attacks may modify their presentation over the years: as they age, some people may still experience the visual or sensory-motor aura but, mercifully, forgo the headache.

Like common migraines, classic migraines affect men and women equally, tend to occur at any age, and often run in families; also, a history of motion sickness is not uncommon. For most sufferers of classic migraines, mild over-the-counter analgesics do absolutely nothing; stronger medications are often needed. As with other forms of migraines, attacks can be precipitated by a variety of things, including stress, bright light, loud noise, caffeine (coffee, tea, cola, chocolate), certain spices and seasonings, certain foods, unusual diets, and medications such as birth control pills. (Identifying the precipitating event is an important part of the treatment, as you may imagine.)

Cluster Migraines

Cluster migraines are five times more likely to occur in men than women, most commonly in middle age. These are often *unilateral* headaches (occurring on only one side), described as excruciating, burning, sharp, or a deep ache. They begin and end quickly, lasting only one or two hours. However, they don't stay away long; on really bad days they can return several times within a twenty-four-hour period (hence the term *cluster*). Eye-related symptoms may include a droopy eyelid, tearing, and a red eye. The droopy eyelid goes away when the headache's gone.

Complicated Migraines

"Complicated migraines" is a general classification for a variety of temporary or permanent symptoms and patterns. The typical migraine headache may not always be present. Complicated migraines are often associated with eye problems; the three forms of complicated migraines most often associated with the eyes are acephalgic, ocular (also called retinal or ophthalmic migraines), and ophthalmoplegic.

Acephalgic migraines usually have visual symptoms but, by definition, don't come with a headache. Visual symptoms can be like those reported in classic migraines but may also include blurred vision, temporary blindness in one or both eyes, and abnormal pupil dilation (which you can see in a mirror). Other symptoms may include numbness or tingling, difficulty with speech or reading, dizziness, confusion, and trouble hearing.

Ocular (retinal or ophthalmic) migraines involve a temporary or even permanent loss of vision in one eye. The vision loss may last from seconds to hours, but it usually goes away in less than half an hour. It tends to affect people under age forty with a strong history of common or classic migraines. *Permanent visual defects are very rare but can occur after repeated attacks.* As with all types of migraines, the associated visual and neurologic aura almost always goes away. Although the retina and optic nerve are usually normal after these attacks, some people go on to develop ischemic optic neuropathy (see chapter 16), central and branch retinal artery occlusions, central retinal vein occlusion, and central serous retinopathy. (As you may imagine, if there's vision loss in one eye but no other evidence of eye damage, this form of migraine can be very difficult to distinguish from amaurosis fugax, discussed above.) Although we don't know why these particular headaches affect vision, some scientists believe that in some people, as the cerebral blood vessels constrict during a migraine, so do the major blood vessels supplying the retina and optic nerve.

Ophthalmoplegic migraines: In this form of complicated migraine, the attack also strikes the nerves that control the eye's muscles, commonly resulting in a droopy eyelid, trouble raising the eyelid, and trouble moving the eye from side to side. Although, as with ocular migraines, these problems are usually temporary, they can in rare cases become permanent after repeated attacks.

Here too, as with other forms of complicated migraines, ophthalmoplegic migraines are a "diagnosis of exclusion." In other words, we need a complete medical and eye evaluation to rule out every other possible cause—including a blood clot, myasthenia gravis, thyroid eye disease, or a tumor—before we can be sure this is what's causing the problem.

Giant Cell Arteritis

Giant cell arteritis can cause headaches, tenderness in the temples, and other symptoms. See chapter 17 for a full description of this medical emergency.

Brain Tumors and Headaches

How do we know it's a brain tumor? We don't, at first. Although headaches occur in an estimated two-thirds of people with brain tumors—and for many, headaches are the first symptom of a problem—there is no "classic brain-tumor headache." In fact, in many cases the pain isn't even on the same side of the head as the tumor.

These chronic headaches characteristically are intermittent, dull (not throbbing), and moderate in severity; they tend to get worse with exercise or positional changes, and they don't respond to headache medications. They may be associated with nausea and vomiting—which, again, makes them tough to distinguish from certain forms of migraine. Some people with brain tumors can be awakened from sleep by their headaches.

Again, we make the "diagnosis of exclusion," which involves a complete medical and eye examination, often including brain imaging. (For more on brain tumors and other visual problems, see below.)

STROKES

Here's what happens in a stroke: Blood, which normally courses through an artery, suddenly can't get where it needs to go. It's blocked by a clog in the artery. Suddenly the tissue on the *other* side of the obstruction—

which needs the oxygen and nutrients in blood to stay alive—begins to die; it becomes ischemic, or oxygen-starved. If the clog opens in time, the tissue survives. If not, it dies.

We've already discussed strokes inside the eye (see "When the Eye's Blood Supply Is Blocked" in chapter 15). These blockages of blood flow can also occur outside the eye, at sites along the visual pathways including the optic nerves, the *chiasm* (the meeting place at which the nerve fibers from each eye come together), and the cerebral cortex. Also, strokes can occur deeper in the brain; of these, the ones most commonly affecting eyesight occur in the parietal, temporal, and occipital lobes.

All strokes are not equal: the location of a blockage is crucial in determining the extent of the damage. A shutoff of blood supply to the retina or optic nerve—such as amaurosis fugax or ischemic optic neuropathy (see below), or a tumor along the optic nerve up to the chiasm—usually results in partial or total loss of sight in one eye. Like two roads that intersect, optic nerve fibers meet at the chiasm before continuing on their journey toward the occipital lobe (see figure 1.8). An injury or stroke here at the chiasm or even deeper in the brain injures visual fibers of *both* eyes—and may result in partial loss of vision in both eyes, also called *bilateral vision loss.*

A blockage or stroke in the parietal or temporal lobe can also result in partial loss of vision in both eyes. To make matters worse, the blow to eyesight usually isn't the only damage. Most strokes here also cause specific neurologic problems, depending on the area of the brain that's damaged. (In fact, the particular symptoms help doctors pinpoint the exact location of the stroke.)

A parietal lobe stroke usually produces a similar pattern of visual field or peripheral vision loss in each eye, concentrated in the lower half of the field of vision. Also, the degree of loss usually varies; one eye may have more damage than the other. After a parietal lobe stroke, someone may also have difficulty with spatial orientation—becoming disoriented in a familiar place, for example, or having trouble reaching for a glass of water.

An occipital lobe stroke usually causes each eye to lose one-quarter or one-half of its field of vision, or to lose sight in the central visual field. Unlike parietal and temporal lobe strokes, this particular loss is often highly symmetrical—the damage in one eye is a carbon copy of that in the other. (This is because in the occipital lobe, both eyes' nerve fibers exist almost side by side and may be equally affected by ischemia.) A temporal lobe stroke can cause partial vision loss, too. As with all strokes, the damage caused by those that affect eyesight may improve somewhat with time. Usually, however, at least some of the damage is permanent.

Tumors

Tumors can also harm eyesight. These, like strokes, may occur anywhere, from the optic nerve in the front to the occipital cortex at the back of the brain. Here too the specific visual and neurologic problems can help pinpoint the area of damage.

Among the most common and significant of the tumors that affect eyesight are *pituitary tumors.* The pituitary gland is located below the optic chiasm, the place where the two sets of optic nerves come together. Think of the optic chiasm as a crossroads: The nerve fibers from one part of each eye's retina (the temporal portion) pass straight through, on their way to the brain's occipital lobe. The fibers from another part of the retina, the nasal portion (the fibers that transmit images from our peripheral vision), cross here.

If a pituitary tumor grows large enough to press on the chiasm, it can disrupt these crossed fibers and cause someone to lose side vision. If your doctor suspects that you might have a pituitary tumor, you'll probably need visual field testing (see chapter 3) and a brain-imaging test such as an MRI scan. The good news here is that there are several good treatments for pituitary tumors, including medication and surgery. Bromocriptine is a medication that is very effective for treating prolactin-secreting pituitary tumors. Many people are able to return to normal activity—including driving and playing sports—and many have a near-complete restoration of their vision.

Collagen Vascular Diseases (Arthritis and Its Relatives)

The broad term *collagen vascular diseases* encompasses many disorders, all linked because they cause inflammation and scarring of connective tissue (the cells and fibers that make up the body's framework and system of support—things like cartilage, bone, and elastic tissue). In many of these disorders the body appears to attack itself. This *autoimmune* reaction usually occurs throughout the body, and it frequently involves the eye—which is why regular eye examinations and prompt attention to any eye problems are essential. Here are some of the most common of these diseases and their consequences in the eye (these symptoms are covered separately elsewhere in this book):

Disease	Symptoms
Rheumatoid arthritis	Dry eyes, episcleritis, scleritis, or an unusual thinning or "melting" of the cornea and/or sclera
Sjögren's syndrome	Dry eyes, uveitis, optic neuritis, inflammation of the retinal blood vessels
Behçet's disease	Uveitis, inflammation of the retinal blood vessels and choroid
Reiter's syndrome	Conjunctivitis, iritis
Psoriatic arthritis	Iritis
Scleroderma	Dry eyes, inflammation of the retinal blood vessels, iritis, cataract
Ankylosing spondylitis	Uveitis
Sarcoidosis	Uveitis, swelling of the lacrimal gland, and localized conjunctival swelling; optic nerve involvement

THYROID DISEASE

The thyroid gland sits in the neck, over the trachea, just below the larynx, or "Adam's apple." It has two halves, one on each side of the trachea, connected by a thin isthmus of tissue. (Most people can't feel their thyroid. But as a diseased thyroid gets bigger, it can become easier to feel, especially when you swallow. A massively enlarged thyroid, also known as a *goiter*, is hard to miss.)

The thyroid gland secretes thyroid hormone, which is crucial for metabolism and body regulation. Its intricate effects on the body are too numerous to describe here, but the thyroid keeps us at an even keel. Basically, producing too much thyroid hormone (a condition called *hyperthyroidism*) makes someone anxious and overactive; producing too little *(hypothyroidism)* makes someone tired and lethargic.

How does the eye become involved? Well, in thyroid disease, as in collagen vascular diseases, the body turns on itself; it creates *antibodies* (cells designed to fight off infection and disease) that act against normal tissue. In thyroid disease, the body's confused immune system attempts to protect or immunize itself against normal thyroid tissue. The consequences of this "mistaken identity" can be serious, for as the body fights its own thyroid gland, it also attacks other tissues—perhaps mistaking them for thyroid tissue as well. Some of these chemical weapons specifically target the eye. This leads to an inflammatory reaction in the connective tissue of the eye's muscles, fat, and soft tissues. The result: fibrous scarring and fluid swelling.

There are many medical names for what's happening in the eye, including Graves' ophthalmopathy, or Graves' disease (after one of the early investigators of this condition), infiltrative ophthalmopathy, endocrine ophthalmopathy, and thyroid eye disease. There are also many symptoms, including bulging eyes (called *proptosis*); edema, or swelling, of the eyelids; retraction of the eyelids; swelling of the conjunctiva; drying and ulceration of the cornea; problems with double vision; and optic nerve damage.

Most people with thyroid eye disease—about 80 percent—are hyperthyroid. (Up to 40 percent of people with hyperthyroidism eventually develop some degree of eye trouble.) The disease affects more women than men, and it usually strikes people in their thirties and forties.

Thyroid eye disease is very unpredictable in its onset, progression, severity, and duration. Often it moves slowly, with remissions and advances lasting from months to years. But sometimes it's fast and relentless. One of the most frustrating aspects of thyroid eye disease—and the most difficult feature for doctors as well as patients to understand—is that *regulating the thyroid gland itself often has little or no effect on the course of the eye disease.* In fact, the eyes can become affected even decades after the thyroid disease has been under control. Thus, if you have thyroid disease, regular eye examinations are crucial!

One means of organizing and cataloging the thyroid's degree of ocular involvement is called the *NOSPECS classification:*

Class 0: **N**o physical signs or symptoms of thyroid eye disease
Class 1: **O**nly signs (but no noticeable symptoms)
Class 2: **S**oft-tissue involvement
Class 3: **P**roptosis (bulging eyes)
Class 4: **E**xtraocular muscle involvement
Class 5: **C**orneal involvement
Class 6: **S**ight loss (due to optic nerve involvement)

In *Class 1* disease, patients don't have any noticeable symptoms, but eye doctors can detect early signs of thyroid eye disease. One such sign is a tightening of the upper eyelid so that it can't close all the way, all the time, producing problems with dryness. Another is "lid lag," in which the eyelid can't close quickly, as in a blink, but seems to shut in slow motion.

In *Class 2*, the soft tissue begins to swell, or have edema. The eyes may look puffy and may appear to have bags below them. The conjunctiva may appear watery, swollen, or thickened.

In *Class 3*, proptosis, or bulging eyes, becomes a problem. (This is largely due to the concentration of the thyroid antibody in the extraocular muscle and the inflammation this causes.) As these muscles enlarge, they push the eye out from behind, making it shift forward so that it appears to be bulging out of the socket. This can happen in both eyes, or in one.

In *Class 4*, as the extraocular muscles become increasingly swollen and inflamed, it becomes harder to move them; it's particularly difficult to look up. Double vision also becomes common as the eyes lose their ability to move together. (Ultrasound, a painless imaging technique, may be helpful in determining the extent of this problem.)

In *Class 5*, severe dryness is common, because the eyelids are no longer able to cover the bulging eye. This causes *exposure keratitis*, which can range from mild dry spots on the cornea to ulcers on an extremely parched cornea. Compounding the dryness problem, the eye's ability to make tears is hampered as inflammation and scarring encompass the lacrimal, or tear-making, glands. Treatment at this stage involves the use of lubricants for the dryness, and sometimes surgery to help the eyelids close.

In *Class 6*—a degree of ocular involvement experienced by fewer than 5 percent of patients with thyroid eye disease—the optic nerve may be damaged by the prolonged inflammation and swelling, and sight may be damaged or lost. (The optic nerve can be damaged even if the eyes aren't noticeably bulging—another reason why regular eye examinations are essential.)

Treatment: The first task is to get the thyroid under control. However, if you have any kind of thyroid irregularity, your eyes may still be at risk; thyroid eye disease can occur even in people with normal or low levels of thyroid hormone. Thyroid eye disease can occur in people with normal thyroid function; in this case it is called *euthyroid Graves'*.

In the early stages of thyroid eye disease, lubrication with tear-substitute drops and ointments, along with increased humidity (see chapter 13), can be very helpful in easing symptoms. More lubrication may be needed if the eyes begin to bulge. Taping the eyelids shut at night may help keep the eyes from drying out during sleep; in some cases, special goggles can help keep the eyes moist. If the eyelid's ability to close is poor, then *tarsorrhaphy*, a surgical technique that partially closes the eye, may also help. In advanced cases, oral steroids, radiation, and surgery for decompression and lid positioning may help.

ACNE ROSACEA

Acne rosacea—a skin condition different from the acne most of us suffered as teenagers—mainly targets the forehead, nose, cheeks, and chin. But the eyelids have skin too, and they're not immune from this annoying problem. (Eyelid acne is often seen in people with facial acne.) The symptoms here can range from mildly irritating to disabling. Many people with this condition develop a chronic blepharitis with a mild conjunctivitis (see the discussion of conjunctivitis in chapter 12); but if the problem isn't treated, it can lead to corneal scarring and new blood vessel growth, which may eventually impair vision.

Rosacea of the eyelids is very difficult to treat, and treatment usually takes months. An oral antibiotic, such as tetracycline, is often prescribed, along with lid "shampoos," warm compresses, and an antibiotic eye drop or ointment. (See the discussion of blepharitis in chapter 10.) Even after the condition is under control, you may need to continue this daily regimen for years.

PARKINSON'S DISEASE

Parkinson's disease is characterized by progressive, involuntary tremors, caused by a loss of chemical-producing nerve cells in the brain.

People with this disease develop a "wooden" face, with decreased blinking, little eye movement, and the appearance of a fixed stare. Because blinking is one of the eye's ways of maintaining moisture, a perpetual lack of blinking causes dryness. Tear substitutes (drops and ointments), along with increased humidity, can be very helpful here. Another problem, stemming from the decrease in head and eye movement, is difficulty in using bifocals. Many people with Parkinson's disease find it helpful to keep two pairs of eyeglasses, one for distance and the other for near vision, on hand.

MYASTHENIA GRAVIS

Myasthenia gravis is a neuromuscular disorder, characterized by intervals of weakness and paralysis. It can occur at any age, and it strikes women twice as often as men. Here too, as in thyroid eye disease, the body inexplicably turns on itself, attacking certain muscles—particularly those in the eye, face, throat, and chest—and interfering with their function. An estimated 90 percent of people with this disease eventually develop some eye trouble; in fact, difficulty moving the eye muscles is the most common early symptom. "Droopy" eyelids (a condition called *ptosis*) and double vision *(diplopia)* are common, and these symptoms seem to wax and wane over the course of the day. Fatigue makes the symptoms worse.

Although the diagnosis of myasthenia gravis is largely based on someone's medical history and the physical exam, we now have a chemical test that can confirm its presence. It's called a *Tensilon test*, and it works by helping to overcome the antibodies' effect on the muscles, causing them to function normally again. (Longer-acting versions of this drug are also used to treat myasthenia gravis.) Other studies can also be important in helping diagnose myasthenia gravis, such as the acetylcholine receptor antibody test (positive in 70–93 percent of people with MG), electromyography, and muscle biopsy.

ACQUIRED IMMUNODEFICIENCY SYNDROME (AIDS)

AIDS is a devastating disease that besieges the body's immune system, destroying its ability to fight off infection. It targets *T-cells*, cellular warriors that attack viruses and bacteria—anything the body perceives as an enemy.

Tears and AIDS

AIDS cannot be transmitted by routine social contact with an infected person. You can't get it from being coughed on, or shaking hands, or using the same computer. As viruses go, HIV's transmission is pretty limited; it can be passed on only by intimate acts: by unprotected sexual intercourse with someone infected with the virus; by contact with infected blood or tissue (via a shared hypodermic syringe, for example, or a transfusion of tainted blood); or by being born to a mother infected with HIV (and even here, the virus isn't passed on to all babies of HIV-infected mothers). Although HIV has been found in the body's secretions—tears, saliva, urine, and bronchial fluids—transmission of HIV from these secretions has not been reported as of this writing.

Having said that: Even though tears are not considered a risk factor, your eye doctor will still (as all doctors should) take precautions to keep the examination and all equipment as sterile as possible. We disinfect tonometers (for intraocular pressure testing) with hydrogen peroxide, alcohol, or a bleach solution. We clean any diagnostic contact lenses that are reused with alcohol-based cleaners and then disinfect them with hydrogen peroxide or heat disinfection to kill HIV. Many of us use disposable contact lenses for diagnostic fitting whenever possible.

AIDS is caused by an insidious virus called *HIV (human immunodeficiency virus)*, and having HIV infection is not the same thing as having AIDS; AIDS represents the late stages of HIV infection. Many people live for a decade or more with HIV before it progresses into AIDS. (About 70 percent of people with HIV develop AIDS within fifteen years.)

When initially infected with HIV, many people experience symptoms of the flu or mononucleosis—such as feeling rundown and having sniffles—for a week or two. Then, nothing. HIV may hibernate for months, years, or even more than a decade before the signs of AIDS begin to appear.

In the eye, the most common manifestation of AIDS is the development of *cotton-wool spots* in the retina. The problem here is that retinal blood vessels get inflamed, decreasing the blood flow to the nerve fiber layer and damaging the surrounding tissue. Cotton-wool spots usually go away on their own within four to six weeks and rarely affect vision.

Most of the HIV-related problems that do affect vision are indirect, the by-product of a compromised immune system that can no longer stave off infections from opportunistic microorganisms (the "bugs" most of us come into contact with, and fight off, every day). Of these, the most serious threat to vision is *CMV,* or *cytomegalovirus.*

CMV attacks the retina in as many as 30 percent of people with AIDS, especially when the number of T-cells in the bloodstream plummets. CMV ravages the retina as it spreads like wildfire, destroying tissue, causing bleeding and retinal detachment. Symptoms of CMV include floating spots or "spider webs," flashing lights, blind spots, and blurred vision. If you have any of these symptoms, see your eye doctor immediately. However, CMV infection can occur in the eye without any symptoms—an important reason for all people with HIV to have regular eye examinations.

There are two drugs used to treat CMV: Gancyclovir and Foscarnet. However, these drugs only slow the infection down; they don't completely eradicate CMV. If CMV is caught early in one eye, these drugs may help to keep the virus from spreading to the other eye.

Other infections common in AIDS are herpes zoster and ocular toxoplasmosis. AIDS complicates the way we treat all of these infections. Usually a drug does only part of the work in fighting a "bug"; the body's immune system shoulders a large part of the load as well. But in AIDS, because the body's immune system is failing, normal dosages of drugs are inadequate. Even megadoses—as much as five times the normal potency—don't always work. Lingering conjunctivitis is also common. Less common is Kaposi's sarcoma, a noncancerous kind of tumor (which doesn't threaten vision). This purple-red bump may appear anywhere on the body, even on the eyelid or sclera (the "white" of the eye), and can be treated with radiation, laser, or cryosurgery (a freezing technique). If you have AIDS, it's extremely important—for the sake of your vision—that you have regular eye checkups to catch and treat any eye problems at their earliest signs.

LYME DISEASE

The culprit in Lyme disease is a deer tick, a minuscule relation—it's about as big as the point of a pencil—of the big dog ticks you may have found on your pets.

Many deer ticks are infected with *Borrelia burgdorferi,* a form of bacteria. The result is Lyme disease—named for Lyme, Connecticut, where this problem was first discovered, although the ticks are found all along the Atlantic coast, from Massachusetts to Maryland, in the upper Midwest in Wisconsin and Minnesota, and along the West Coast in California and

Oregon. It's characterized by distinctive skin lesions, most commonly a round red "bull's-eye" rash at the site of the tick bite. Its effects can be widespread; early symptoms can include malaise, fatigue, fever, headache, stiff neck, myalgia (muscle soreness), migratory arthralgia (joint soreness), and lymph adenopathy (swollen glands). *Note:* Lyme disease is not contagious; you can't get it from someone who has it. You can only get it from being bitten by a tick.

In the eye, most commonly Lyme disease can cause a relatively mild problem, conjunctivitis (see chapter 12). More significantly, it can also cause an anterior uveitis (see chapter 14). If not treated, Lyme disease can drag on for months or even years—a terrible thing, when you consider that Lyme disease is easily treated with antibiotics (usually doxycycline or amoxicillin, usually taken for three to four weeks). Similarly, the conjunctivitis can be treated with tetracycline eye drops, along with other medications.

Treatment of the uveitis depends on its severity. A mild case of uveitis may not need any specific treatment; if you're already taking antibiotics to treat the Lyme disease, the problem should go away as soon as the infection is gone. In some people the disease is localized in the eye. We know this because although their systemic tests for Lyme disease are negative, the borrelia organism is found in the vitreous. If this is the case, a diagnostic and therapeutic vitrectomy may be needed.

19

Coping with Low Vision

With Dena Zorbach, M.S.E.

The American Academy of Ophthalmology defines low vision as what results "if ordinary eyeglasses, contact lenses, or intraocular lens implants don't give you clear vision." But that's a woefully inadequate way of describing one of the greatest challenges—if even that word isn't too simplistic—to the quality of life.

Low vision means that the simplest, most mundane things you do—reading the newspaper, making coffee, or finding the right bills to pay for a hamburger at a restaurant—become ordeals. It means that because you can't see well, life gets unnecessarily complicated and ridiculously frustrating.

It may be some comfort to know that you are not alone. At least twenty million people over age forty have some serious visual impairment. Ninety percent of these people have some vision, often called *residual vision*. Most of them have what is termed *low vision*, which can include decreased side vision (peripheral vision), loss of color vision, or loss of the ability to adjust to light, contrast, or glare. Again, low vision is defined in the most general terms as the absence of sharp sight even when wearing ordinary glasses, contact lenses, or intraocular lenses.

HOW LOW VISION IMPACTS EMOTIONS

Loss of vision has a profound effect on the individual, family members, and the community. Next to cancer, older people fear vision loss most. Many people associate low vision with being blind, and many people feel that there is a stigma to being blind. This stigma may be a difficult issue to work through, and it may seem impossible when someone is just beginning the rehabilitation process.

As with any loss, the person with vision loss can be expected to express normal emotions of denial and disbelief, anger, frustration, depression, and fear. The person with vision loss may also experience a loss of mobility, which may make him or her withdraw from social activities and become isolated. And when financial and other personal matters must be handled by others, the resulting loss of autonomy and privacy can be devastating to the person who is used to doing these things for himself or herself.

An overall loss of independence is often a catalyst for reduced self-esteem, productivity, and motivation. Although the period for passing through the emotions of loss varies in length, almost everyone eventually moves from saying "I won't" through believing "I can't" to learning "I *can.*" A successful adjustment and rehabilitation of the person experiencing new sight loss will involve family, friends, and significant others. The key to coping with this loss is to accept the reality of the new situation. Once this has happened, the person can begin seeking solutions to life's new challenges. During this critical period, family and friends need to be encouraging and find ways to help the person become more independent.

SOME DEVICES THAT MAY HELP

There is life beyond normal reading glasses. If your vision is reduced to a level where regular print is difficult to read with normal reading glasses, there are several "low-vision devices" that can help make books, magazines, newspapers, and mail easier to read. They're worth considering, and they really can help.

There are five main types of devices: hand-held magnifiers, extra-powerful reading glasses (much stronger than ordinary reading glasses), stand magnifiers, telescopes, and electronic magnifiers. In the future there are likely to be even more helpful devices available, as scientists and engineers collaborate to design and produce rehabilitative devices. One promising new device is the low-vision enhancement system (LVES) developed by Robert Massof and his colleagues at the Wilmer Eye Institute and NASA, which should soon become more widely available.

Hand-held magnifiers come in a variety of shapes and sizes. One advantage here is that whatever you're reading—a book, a newspaper—can be held at the normal reading distance. You can buy low-power magnifiers, which magnify by about one time (1x) to three times (3x), at most drugstores. Higher-powered models are available at specialized low-vision centers—for help finding one in your area, see "For More Help" at the end of this chapter—or possibly through your eye doctor.

High-powered reading glasses are stronger than your normal reading prescription. One drawback is that because the prescription is so strong, the print must be held very close (or else it looks distorted). For some, this working distance may be uncomfortable, but it does mean that you don't have to use your hands to hold the vision device, so they're free to hold the printed page. An adjustable direct-source light, beamed directly at whatever you're reading, may also help.

Stand magnifiers rest directly on the printed page. They provide a comfortable working distance but a somewhat limited field of view (you can't scan an entire magazine page at once, for example).

Telescopes can help you see objects farther away. For many people they're invaluable for seeing bus numbers, street signs, chalkboards, a computer screen, or a baseball game. These can be hand-held, clipped on, or permanently attached to eyeglasses. In thirty states it's even legal to drive while wearing these telescopes mounted to glasses, called *bioptics.* Requirements vary: in Maryland, for instance, people with mild visual impairment (20/100 or better) may be eligible; they must also have a visual field of 150 degrees horizontally, if they have functioning vision in two eyes, or of 100 degrees if they can see out of only one eye. (Check with the Motor Vehicle Administration for the specific requirements in your state.) It may take some training and time to master driving with bioptics, but many people find the continued independence well worth the effort.

Electronic magnifiers: Closed-circuit television has been adapted for use by people with low vision. This system scans reading material and projects an enlarged image onto a television screen, allowing for enhanced magnification, brightness, and contrast. These systems are costly to buy, but they can be leased. They have proved invaluable for some of our patients.

HELP FROM LOW-VISION CENTERS

There's no "right" way of using low-vision devices. Some of them, frankly, may drive you crazy or seem more trouble than they're worth. But

Tips for Dealing with People Who Are Blind or Visually Impaired

Some of our patients say they feel awkward when meeting a blind or severely visually impaired person. Suddenly, they say, every conversational gambit becomes a potential foot in the mouth. Our first bit of advice? Relax. Don't worry if you mention the ballgame you (oops) *watched* last night, or the movie you just *saw*. Talking about everyday things isn't going to make you seem insensitive. Just be yourself.

Having said that, however, there certainly are some things you *can* do to make things easier for both of you:

- When you start up a conversation, even if you've met before, introduce yourself by name. It can be hard to recognize voices, especially in a crowd.
- Make eye contact, just as you would when talking to a sighted person. It's obvious, from the way your voice sounds, when you're looking around the room instead of at the person you're talking to.
- For heaven's sake, don't speak louder than normal. This happens more often than you might think; some people have a tendency to shout at blind people, as if a certain decibel level were all that's needed to penetrate the vision problem. Remember, it's their vision that's impaired, not their hearing. Chances are, their ears work just fine.
- Because your hand gestures won't be seen, be more descriptive in your conversation; take time to draw a verbal picture.
- If you're ending a conversation, say something to that effect.
- Always announce yourself when you are entering or leaving a room. Your acquaintance won't be able to see you come in or walk away.
- When walking with a visually impaired person, offer your arm for assistance. *Never* pull or steer; this can lead to accidents. When you're approaching a chair to help the person sit down, gently take his or her hand and touch it to the seat, arms, and back of the chair for orientation. At a meal, describe the table and the location of the plate, glass, and utensils. Some people appreciate it if someone tells them where the food is located on the plate as it relates to a clock face (for example, "The chicken is at six o'clock").
- Just rearranged your living room? Speak up; your visually challenged friend will need to make a new mental picture of the room he or she will be navigating.
- Finally, be honest. If you feel awkward in a new situation and are not sure how to act or be of help—a crowded train or street corner, for instance—just say so. Chances are, you'll both be glad you did.

in all of the categories mentioned above, there are several models to choose from—so don't rule something out until you've exhausted all the options.

To this end, low-vision centers—and there are many of them throughout the country—can be invaluable. They can also help you learn other "tricks of the trade" to help make everyday activities—such as cooking, identifying money, and writing checks—more doable and less frustrating.

Most of these centers are staffed by an interdisciplinary team that might include an ophthalmologist, optometrist, nonphysician low-vision specialist, and experts in rehabilitation who can show you how to perform your daily tasks and use the low-vision devices prescribed by your eye doctor. For example, a rehabilitation teacher can make a house call to show you, on your home turf, the specifics involved in setting up a "low-vision-friendly" kitchen, medicine cabinet, and home. This visit may also result in helpful recommendations for eliminating glare, improving the lighting, and generally making life easier.

SOME HANDY TIPS TO GET YOU STARTED

There's no big secret as to what the problem is: you can't see very well. Now, let's start working on the solution: how you can maximize the vision you have and make your home a "low-vision-friendly" place. Here are some tips, based on the experiences of many people who are in the same boat, that may help. Remember: high-contrast means it's easier to see!

In the Kitchen

- Use an easy-to-see marker, or brightly colored tape, to highlight the dials of your oven, washing machine, and thermostat. A rehabilitation teacher can also mark your dials tactilely, so that you can *feel* the settings rather than be forced to rely on vision.
- For meals, use a white plate on a black placemat, or vice versa.
- When the meal consists of light-colored foods, use a solid black plate. (Mashed potatoes, for example, stand out just fine on a black plate but magically disappear on a white plate.)
- For black coffee, use a white cup.
- When pouring any drink, line up the spout of the pitcher so that it makes contact with the rim of the cup or glass. Then, so you don't spill, place an index finger just inside the rim. Stop pouring when you feel the liquid. (This

may take some getting used to if you like your coffee piping hot!)

- It's easier to feel the skin of the vegetables you're about to peel when they're wet.
- Force yourself to keep your cabinets and pantry organized. It's infinitely easier to find items that are always kept in the same place.
- Label your spices with a thick permanent marker. For example, write the name, or an easy abbreviation, such as "CINN," in very large letters on an index card. Punch a hole in the card and run a rubber band through it, then attach it to the cinnamon bottle. Another way to make spices easier to tell apart is to put different spices in different-sized containers.

Lighting

- Too much glare from the windows? Try diffusing the light with sheer ivory curtains.
- Too dark? Buy higher-powered bulbs. There's a world of difference between 60 and 150 watts. Lamps with dimmers, which allow you to adjust the level of light, are effective; also, a torchiere lamp (one that provides indirect lighting by shining the light up onto the ceiling) is a great way of providing more light to a large room. (These are available at most office-supply and department stores.)
- For reading, think *direct beams of light.* Aim a gooseneck lamp right at what you're reading. (An incandescent 75-watt bulb may work best for this.)
- Need more light? Keep several large flashlights around the house to help when the room lighting is just not enough.

Miscellaneous Tips

- Why make doing business harder with regular checks? Large-print checks are available at most banks; they're usually yellow and black, with raised lines that act as guides. (Your bank can also order large-print checks for you through the Deluxe Checking Company at 1-800-451-1455.)
- Throw out your pencils. Instead, use bold black markers to jot down phone numbers or make your grocery list. Write on yellow paper for maximum contrast.
- For correspondence, use bold-lined paper. Also, page-writing guides and check, envelope, and signature templates are available at most low-vision centers.
- Call for help. Some local phone companies provide free directory assistance

and dialing to visually impaired persons. Many long-distance carriers also offer free long-distance dialing assistance for people who are visually impaired.

- Walk with care. Place a nonskid, brightly colored strip of tape on the edge of each step to help you negotiate stairs.
- Don't use direct lamps just for reading; aim a gooseneck lamp wherever you need extra light. For example, put one on your kitchen counter, to help you fix meals.
- Take advantage of free services. Every state has at least one Library for the Blind and Physically Handicapped that provides books on tape, large-print books, and magazines on disk—*all for free*. They can also help you find many everyday items such as wrist watches, table clocks, and telephone dials that also are made in large print. And for you bridge players, there are even large-print playing cards. Talking computers, clocks, watches, and timers are also available. So are machines that can scan a page and read it to you!

FOR MORE HELP

For starters, consider trying one of these agencies, or ask your doctor to recommend helpful resources in your area:

American Foundation for the Blind (AFB)
11 Penn Plaza, Suite 300
New York, NY 10001
(800) 232-5463

This is a nonprofit organization with five regional centers, which publishes the *Journal of Visual Impairment and Blindness*. It also offers many educational programs and acts as a national clearinghouse for information and referrals.

Association for Macular Diseases
210 East 64th Street
New York, NY 10021
(212) 605-3719

This group provides information and educational services, sponsors support groups, offers counseling, and publishes a newsletter.

**Association for Education and Rehabilitation of
 the Blind and Visually Impaired (AER)
4600 Duke Street, #430
P.O. Box 22397
Alexandria, VA 22304
(703) 823-9690**

This association promotes education and work for blind and visually impaired persons and offers training programs through colleges and universities.

**The Foundation Fighting Blindness
Executive Plaza I, Suite 800
11350 McCormick Road
Hunt Valley, MD 21030
(410) 785-1414**

This is a consumer organization providing public education and awareness for people with retinal degenerative disease. It conducts workshops and research and publishes a newsletter called Fighting Blindness.

**National Association for the Visually Handicapped
22 West 21st Street
New York, NY 10010
(212) 889-3141**

Helps people with low vision. Supplies low-vision aids (lamps, mirrors, magnifiers). Publishes a quarterly newsletter.

**National Center for Vision and Aging
The Lighthouse
111 East 59th Street
New York, NY 10022
(800) 334-5497**

Acts as a national network and referral resource.

**National Federation of the Blind
1800 Johnston Street
Baltimore, MD 21230
(410) 659-9314**

Strives to improve social and economic conditions of people who are blind. Provides education and scholarships.

National Library Service for the Blind and Physically Handicapped
Library of Congress
1291 Taylor Street N.W.
Washington, DC 20542
(800) 424-8567

A source of large-print and Braille materials; talking books such as *Reader's Digest* and *Newsweek Magazine*; and educational aids, tools, and supplies.

The following organizations supply a variety of products for people who are visually impaired. You can contact them to ask about their catalogs, mail-order services, and equipment:

American Printing House for the Blind
1839 Frankfort Avenue
Louisville, KY 40206
(800) 223-1839

Lighthouse Low Vision Products
36-20 Northern Boulevard
Long Island City, NY 11101
(800) 829-0500

LS&S Group
P.O. Box 673
Northbrook, IL 60065
(800) 468-4789

Maxi-Aids
42 Executive Boulevard
P.O. Box 3290
Farmingdale, NY 11735
(516) 752-0521

The following companies produce materials in Braille and large-print versions as well as audio cassettes and computer-access equipment:

Arkenstone
1390 Borregas Avenue
Sunnyvale, CA 94089
(800) 444-4443
http://www.arkenstone.org

Doubleday Large Print Home Library
6550 East 30th Street
P.O. Box 6375
Indianapolis, IN 46206-6375
(317) 541-8920

New York Times Large Type Weekly
P.O. Box 9564
Uniondale, NY 11555-9564
(800) 631-2580
Two and a half times the size of a regular newspaper; thirty-six pages; full-page crossword puzzle.

Reader's Guild—Large Print Books
Thorndike Press
P.O. Box 159
Thorndike, ME 04986
(800) 223-2348 (customer service is through Simon and Schuster)

TeleSensory Corporation
Low Vision Products Division
P.O. Box 7455
Mountain View, CA 94039-7455
(415) 335-1800 or (800) 804-8004
http://www.telesensory

20

Common Medications That Affect the Eyes

Very few medications work like a rifle, taking aim at a particular target and hitting it with elegant precision. Instead, most take the shotgun approach—generally hitting the mark, but scattering plenty of buckshot in the process.

Thus the concept of *side effect*—medicine's unintended impact on various parts of the body, including the eyes. Taking just about any kind of medication usually means a trade-off—weighing the good that the medicine does, particularly for serious illnesses, versus the extra mischief it causes.

For most medications the side effects are minimal—a little drowsiness, for example, or changes in appetite, or dryness in the mouth. In fact, sometimes a drug's manifestations, particularly those that affect the eye, are so subtle that it takes us days or weeks to figure out the connection (if we ever do). This is why when you seek medical help for such symptoms as blurry, distorted, or double vision, red eyes, dry eyes, or light sensitivity, it's extremely important to discuss your medical history, including any medications you're taking. If the medicine is indeed to blame—and if it's not possible to switch to an alternative drug to avoid these unwanted effects—then your eye doctor may need to monitor your eyes as long as you're taking that particular drug.

Of the thousands of medications available today, there are a few—many of them prescription drugs—that cause problems for many people. These include antibiotics, antidepressants, antihistamines, appetite suppressants, blood pressure medications, daily hormone supplements, and steroids. Chloroquine, Plaquenil, lovastatin, and tamoxifen can also cause eye problems that you need to be aware of. In the rest of this chapter you'll find a roundup of the most common drugs that affect the eyes, and their side effects.

ANTIBIOTICS

Antibiotics applied to the eye (used topically) have the potential to cause allergic conjunctivitis, which shows up as red conjunctival injection, tearing, and itching. Occasionally there will be associated orbital redness and swelling of the skin around the eyes due to an allergic dermatitis brought on by the eye drops. Topical neomycin eye preparations cause an allergic reaction in a high percentage of the people who use them.

Systemic (oral, intramuscular, or intravenous) antibiotics used in treating an acute bacterial infection generally produce few side effects in the short term. However, when they're used for weeks or months to treat chronic infections, they can cause eye problems. Fortunately, most of these side effects are rare, and they go away when you stop taking the drug.

Synthetic penicillins (amoxicillin and ampicillin): These drugs are known to cause an allergic reaction in the eyes that shows up as mild redness of the conjunctiva, itching, and dry eyes in some people who take them. They can also cause a drug-induced anemia that can lead to subconjunctival and retinal hemorrhages. These hemorrhages usually are not harmful, do not affect vision, and require no treatment.

Tetracycline: This antibiotic can cause the same side effects as synthetic penicillin, plus blurred vision and increased sensitivity to light.

Sulfonamides: Many people are allergic to "sulfa drugs," and these allergies can manifest themselves in a variety of side effects. In the eyes, these may include blurred vision (secondary to a transient myopia that resolves with discontinuation of the drug), eye irritation (resulting in watery eyes that are extra-sensitive to light), and hemorrhages similar to those caused by penicillin.

ANTIDEPRESSANTS

Antidepressants are a group of medications designed to change how information is processed in the nerves, or neurons, in the brain. Some of these drugs are used to treat other problems, such as migraine headaches. *And any medication that alters neurological function has the potential to affect the eye.* (Fortunately, the most recent antidepressants, such as Zoloft, have few significant eye-related side effects.) Antidepressant medications include the following:

Tricyclic antidepressants: This is the class of antidepressants (including such drugs as amitriptyline, desipramine, imipramine, and nortriptyline) that causes most of the unwanted side effects in the eye, including blurred vision, loss of accommodation (the ability to focus your eyes), dilated pupils, double vision (caused by loss of function in the eye muscles), and dry eyes. If these side effects are intolerable, there are other medications to try that may be as effective with less severe side effects—or even none.

Fluoxetine hydrochloride (Prozac): Prozac is an antidepressant, but it's not in the tricyclic group. However, because Prozac does influence neural pathways, it can cause some similar side effects, including blurred vision, dilated pupils, double vision, and dry eyes. It also can cause eye pain, eyelid infection (blepharitis), ptosis, cataracts, glaucoma, and iritis. These side effects can't be avoided except by discontinuing the medication. This is a "risk-versus-benefit" situation that can be resolved only by the patient and his or her doctor talking the situation over and making a decision based on the patient's needs.

ANTIHISTAMINES

Almost everyone has taken antihistamines at one time or another, particularly during hay-fever season. The racks at any drug, grocery, or even convenience store have a dazzling array of choices—some with decongestants, some that make you drowsy, some that don't, some that also fight cold symptoms. One thing they have in common is that most of the antihistamines have a drying effect on the eye, just as they do on a runny nose. And drying, as discussed in chapter 13, often makes vision blurry, lights seem too bright, and contact lenses much less pleasant to wear. If a decongestant—another drying agent—is added to the pill, these symptoms are often made worse. In very rare instances antihistamines can cause the pupils to dilate or become unequal in size. This can make the light sensitivity even worse for many people. But for people with "narrow angles" (see chapter 8), dilated pupils can lead to something far more serious: closed-angle glaucoma. Most of these side effects go away when you stop taking these drugs, with the exception of closed-angle glaucoma, which will persist and require treatment.

APPETITE SUPPRESSANTS

Appetite suppressants include amphetamines, dextroamphetamines, methamphetamines, and phenmetrazine compounds. These drugs are marketed under many different names throughout the world. Systemic use of these appetite suppressants can cause such side effects in the eye as impaired vision, pupil dilation, a widening of the palpebral fissure, and decreased accommodation and convergence—making it difficult to read. In people who have narrow anterior chamber angles—many farsighted people, for example, and those with a family history of an acute onset of painful glaucoma—the use of appetite suppressants can lead to closed-angle glaucoma.

BLOOD PRESSURE MEDICATIONS

Imagine a hose with water running through it so fast that it's about to burst. You need the water, but you want to lower the pressure. One way to do this is to adjust the *volume*, so that there's less water running through the hose at all times; or you could adjust the *rate*, so that only a certain amount of water can go through the hose at any given time; you could also use a bigger hose, so that there's more room for the water to flow. That's pretty much the situation with the drugs used to control hypertension, or high blood pressure: they can deplete the fluid volume in the body, regulate the heart rate and pumping volume, or dilate the blood vessels that carry the blood.

However they work, antihypertensive medications can produce some side effects in the eyes. These go away when you stop taking the drugs; however, because these high-powered medications are also life-saving, you should never stop taking them without talking to your doctor first! Stopping "cold turkey" could cause much more harm than having never started to take them at all.

Diuretics: Diuretics cause the body to excrete excess fluid (which is why many women take them to ease premenstrual and menopausal symptoms). In the blood vessels, less fluid means less pressure. But in the eyes, less fluid means dry eyes, increased light sensitivity, and blurred vision. These symptoms are reversible when the medication is discontinued. *Note:* Women seem particularly susceptible to dry eyes because of hormonal changes as they get older, and diuretics may make this problem worse.

Regulators: These drugs, typically beta-blockers like Inderal and Tenormin, work via neural pathways—and again, whenever the neural pathways are affected, the eyes are also at risk for side effects. Eyes may feel dry; the pupils may be dilated (just like the blood vessels); blurry vision and increased light sensitivity can result from either of these. (In rare instances this dilation of the pupil can bring on a bout of closed-angle glaucoma; see chapter 8.) Because neural pathways in the eye also control eye muscles, these drugs can create double vision by interfering with how the eyes work together. If necessary, another medication can be substituted that may have less troublesome side effects.

HORMONAL SUPPLEMENTS

Because these hormones can do so much good (reducing the risk of heart attack, osteoporosis, and cervical cancer, among other things), estrogen and progesterone are being taken (individually or in combination, in a variety of dosages) by more women than ever before.

For women on supplemental hormones, dry eyes are a common and annoying problem; however, changes on the surface of the cornea are to blame for this. Supplemental hormones can cause the cornea's curvature to steepen and its surface to become pockmarked from dryness, known as *superficial punctate keratitis,* or *SPK.* The result of these latter changes? Eyes that can burn, or feel dry, gritty, irritated, and tired. If these corneal changes are significant enough, they can make wearing contact lenses an unpleasant chore. SPK also heightens a person's sensitivity to bright light as the dry spots scatter light and cause glare. Artificial tear supplements help to resolve SPK and its symptoms. Other hormone-caused complications—which actually affect the central nervous system, the brain and spinal cord—may seem like eye problems, including headaches, fatigue, dizziness, and difficulty concentrating. Many people wrongly blame these symptoms on eyestrain—from, for instance, a bad prescription for glasses or contact lenses—when they are actually caused by the hormones' effect on the body.

Still other eye-related complications of supplemental hormones may spring from side effects in the vascular system (the heart and blood vessels). One of the most serious of these is thrombosis, or formation of a blood clot. Sometimes a blood clot breaks free, blasts into the bloodstream, and lodges somewhere else (this is called an *embolism*), blocking blood flow in that area. Embolisms that reach the retina can cause oxygen-deprived tissue there to die; this in turn may lead to vision loss (see the discussion of artery occlusions in chapter 15). *Note:* If you have any pain—in your leg, for example—that you think might be caused by a blood clot, call your doctor immediately. Prompt treatment may save your vision—as well as your life!

Finally, in rare instances hormone supplements can cause other side effects, including double vision (caused by loss of function of the extraocular muscles, the muscles that move our eyes); optic neuritis (inflammation of the optic nerve); increases in myopia (nearsightedness); and damage to the macula (the part of the retina that provides central vision) secondary to fluid swelling. Except when there has been retinal photoreceptor damage, these side effects are reversible when the medications are discontinued. Women taking hormonal supplements should see their eye doctor routinely.

STEROIDS

Steroids, such as prednisone, mimic the action of the body's own hormones (particularly those produced by the adrenal glands to control inflammatory reactions in the body). They're most often prescribed for diseases in which there's major inflammation in multiple areas of the body—including rheumatoid arthritis, giant cell arteritis, Crohn's disease, sarcoidosis, and systemic lupus erythematosus. Long-term steroid use can cause many other problems, including posterior subcapsular cataracts and changes in intraocular pressure.

Posterior subcapsular cataracts occur in 30 to 49 percent of the people taking 10 to 15 milligrams of prednisone daily for one to two years. These cataracts can be very dense and cause a rapid loss in vision. Even worse, they don't go away if you stop taking the medication, and they are only treatable by surgical removal (see chapter 7).

Changes in intraocular pressure, although not as common as cataracts, are still a serious problem. Steroids—whether taken orally or topically, or injected around the eye—can lead to glaucoma by causing an elevation in eye pressure, usually after prolonged use. When the eye's fluid pressure builds beyond the normal range, this can cause significant damage to the nerves in the retina that process visual images and can lead to glaucoma (see chapter 8). The good news is that this intraocular pressure usually returns to normal if the steroid is discontinued. The bad news is that any damage caused by the increased intraocular pressure remains.

Steroids can also damage the eyes indirectly. For example, prolonged steroid use can raise someone's blood sugar, causing diabetes. Skyrocketing levels of sugar in the blood can produce a shift in the focusing power of the eye's crystalline lens, making nearsightedness worse (or actually causing farsightedness to improve); it may also cause vision to fluctuate. Other ocular changes from diabetes can result as well. (For more on the ocular effects of diabetes, see chapter 18.)

Steroid use can raise someone's blood pressure, and as we discussed in chapter 18, this can damage blood vessels within the retina, causing hemorrhaging and damaging nearby nerve tissue. People on high doses of steroids should see their eye doctor every three to six months.

OTHER MEDICATIONS THAT CAN CAUSE PROBLEMS IN THE EYE

Chloroquine and Plaquenil

As far as the eye goes, chloroquine and hydroxychloroquine (Plaquenil) are serious, potentially toxic drugs (although Plaquenil seems to cause considerably fewer eye problems than chloroquine), and if you're taking one of these medications, such as chloroquine for malaria or Plaquenil for arthritic problems, we recommend that you be checked thoroughly for any signs of side effects *at least every six months.*

The big worry here is retinal toxicity (drug-caused damage to the retina). Fortunately, regular eye exams can detect changes in the retina (mainly in the pigmentation) very early; and these changes can diminish or go away altogether after you stop taking the drugs.

Regular eye exams are so important because in their earliest stages these retinal changes cause no symptoms. (Rarely, the visual field can be damaged even if there aren't any obvious retinal changes.) The most common vision problems attributed to the retinopathy, or retinal changes, include difficulties with reading and seeing (such that words, letters, or parts of objects appear to be missing), blurred distance vision, missing or blacked-out areas in the central or peripheral vision, light flashes, and streaks. Difficulty seeing red targets (sometimes called *premaculopathy*) may also be an early warning sign; this usually goes away when therapy is stopped. In fact, most of these side effects seem to be reversible. (However, for some people they actually continue to progress, and unfortunately, there's nothing that can be done.)

Another unfortunate twist is that in a few people taking chloroquine, retinal damage has shown up *several years* after the antimalarial drug therapy was stopped—another reason why regular eye exams are so important, whether you're having symptoms of any trouble or not!

Lovastatin (MEVACOR, MSD)

Lovastatin works by specifically inhibiting an enzyme in the liver needed to synthesize cholesterol, and its goal is to lower someone's risk of having a heart attack or stroke by reducing levels of "bad" cholesterol in the blood. But many patients have recently begun to worry that taking these drugs might cause other problems—namely, the development of cataracts.

The good news is that they probably don't. So why all the fuss? It seems to have started when lovastatin was in the "clinical evaluation" stage of testing, being put through its paces in humans after laboratory and animal tests, to make absolutely certain that the drug was safe. Part of the battery of tests included checking the eyes. Early studies on lovastatin seemed to suggest an association between its use and the development of cataracts; however, because the tests were highly subjective, this link remained unclear. Later, after a three-year double-blind controlled trial, investigators were *not* able to show any clear tie between the drug and the development or progression of cataracts.

Tamoxifen (NOLVADEX, Zeneca)

As part of their treatment for breast cancer, some people take the chemotherapy drug tamoxifen. In a very small segment (less than 1 percent) of them, tamoxifen produces certain side effects in the eyes.

The most common eye problem tamoxifen may cause is a retinopathy, characterized by small deposits—thought to be by-products of retinal nerve tissue dysfunction—found in the retina's inner layers. Although not particularly troublesome by themselves, these deposits often serve as signposts of more significant trouble, because they are sometimes linked with macular edema and retinal hemorrhages that may compromise vision. *These retinal lesions usually go away once a person stops taking the drug.*

Other side effects can include corneal and lens changes. In the cornea, tamoxifen deposits can build up, leaving superficial erosions and opacities; these usually regress when tamoxifen is stopped. In the lens—again, very rarely—these tiny deposits may cause irreversible cataracts, which may require surgery.

All of these side effects seem to be dose-dependent: people who take conventional doses of tamoxifen have much fewer, *and much more minor,* drug-related eye problems than those taking higher doses.

A Guide to Eye Medications and Their Side Effects

This table provides an overview of the more common medications used to treat eye conditions. It will help put in perspective some of the drops, ointments, and pills you may use or hear about. Using this table, you will be able to identify these medications by category (such as antibiotics or glaucoma medications) and by their generic names as well as their aliases, or "brand names." You will also have a pretty good idea of the potential side effects of these medications.

Our side-effect list might appear formidable at first glance. In fact, after looking over this list of potential side effects, you may even ask why anyone would want to take any of these medications at all! And we have not even listed every side effect that has been attributed to each medication—only those we believe are the most important. The reality, however, is that most of these side effects are not common; they occur infrequently. Moreover, your doctor would not prescribe a medication for you unless she or he felt that the benefit of the treatment far outweighed the risk of developing a reaction. Of course, if you are allergic to sulfa or have a history of reactions to any of these drugs, you should discuss this with your doctor. Package inserts and information provided at the time of drug dispensing are also very important, and you should read such information carefully to check the safety of the medication for you. After all, the best person to watch out for you is you. Don't be afraid to ask questions if something does not sound right or if something concerns you.

There are basically two types of reactions to medications: allergic and toxic. In *allergic reactions* the eye recognizes the medication as foreign and attacks it. These reactions are generally mild, causing symptoms of eye irritation and itching that are often accompanied by conjunctival redness and swelling. Once the medication wears off or is washed out, the eye feels a lot better. *Toxic reactions*, on the other hand, are usually more severe and may damage or inhibit function of the eye or other organs. Many toxic reactions are reversible once there is no longer any contact between the tissue and the medication, but recovery from a toxic reaction—such as a reaction that causes damage to corneal epithelial cells or retinal pigment epithelium, for example—can take days or months. Fortunately most ocular side effects from a medication, whether allergic or toxic, usually go away without doing permanent damage to a person's sight.

When taking any medications, it is essential that you discuss any unusual signs or symptoms with your prescribing doctor as soon as you notice them.

Type	Generic Name	Brand Name	Potential Side Effects
ANESTHETICS			
	Bupivacaine		Same as lidocaine (below).
	Lidocaine		*Systemic:* Allergic reactions (ranging from mild swelling and redness around the injection site to severe anaphylaxis), convulsions, heart rate changes, and respiratory arrest.
	Proparacaine	AK-Taine Alcaine Ophthaine Ophthetic	Same as tetracaine (below) but not as significant.
	Tetracaine	AK-T-Caine Pontocaine	*Ocular:* Stinging on insertion that lasts 20–30 seconds, delayed healing of corneal wounds, and (rare) mild allergic reactions causing eyelid and conjunctival swelling and tearing.
ANTI-INFECTIVES			
Antibacterials (also known as antibiotics; see also "Combination drugs")	Bacitracin		*Ocular:* Allergic reactions causing redness and itching.
	Chloramphenicol	Chloromycetin	*Ocular:* Allergic reactions causing burning or stinging.

	Chloroptic	*Systemic:* (Very rare) aplastic anemia from bone marrow depression.
Ciprofloxacin	Ciloxan	*Ocular:* Burning on insertion of the drop, foreign-body sensation, itching, redness, and photophobia. *Systemic:* Nausea, headache, dizziness, rash, and bitter taste.
Erythromycin	Ilotycin	*Ocular:* (Rare) mild allergic reactions.
Gentamicin	Garamycin Genoptic Gentacidin	*Ocular:* Dryness, irritation, foreign-body sensation, and photophobia; conjunctival swelling and redness.
Neomycin		*Ocular:* Same as gentamicin, but allergic reactions are much more common.
Norfloxacin	Chibroxin	Same as ciprofloxacin.
Ofloxacin	Ocuflox	Same as ciprofloxacin.
Polymyxin B		*Ocular:* (Rare) mild allergic reactions.
Sulfacetamide	Bleph-10 Cetamide Ocusulph-10	*Ocular:* Allergic reactions, increased sensitivity to UV radiation causing a sunburn on the eyelids, and deposits of small white plaques in

(Continued)

Type	Generic Name	Brand Name	Potential Side Effects
		Sodium Sulamyd Sulph-10	the cornea and conjunctiva. Not to be used if there is a known sensitivity to PABA (found in sunscreens) or any sulfa medication.
	Sulfisoxazole	Gantrisin	Same as sulfacetamide.
	Tobramycin	Tobrex	Same as gentamicin.
Antifungals	Amphotericin B	Fungizone	*Systemic:* Headaches, chills, fever, and vomiting with intravenous administration. Also kidney malfunction, anemia (reversible with discontinuation of the drug), and gastrointestinal cramping.
	Miconazole	Monistat	*Ocular:* (Rare) mild allergic reactions.
	Natamycin	Natacyn	Same as miconazole.
	Nystatin	Mycostatin Nilstat Nystex	Same as miconazole.
Antivirals	Idoxuridine	Herplex	*Ocular:* (Common) redness and swelling of the conjunctiva and eyelids, with irritation of the cornea.

Trifluridine	Viroptic	*Ocular:* Same as idoxuridine but less frequent reactions than with any of the other ocular antiviral drugs. Additional side effects include burning or stinging on insertion, dry eye, increased intraocular pressure, conjunctival scarring, and ptosis.
Vidarabine	Vira-A	*Ocular:* Same as idoxuridine. Additional side effects include burning or stinging on insertion, tearing, foreign-body sensation, dry eye, and corneal swelling and erosion.

ANTI-INFLAMMATORY DRUGS

Steroids (also see "Combination drugs")

Dexamethasone	Decadron Phosphate Maxidex	Same as prednisolone (below). Of the topical steroid drugs, dexamethasone has the greatest effect on intraocular pressure.
Fluorometholone	Flarex Fluor-Op FML FML Forte	Same as prednisolone (below).
Loteprednol	Lotemax	Same as prednisolone (below).
Medrysone	HMS	Same as prednisolone (below). Of the topical steroid drugs, medrysone has the least effect on intraocular pressure.
Prednisolone	Inflammase Forte Inflammase Mild	*Ocular:* Increased intraocular pressure, posterior subcapsular cataracts, secondary

(Continued)

337

Type	Generic Name	Brand Name	Potential Side Effects
		Pred Forte	ocular infection, retarded corneal healing, pupil dilation, ptosis, visual blurring, and ocular discomfort.
		Pred Mild	
	Rimexolone	Vexol	Same as prednisolone.
Nonsteroid anti-inflammatories	Diclofenac	Voltaren	Same ocular effects as flurbiprofen (below).
	Flurbiprofen	Ocufen	*Ocular:* Stinging, burning, and conjunctival redness on insertion. Allergic reactions are rare. *Systemic:* Reduced ability for blood to clot, so to be used with caution by those taking other blood thinners.
	Suprofen	Profenal	Same ocular effects as flurbiprofen.
	Ketorolac	Acular	Same ocular effects as flurbiprofen.
OCULAR DECONGESTANTS	Naphazoline HCl	Albalon	Same ocular effects as phenylephrine HCl (below).
		Allerest Eye Drops	
		Clear Eyes ACR	
		Naphcon	
		Opcon	
		Vasoclear	
		Vasocon	

Drug	Brand names	Effects
Oxymetazoline HCl	OcuClear, Visine LR	Same ocular effects as phenylephrine HCl (below).
Phenylephrine HCl	AK-Nefrin, Efricel, Eye Cool, Isopto Frin, Prefrin Liquifilm Relief	*Ocular:* Pupil dilation that can lead to closed-angle glaucoma (in those susceptible) and a "rebound reaction" where blood vessels dilate rather than constrict, causing the eye to appear redder after insertion of the drop. *Systemic:* Heart rate changes.
Tetrahydrozoline HCl	Collyrium Fresh, Eyesine, Murine Plus, Soothe, Tetracon, Visine	Same ocular effects as phenylephrine HCl.

ANTIALLERGY

Drug	Brand names	Effects
Antazoline phosphate with naphazoline	Vasocon-A	*Ocular:* Same as the ocular decongestants. *Systemic:* Topical antihistamines can have a sedative effect and can exacerbate sedative effects of oral antihistamines.
Cromolyn sodium	Crolom	*Ocular:* Burning and stinging on insertion, conjunctival redness, dry eyes, puffy eyes, and hordeolum.
Ketorolac	Acular	See "Anti-inflammatory drugs" (above).
Levocabastine	Livostin	*Ocular:* Burning and stinging on insertion. *Systemic:* Sedation.

(Continued)

Type	Generic Name	Brand Name	Potential Side Effects
	Lodoximide	Alomide	*Ocular:* Burning and stinging on insertion. *Systemic:* (Very rare) nausea, dizziness, and sedation.
	Olopatadine hydrochloride	Patanol	*Ocular:* Burning and stinging on insertion, dry eye, foreign-body sensation, conjunctival redness, puffy eyes. *Systemic:* Headaches, coldlike symptoms, taste change.
	Pheniramine maleate with naphazoline	Naphcon-A Opcon-A	Same as antazoline phosphate with naphazoline.
CORNEAL EDEMA			
	Sodium chloride	Adsorbonac Muro-128	*Ocular:* Burning and stinging on insertion. Adsorbonac contains the preservative thimerosal, which can cause an allergic reaction.
COMBINATION DRUGS (A mixture of more than one medication; for side effects, see the individual components of these drugs and additional notes here.)	Gentamicin and prednisolone	Pred-G	

Neomycin and dexamethasone	Neodecadron, Neodexair	
Neomycin, polymyxin B, and dexamethasone	Maxitrol, Dexacidin, Dexasporin	
Neomycin, polymyxin B, and hydrocortisone	Cortisporin	Hydrocortisone is a topical steroid with side effects similar to prednisolone.
Neomycin, polymyxin B, and prednisolone	Poly-Pred	
Oxytetracycline and hydrocortisone	Terra-Cortil	
Polymyxin B and bacitracin	Polysporin	
Polymyxin B, neomycin, and bacitracin	Triple Antibiotic, Neonatal, Neosporin	
Polymyxin B, neomycin, and gramicidin	Ocutricin, Neosporin, Neocidin	Gramicidin in combination with polymyxin B and neomycin is rarely irritating.
Polymyxin B and oxytetracycline	Terramycin	Oxytetracycline in combination with polymyxin B rarely causes allergic or inflammatory eye reactions.

(Continued)

Type	Generic Name	Brand Name	Potential Side Effects
	Tobramycin and dexamethasone	TobraDex	
	Trimethoprim and polymyxin B	Polytrim	Trimethoprim can cause local eye irritation including redness, burning, stinging, and itching.
DRUGS USED TO DILATE THE PUPILS			
	Atropine sulphate		*Ocular:* Irritation, allergic dermatitis, pupil dilation, increased intraocular pressure, and closed-angle glaucoma in those susceptible. *Systemic:* Central nervous system effects, including convulsions, cognitive impairment, and delirium. Dry mouth due to a decrease in saliva production is an early sign of an adverse reaction.
	Cyclopentolate hydrochloride	Cyclogyl	Same as scopolamine hydrobromide (below). Additional central nervous system side effects include hallucinations, speech and motor impairment, disorientation, restlessness, and emotional disturbances.
	Homatropine hydrobromide		Same as atropine sulphate.
	Hydroxyamphetamine	Paremyd	*Ocular:* Irritation on insertion. *Systemic:* Hypertension.

342

Phenylephrine HCl	Mydfrin NeoSynephrine	*Ocular:* Pupil dilation, irritation on insertion, corneal swelling, and rebound conjunctival reaction. *Systemic:* Hypertension, change in heart rate, and headaches.
Scopolamine hydrobromide		Same as atropine sulphate, but the risk of central nervous system side effects is greater.
Tropicamide	Mydriacyl	*Ocular:* Irritation, allergic dermatitis, increased intraocular pressure, and closed-angle glaucoma in those susceptible.

DYES

Fluorescein sodium		*Ocular:* Topical use can cause mild stinging and redness. *Systemic:* Injected fluorescein can cause nausea, vomiting, and respiratory edema, and can lead to myocardial infarction.
Rose bengal		*Ocular:* Pain and irritation on insertion is usually significant, so a topical anesthetic is usually used before insertion of rose bengal.

GLAUCOMA MEDICATIONS

Beta-blockers		
Betaxolol	Betoptic	Same as timolol maleate (below), but with less severe pulmonary side effects.
Carteolol	Ocupress	Same as timolol maleate (below).

(Continued)

Type	Generic Name	Brand Name	Potential Side Effects
	Levobunolol	Betagan	Same as timolol maleate (below).
	Metipranolol	OptiPranolol	Same as timolol maleate (below), but with less severe systemic side effects.
	Timolol hemihydrate	Betimol	Same as timolol maleate (below).
	Timolol maleate	Timoptic	*Ocular:* Redness and irritation and reduced tear production.
			Systemic: Changes in heart rate, asthma, loss of libido, dizziness, depression, and skin sensitivity.
Miotics			
	Carbachol	Isopto Carbachol	Same as pilocarpine (below), but side effects can be more severe.
	Demecarium bromide	Humorsol	Same as echothiophate iodide (below); in addition, may cause cysts to form in the iris.
	Echothiophate iodide	Phospholine Iodide	Same as pilocarpine (below), but side effects can be more severe. More likely to cause a cataract than other similar drugs.
	Isoflurophate	Floropryl	Same as demarcarium bromide.
	Physostigmine	Eserine sulfate	Same as demarcarium bromide; in addition, allergic reactions are likely.
	Pilocarpine	Isopto Carpine	*Ocular:* Stinging, burning, blurred vision,
		Pilagan	induced nearsightedness, pupil constriction,
		Pilocar	poor night vision, tearing, cataracts, and retinal detachment.

Drug class	Generic	Brand	Side effects
			Systemic: Headaches (browaches), hypotension, change in heart rate, difficulty breathing, pulmonary edema, nausea, salivation, sweating, cramps, and diarrhea.
Alpha-adrenergic agonists			
	Apraclonidine	Iopidine	*Ocular:* Same as epinephrine (below) and including abnormal upper eyelid movement. *Systemic:* Heart symptoms, as with epinephrine, but less likely; dry mouth, dry nose, fatigue.
	Brimonidine	Alphagan	Same as apraclonidine. Less likely to cause cardiovascular side effects than apraclonidine.
	Dipivalyl epinephrine	Propine	Same as epinephrine (below), but side effects are less common. However, dipivalyl epinephrine is more likely to cause an allergic conjunctivitis.
	Epinephrine	Epifrin	*Ocular:* Eye pain or eye ache, browache, pupil dilation, allergic conjunctivitis, tearing, dark-pigmented conjunctival deposits, cystoid macular edema in people who have had cataract surgery, and closed-angle glaucoma in those susceptible. *Systemic:* Increased heart rate and heart palpitations.

(Continued)

345

Type	Generic Name	Brand Name	Potential Side Effects
Carbonic anhydrase inhibitors			
	Acetazolamide	Diamox	*Systemic:* "Tingling" in extremities, ringing in ears, poor appetite, malaise, depression, gastric upset, respiratory failure, aplastic anemia, and kidney and liver malfunction. Not to be taken if there is an allergy to sulfa.
	Dichlorphenamide	Daranide	Same as acetazolamide, but side effects are much more likely.
	Dorzolamide hydrochloride	Trusopt	*Ocular:* Stinging on insertion, itching, transient blurring, and allergic conjunctivitis (especially if there is an allergy to sulfa).
	Methazolamide	Neptazane	*Systemic:* Headaches and diarrhea. Same as acetazolamide; (rarely) causes kidney stones.
Hyperosmotic agents			
	Glycerin	Osmoglyn	*Systemic:* Headache, nausea, vomiting, dehydration, confusion, disorientation. Because glycerin is glucose-based, it is not to be used by anyone who has diabetes.
	Isosorbide	Ismotic	Same as glycerin. Not glucose-based, so can be used by people with diabetes.

	Mannitol	Osmitrol	*Systemic:* Dehydration, headache, chills, and chest pain.
	Urea	Ureaphil	*Systemic:* Dehydration, confusion, disorientation, severe headache, arm pain, and liver and kidney involvement.
Antimetabolites			
	5-fluorouracil	5-FU	*Ocular:* Conjunctival and corneal edema, conjunctival redness, lacrimation, ocular pain.
	Mitomycin-C	MMC	*Ocular:* Cornea, iris, ciliary body, and retina toxicity; and cataract.
Prostaglandins			
	Latanoprost	Xalatan	*Ocular:* Can cause temporary conjunctival redness. Other temporary side effects include dryness, itching, burning, blurred vision, and photophobia. In addition, the iris can change color, usually from green or hazel to brown, darkening centrally. The color change can be permanent. *Systemic:* (Rare) upper respiratory tract infection; pain in muscles, joints, back, and chest; and skin allergies.

(Continued)

Type	Generic Name	Brand Name	Potential Side Effects
LUBRICATING			
	Acetylcysteine	Mucomyst	*Ocular:* Stinging on insertion.
	Artificial tear inserts	Lacrisert	*Ocular:* Blurred vision and foreign-body sensation.
	Artificial tears	Aquasite	*Ocular:* Stinging, itching, and redness associated with allergy to any components in the drops or ointments. Unpreserved preparations are less likely to cause these side effects. Ointments also cause blurring because of their thick consistency.
		Hypotears	
		Liquifilm Tears	
		Moisture Drops	
		Refresh Plus	
		Tears Naturale	
		and many generics	
	Hydroxypropylmethyl-cellulose	Goniosol	*Ocular:* Transient blurring of vision due to the thick consistency of the drop.
REVERSE DILATING DROPS			
	Dapiprazole HCl	Rev-Eyes	*Ocular:* Blurred vision, conjunctival redness and swelling, dryness, itching, lid swelling and drooping, and browache.

Sources: J. D. Bartlett and S. D. Jaanus, *Clinical Ocular Pharmacology* (Newton, Mass.: Butterworth-Heinemann, 1995); *Physicians' Desk Reference* (Montvale, N.J.: Medical Economics Data, 1997).

Signs and Symptoms Index

Pages cited which are followed by *f* contain an illustration

General Index

Pages cited which are followed by *f* contain an illustration

multiple sclerosis, 262–63
Murine Plus, 339
Muro-128, 340
muscles, eye, 4f, 5f, 6, 13f, 52; and binocular fusion, 27, 29; and contact lenses, 85; and double vision, 32, 130; extraocular, 13–14, 306; eyelid, 210, 211, 212; and focusing, 10, 19–20, 22, 65; in iris, 9; and systemic disorders, 276, 308
myasthenia gravis, 212, 301, 308
Mycostatin, 336
Mydfrin, 343
Mydriacyl, 343
myocardial infarctions, 168, 181–82, 343
myokymia (twitching eyelid), 213–14
myopia. See nearsightedness
myopic shift, 134

nadolol, 179
naphazoline, 338, 339, 340
Naphcon, 338
Naphcon-A, 340
NASA, 313
nasolacrimal ducts, 5f, 234, 235f. See also tear ducts
nasolacrimal sac, 5f, 242, 243
Natacyn, 336
National Association for the Visually Handicapped, 319
National Center for Vision and Aging, 319
National Eye Institute (of NIH): on macular degeneration, 198; studies by, 121, 200, 202, 263, 285–88
National Federation of the Blind, 319
National Institutes of Health (NIH), 121, 135, 189, 198
nearsightedness (myopia), xv–xvi, 17–18, 18f, 19f; and aging, 24–25, 30; correction of, 76, 82, 114; and glaucoma, 167, 171, 175, 183, 190; and headaches, 297; and myopic shift, 134; and refractive surgery, 116–19, 120f, 122, 123; and retinal detachment, 251; as side effect, 323, 327, 328
Neocidin, 341
Neodecadron, 341
Neodexair, 341
neomycin, 323, 335, 341
Neosporin, 341
NeoSynephrine, 343

neovascularization, 307; corneal, 98, 101; and glaucoma, 257, 258, 293–94; retinal, 277, 281–83
neovascular membranes, subretinal, 196f, 198, 199, 201–4, 274
Neptazane, 183, 346
nerve fibers, 193, 214, 218–19, 261
neuralgia, post-herpetic, 214
nevi, 246–48
night vision, 194, 289
nocturnal lagophthalmos (open-eye sleep), 238
"no-line" bifocals. See progressive addition lenses
NOLVADEX, 329–30
norepinephrine, 179
norfloxacin, 335
nortriptyline, 237, 324
nuclear sclerotic cataracts, 25, 26, 129–32, 130f, 136
nutrition, 246, 273; and cataracts, 132, 134–35; and glaucoma, 189–90; and macular degeneration, 199–200; and migraines, 298, 299
Nystex, 336

occlusion (blockage), 255, 292, 300, 327
OcuClear, 339
Ocufen, 338
Ocuflox, 335
Ocular Hypertension Study, 189
ocular ischemia, 293–94
Ocupress, 180, 343
Ocusulph-10, 335
Ocutricin, 341
ofloxacin, 335
ointments: antibiotic, 272; for dry eyes, 236, 240; for eyelids, 207, 210, 212; hypertonic, 221; side effects of, 348; and systemic disorders, 307, 308. See also eye drops
olopatadine HCl, 340
opacified posterior capsule, 156–57, 160
Opcon, 338
Opcon-A, 340
Ophthaine, 334
ophthalmic artery, 253, 255, 291
ophthalmodynamometry, 294
ophthalmologists, 37–38, 201, 316; choice of, 73–75, 158–59; and contact lenses,